D0906414

Organizational Ethics
in Health Care

Organizational Ethics in Health Care

Principles, Cases, and Practical Solutions

Philip J. Boyle

Edwin R. DuBose

Stephen J. Ellingson

David E. Guinn

David B. McCurdy

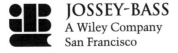

JOSSEY-BASS
A Wiley Company
San Francisco

press

Published by

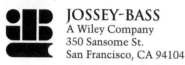

JOSSEY-BASS
A Wiley Company
350 Sansome St.
San Francisco, CA 94104

www.josseybass.com

Jossey-Bass books and products are available through most bookstores. To contact Jossey-Bass directly, call (888) 378-2537, fax to (800) 605-2665, or visit our website at www.josseybass.com.

Substantial discounts on bulk quantities of Jossey-Bass books are available to corporations, professional associations, and other organizations. For details and discount information, contact the special sales department at Jossey-Bass.

We at Jossey-Bass strive to use the most environmentally sensitive paper stocks available to us. Our publications are printed on acid-free recycled stock whenever possible, and our paper always meets or exceeds minimum GPO and EPA requirements.

Library of Congress Cataloging-in-Publication Data

Organizational ethics in health care : principles, cases, and practical solutions / Philip J. Boyle ... [et al.]. — 1st ed.
   p. ; cm. — (The Jossey-Bass health series)
   Includes bibliographical references and index.
   ISBN 0-7879-5558-2 (alk. paper)
   1. Health services administration—Moral and ethical aspects.
2. Medical ethics.
   [DNLM: 1. Ethics, Institutional.   2. Health Facilities.   3. Organizational Case Studies.   WX 150 O693 2001]   I. Boyle, Philip.   II. Series.
   RA427.25 .O74 2001
   174'.2—dc21
                                                 2001001349

HB Printing   10 9 8 7 6 5 4 3 2 1

The Jossey-Bass Health Series

Contents

Part Three: Appendixes

To the memory of Angela Schneider-O'Connell

Angela was a pioneer in bridging the fields of bioethics and business and organizational ethics. More than that, her keen intellect, sense of humor, and warm personality were a joy to all who knew her.

Foreword

Complexity is the hallmark of contemporary health care organizations. The emergence of multisystem hospitals and even larger integrated delivery networks throughout the United States has radically altered and indeed reordered the landscape of health-related services. Sources of influence and incentive have shifted as various constituencies struggle to adapt to the dynamics of a largely market-driven environment that is characterized by instability and exposure to rapidly shifting political priorities. Health care organizations are forced to make more critical decisions, and more rapidly and decisively, than ever before. Given the complexity of the environment and the relatively small margin for mistakes that can take down an entire organization, a serious question emerges with particular relevance: How does an organization safeguard its moral integrity while responding to the incessant, voluminous, and immediate demands of day-to-day operations?

Although the problems associated with the emergence of new modalities of health care delivery have been proliferating for some time, the Joint Commission on Accreditation of Healthcare Organizations (JCAHO) has now explicitly acknowledged the increasing potential for serious ethical consequences. The JCAHO now mandates that health care organizations seeking its prestigious imprimatur develop mechanisms for identifying and addressing organizational ethics. The complex and rapidly moving pace of today's health care environment simply lends itself to too much ethical ambiguity, which, if left generally unexamined and largely untouched, may threaten the well-being of innocent individuals and unsuspecting communities. The JCAHO standards are, however, just what they appear to be: statements of principle that demand concrete expression in the practical order.

The need to move from statements of theoretical principle to the lived experience of organizations and of the persons who are responsible for the moral character of those organizations provides the rationale for our volume on organizational ethics in health care. Applied ethics usually lags behind the emergence of practice patterns that it eventually recognizes, analyzes, and tries to influence in the public square. It is not surprising, then, that little substantive work has appeared in the field of applied health care ethics as it relates to institutional or organizational ethics.

Given the sometimes overwhelming demand from health care organizations for assistance in complying with JCAHO standards, and our unique approach to health care ethics, the Park Ridge Center for the Study of Health, Faith, and Ethics is responding with this comprehensive, practical guide to understanding and implementing the requirements of organizational ethics at a turbulent time in the history of U.S. health care. In this way, we hope to advance the field of organizational ethics as it applies to health care, while at the same time making a modest contribution to improved quality. Finally, we hope our efforts ease at least some of the burdens experienced by our colleagues in health care leadership and governance as they strive to do their best under damnably difficult circumstances.

LAURENCE J. O'CONNELL
President and Chief Executive
The Park Ridge Center for the
Study of Health, Faith, and Ethics

Preface

Why we wrote this book, and not some other book on health care organizational ethics, is best understood by examining the research process we carried out to gather and reflect upon the stories collected herein. The process was about as simple as the transformation of modern health care itself. Anyone who inhabits the vast territory called health care ethics could not have remained untouched by the last decade's chaotic, and at times opportunistic, restructuring of health care. HMOs, PPOs, PSOs, and "E-I-E-I-O-s" have made health care ethicists think differently about health care and the positions from which they reflect upon it. Thirty years ago, when bioethics was in its infancy, ethicists could follow doctors and nurses around and watch them in their natural habitats. The problems ethicists observed seemed daunting at first, but after years of public conversation, debate, and clarification many dilemmas seemed less imposing, and it became easier to resolve at least some issues.

Today ethicists find it less easy to observe the new organizational ethical dilemmas that can entangle an entire health care institution, from the boardroom to the mailroom. Ethicists can no longer simply observe clinicians to identify the moral problems within health care. They must approach the task from many perspectives to see how a health care organization works, and talk with every person who works within and with the health care organization (executives, housekeepers, and vendors, to name only a few) as well as visit every kind of health provider (acute-care hospital, home care agency, physician practice, and more). At a minimum, this observation requires a revised method for gathering information, and new tools to dissect the ethical problems. The impetus for this book was our own experience of wrestling with this transformation.

The Park Ridge Center team has been fortunate to work within the many nooks and crannies of the health care system. The Center's staff provides ethics consultation and education services to a range of local and regional health care organizations—from acute care to home care—including our parent organization, Advocate Heath Care, an integrated delivery system of eight hospitals and two hundred sites of care in the Chicago region. Through these experiences and several dozen semistructured interviews with informants in many health care organizations, we gathered and analyzed lists of problems and tentative solutions.

Organization of the Book

Armed with data, the authors of this book imagined many ways of capturing an adequate and cohesive picture of health care organizational ethics. We decided to give moral snapshots of an organization at short and long range. In Chapter One, we offer a big picture: how organizational ethical problems span the institutional landscape, lurk in the woodwork of organizations, and touch many moral actors. Chapter Two takes a sociological picture of the formal and informal structure of health care organizations, produces practical insight into organizational complexity, and applies these insights to ethical analysis. Chapter Three also explores the overall picture by enumerating and investigating the possible "ethics mechanisms" an organization can use in promoting acceptable behavior.

Chapters Four through Ten offer different perspectives from which to analyze organizational ethics. The relationship of the law to ethical requirements is a puzzle in all applied ethics, but this relationship has a fresh twist in health care organizational ethics. Just as the latter became a specialized topic of discussion, legal concerns about fraud and abuse in health care finance also began to grow. Chapter Four seeks to untangle this complicated picture.

As our research group discussed how to capture an image of organizational ethics, we thought it might be useful to examine functional units in an organization, such as executive, managerial, and departmental functions. Indeed, future books might approach organizational ethics by investigating health care organizations department by department. Chapter Five presents an analytic model of organizational function by examining the management of human resources.

Another way to depict organizational ethics is to explore choices that span the organization. One issue that affects every member of the organization is the potential for conflict of interest (Chapter Six). Another such issue that affects each member of the organization is using discretion in carrying out job responsibilities (Chapter Seven). Still another issue that touches every member and that partially reveals the moral nature of the organization is policy development and implementation. Chapter Eight uses a resource allocation policy to model the moral method described in Chapter One; in so doing it illuminates how policy reflects the moral nature of the organization. Chapters Nine and Ten approach issues that often remain in the background of discussion of organizational ethics, issues that most ethics mechanisms find difficult to approach. Chapter Nine addresses how resource allocation shapes the moral culture of an organization, and how an organization's external culture affects resource allocation. Finally, Chapter Ten addresses the perennial chestnut of ethics and the business of health care: Is it an oxymoron to be an ethical health care business?

Although we have included twenty cases and accompanying commentaries in Part Two, all the chapters include a mix of practical cases and sample policies. Space limitations forced us to be selective about cases. The selection hardly represents the entire organizational ethics picture, but the cameos do add ways to identify, analyze, and address organizational ethics issues practically.

Acknowledgments

This is an appropriate place to thank the many anonymous informants who provided some of the background for the cases. To ensure confidentiality, the storytelling is ours, not theirs. We obtained the cases from so many informants across so many health care organizations that, in the final depiction, we ourselves are hard pressed to identify the original case—so don't even ask.

This book would not have been possible but for the many friends and colleagues who directed us. Many editorial eyes looked at this book; we are especially grateful to Bette Crigger, Margaret Brennan, and Ann Rehfeldt. Our colleague Joal Marie Hill contributed to the cases, and she and Martha Holstein offered practical insights into resolving organizational ethics conflicts. Final manuscript preparation was made extremely easy thanks to the earlier work of Regena Jackson and Bernice Chantos. Last but not least, we are deeply grateful to the informants—friends in health care systems near and far—who allowed us to use the stories in this book.

The Authors

Philip J. Boyle is chief operating officer of the Park Ridge Center for the Study of Health, Faith, and Ethics. He earned his Doctor of Philosophy in theology at St. Louis University and Master of Divinity and Sacred License of Theology from Pontifical Faculty of Immaculate Conception, Washington, D.C. He comes to the Park Ridge Center from the Hastings Center, where he was the associate for medical ethics. In that capacity, he developed and directed multiyear, multidisciplinary research projects on ethics and public policy, including ethical and public policy issues in health care resource utilization, managed care, managed mental health care, technology assessment, outcomes data, employee health benefit plans, and values dilemmas in corporate science policy. He has also worked on research projects in genetics, ethics committees, and the 1991 federal Patient Self-Determination Act. Before going to the Hastings Center, he taught at St. Louis University Medical School in the Department of Internal Medicine. While there, he served four years as the associate director of the Center for Health Care Ethics and had appointments in the departments of Internal Medicine and Hospital and Health Care Administration. He lectures and consults widely on his areas of interest. He is the coauthor of *Medical Sources of Catholic Teaching* and the *Handbook for Nursing Home Ethics Committees,* coeditor of *What Price Mental Health? The Ethics and Politics of Setting Priorities,* and editor of *Getting Doctors to Listen: Ethics and Outcomes Data in Context.*

Edwin R. DuBose is a research associate at the Park Ridge Center. He holds a Ph.D. from Rice University and an M.Div. from the Harvard Divinity School. Before coming to the Park Ridge Center in 1990, he was a fellow in religious ethics at the Foundation for Interfaith Research and Ministry in Houston, where he served as director of the foundation's AIDS education programs and taught as an adjunct professor at the University of Houston. Presently, he holds an adjunct position in the Department of Religion, Health, and Human Values at Rush University, Chicago. His articles have appeared in medical, public health, and religious journals, among them the *American Journal of Public Health, Pediatric AIDS,* and *Christian Century.* He is coeditor of *A Matter of Principles? Ferment in U.S. Bioethics* and *Must We Suffer Our Way to Death? Cultural and Theological Perspectives on Death by Choice.* He is the author of *The Illusion of Trust: Towards a Medical Theological Ethics in a Postmodern Age.* He chaired the planning committee for the 1996 and 1997 Advocate Health Care Clinical Ethics Conference and in 1997 organized the first Park Ridge Center bioethics intensive course.

Stephen J. Ellingson is an assistant professor of the sociology of religion, Pacific Lutheran Theological Seminary. His Ph.D. in sociology is from the University of Chicago, and his M.A. in theology is from Luther Northwestern Theological Seminary. He held a visiting professorship in the sociology department at the University of Chicago and served as the book review editor for the *American Journal of Sociology.* He was also a research associate at the National Opinion Research Center at that university. He was part of the Chicago Health and Social Life study led by Edward Laumann, studying how religious, health care, and social service organizations understand and address the causes and consequences of high-risk sexual behavior. As a graduate student, he was a member of the research team that conducted the national survey of sexual behavior and attitudes. He has published articles in the *American Journal of Sociology* and the *Review of Religious Research.* He is preparing a monograph based on his dissertation, titled *Discourse, Action, and Social Change: The Politics of Race and Slavery in Antebellum America.*

David E. Guinn is a research associate at the Park Ridge Center. He earned his Ph.D. in ethics and philosophy of religion at McGill University, his A.M. in constructive studies of religion at the University of Chicago Divinity School, and his J.D. at Fordham Law School. He joined the Park Ridge Center in 1997. Among other areas, he is interested in issues of religious freedom, pluralism, legal and moral philosophy, and political theory. He is coeditor or

contributing author for a number of books in press or in preparation, including *Religion and Law in the Global Village; Bioethics and
Law: An International View; Organizational Ethics*; and *Religion and
Civil Discourse*. Prior to commencing his study of religion and ethics,
he worked for many years in the professional theater and practiced
as a lawyer specializing in the areas of entertainment and intellec-
tual property law, during which time he authored numerous articles, was coauthor of a two-volume treatise on entertainment law,
and wrote two books on international collective administration of
copyrights and neighboring rights.

Rev. David B. McCurdy is a research associate and editor at the Park
Ridge Center. His D.Min. is from Bethany Theological Seminary
and his M.Div. from Union Theological Seminary (New York). He
came to the Park Ridge Center in 1995, following fifteen years as
a chaplain, clinical pastoral educator, and vice president of religion
and health at Good Samaritan Hospital (Advocate Health Care) in
Downers Grove, Illinois. Previously, he served as a parish pastor
and later as college chaplain at Elmhurst College. He continues as
an adjunct faculty member in the department of theology and religion at Elmhurst, where he has taught courses in health care
ethics since 1985. He has published articles, reviews, sermons, and
correspondence in numerous journals and periodicals.

The Park Ridge Center explores and enhances the interactions of
health, faith, and ethics through research, education, publications,
and consultation to improve the lives of individuals and communities. It is an independent, not-for-profit organization supported
by grants and gifts from foundations, corporations, and individuals. Additional information may be obtained by writing to the Park
Ridge Center, 211 E. Ontario, Suite 800, Chicago, IL 60611-3215,
or contacting www.prchfe.org.

Organizational Ethics
in Health Care

Part One

Chapter One

The Moral Ecology of Health Care Organizations

Why read this book? The Joint Commission on Accreditation of Health Care Organizations (JCAHO) now requires health care organizations—hospitals, nursing homes, home care agencies, hospices, and integrated delivery systems—to identify and address what it calls "organizational ethics" if they seek JCAHO accreditation (see Appendix One). One threshold problem exists: organizational ethics, sometimes referred to as institutional ethics, is an underdeveloped and underexamined topic in the literature of applied ethics. This book is one contribution meant to help fill that gap. It offers those within health care organizations who are interested in, and responsible for, addressing organizational ethics the tools to identify, analyze, and respond to its broad range of issues.

Although JCAHO accreditation motivates many health care organizations to establish ethics mechanisms (by which term we suggest, among other possibilities, an ethics committee or an ethics consultation team) to respond to patient and organizational ethics, those responsible for implementing such a mechanism may feel inadequately prepared to respond. This is not uncommon; in many areas of applied ethics those responsible for addressing ethical issues do not feel competent to "do ethics"—whatever that is. Those responsible for organizational ethics may have had experience in clinical health care ethics, but if they apply whole cloth, common methods of clinical ethics (perhaps moral reasoning based on autonomy and beneficence) to organizational problems, they quickly become dissatisfied. Clinical ethics only partially illuminate the ethical problem and resolution. Even if handy tools to sort out moral problems in organizational ethics existed, questions would remain: What is the scope of study in organizational ethics? What do the problems look like? Which are the most pressing problems? Who is the best person, or persons, and what is the best way to address these problems?

The challenges are real, but any ambivalence about moving forward should be tempered by the potential gains to be had from wading into this problem area. One benefit is obvious: fulfilling the requirements for accreditation and taking steps to avoid liability by bolstering compliance with the Federal Sentencing Guidelines of 1991 (see Chapter Four). Other benefits to investing time in organizational ethics are less clear but no less important if an organization is to flourish. Take, for example, the ability to identify and reduce the potential for conflict of interest. Such conflict emerges where employees make judgments that challenge their professional responsibility.

An obvious and frequent example occurs when a clinician must balance business and patient care concerns in the same decision. If professionals fulfill their clinical responsibilities, they protect their patients; at first blush, this appears to contribute to fulfilling the organization's mission, since serving the patient is strongly connected to the mission of health care. It is less clear to the professional what obligation there is to meet business demands. Implementing organizational ethics in this case might mean identifying what checks and balances exist within an organization to ensure that the professional appropriately balances competing interests.

These and similar benefits that can emerge from helping the eyes to see, the consciousness to understand, and the will to respond to problems in organizational ethics become apparent in the pages that follow. Anyone who is committed to the success of a health care organization will see throughout this book clear examples of how inattention to problems and poor response to them can undercut a health care organization's mission.

A Snapshot: What's in This Book?

Organizational ethics in health care is a story about the moral lives of individuals within health care institutions and about the moral life of the health care institution as an institution. In contrast, the literature of business ethics addresses, with little controversy, the moral issues individuals face within institutions, but it rarely addresses the moral life of an institution as an institution. When it does, the discussion is far less agreed upon. Is an institution a moral agent? Is it morally accountable? If an organization is a moral agent, with which moral problems should it be concerned? How does the organization identify, analyze, and resolve moral problems? Who in the organization is responsible for this task? This book takes on the challenge of describing health care organizational ethics and offering insights about how an institution can respond to growing concerns about organizational ethics.

This first chapter paints the big picture of organizational ethics: What is the context, who are the actors, what are the generic problems found across organizational units, what method(s) can guide thinking about the complexity of issues, and which mechanisms should be established to resolve them? Chapter One also characterizes organizations, especially health care organizations, and the focus of organizational ethics. In short, it offers a view of the moral ecology of organizational ethics by mapping the forest; the trees come into view in subsequent chapters.

One can glimpse the moral ecology of health care organizational ethics by walking through any health care organization facing a range of ethical dilemmas. It may resemble yours in some important ways, but it may also differ (at least in culture). For now, suspend disbelief and enter the world of that health care organization as we explore in each chapter the case of Partnership Health Care.

> Partnership Health Care, or PHC (a composite of several actual organizations), is a nonprofit, secular organization formed several years ago through the merger of five hospitals and their related institutions. Situated in a large urban area that was experiencing the first wave of managed care competition and consolidation, three faith-sponsored organizations and two community hospitals completed a full-assets merger.
>
> The largest teaching hospital in the merger, St. Somewhere, was founded by a Catholic religious congregation to serve the inner-city poor. The dwindling religious congregation later decided to sell St. Somewhere to focus efforts on another hospital they owned in another city. Another partner in the merger, Deaconess Hospital, was located in an affluent neighborhood of the city and had solid support from its United Church sponsor. The other faith-based

partner, Jewish Health Care, had seen its original patients and health care providers migrate to the suburbs and was financially floundering. The two suburban community hospitals in the system—Suburban and Outwest— were rapidly growing.

The PHC partnership created a small integrated delivery system by consolidating two dozen physician practice groups into the PHC Physician Plan; by acquiring five nursing homes; and by launching a home health organization, a small HMO plan, and several for-profit subsidiaries. It also developed direct contracting with small and midsize local employers.

PHC faced JCAHO accreditation at all its sites. The ethics committee mechanisms across the system functioned at different levels, some well, others not well at all. The JCAHO survey bolstered the system CEO's commitment to organizational ethics; however, she had already faced a range of value conflicts (to be described later) that threatened to undermine the system's market share. She suspected that the dilemmas predated the merger and believed that a cultural transformation could address the administrative nightmares rampaging through the system at varying levels of complexity and influence. The cases that follow are not isolated incidents.

The twenty-member board comprises three representatives from each of the original sponsors and five new members. Recently, they have been in a protracted conflict over employee health benefits and benefit products. Among the benefit products to be sold directly to small employers were reproductive services the Catholic board members rejected. Additionally, the benefits offered to PHC employees needed to be standardized regarding some sensitive issues. Before the merger, Deaconess offered domestic-partner benefits; however, those benefits were now on the chopping block for financial reasons and because of potential adverse public opinion. Yet retracting the benefits was also likely to cause a public backlash (see Case Seven in Part Two of this book).

The PHC's medical director faced challenges in retaining site medical directors and physicians as well. Many of the medical group physicians were frustrated by the practice parameters that the system was introducing to reduce inpatient length-of-stay. The medical group was upset because reduced length-of-stay would be imperative if they were to receive the 10 percent of their annual compensation that was withheld until they met financial targets. They were wondering aloud who had made the decision and what was driving the decisions—patient outcomes or profits. Department heads in particular were demoralized by internal conflict between their obligations as managers and their duty as physicians (see Case Sixteen).

Nurses at Jewish Hospital, the only ones unionized in the system, were prepared to strike. Prior to the merger, they had agreed to a pay freeze to ensure institutional solvency as well as continued access for indigent patients. After the merger, nurses at Jewish were upset that their average salary was significantly less than those at other sites, and that it would take them four years to achieve parity in compensation among nurses at all sites. If parity could not be realized in a shorter time, the nurses would strike. Board members and upper management thought that this might be an opportunity to break the union (see Case Two).

An internal audit had uncovered irregularities in coding and billing at St. Somewhere, where lax employee practices gave the appearance of misconduct. The auditors' report to the board spurred members to pressure the CEO to ensure PHC would not violate federal Medicaid reimbursement law and consequently be subjected to the 1991 Federal Sentencing Guidelines (see Chapter Four), or to risk whistle-blowing by an employee that might ultimately jeopardize federal health reimbursements, upon which PHC depended (see Case Twenty).

These concerns (and those examined throughout this book) are the source of the PHC chief executive's drive to identify, disentangle, understand, prioritize, and address the risks that can slow unification of the system and pose financial and legal threats. These and similar conflicts suffusing the organization make the CEO question her own moral responsibility and integrity and that of her organization as an organization. She wonders whether and to what extent organizational ethics assist in effecting a cultural transformation. What are the truly important questions within organizational ethics? Who should be responsible to identify and analyze the problems? What is the best way to operationalize responses to problems?

Before she can move forward, she has to understand the scope of the problem.

Health Care Ecology: A Moral Perspective

In many ways PHC, like other health care organizations, can be considered an ecosystem, and its study an ecology—that is, the study of the complex relationships between living organisms and their environment. Ecology is a helpful analogy for thinking about organizational ethics because of similar complexities in the study of the two. Ecology takes into account interactions among cells; individual organisms; and groupings of individuals, ecosystems, and the entire biosphere. Similarly, organizational ethics takes into account interaction among individuals, teams of health care workers, institutions, integrated delivery systems, and the entire health care environment. Any account of organizational ethics that focuses only on one level of the environment, such as the team or the institution, without examining and accounting for interaction among the levels of the environment, is inadequate.

Ecological thinking also contributes an emphasis on perspective; depending upon the moral vantage point within the ecosystem, certain issues come to the foreground and others recede. Viewing global warming from the biosphere perspective, for example, may not help one notice cellular mutations. Similarly, focusing on a single health care department might reveal an organizational ethics problem such as noncompliance with policies, but this perspective might not see that the practice is rooted in an organization's culture. Any mechanism that is responsible for addressing organizational ethics must be self-conscious about which perspective it is adopting. The first attempts to examine organizational ethics are likely to occur at a departmental level; however, it is important to keep clear a sense of the problems that could go unobserved and unaddressed.

Ecological analysis also brings to organizational ethics the conceptual troubles of environmental ethics. Are any levels of moral analysis most important? Which level of analysis constitutes an adequate moral analysis? Must the analysis encompass all levels, or some mix of them—individuals, teams, institutions, health care systems, and the organization of health care across the country? In ecology, if some ethicists highly value endangered species such as the spotted owl, then other parts of the ecosystem—the quality of life for the environment—take on a different, and probably lesser, weight. Alternatively, where the entire ecosystem is highly valued, the spotted owl simply becomes one value competing among other values. The same applies to health care organizational ethics; focusing on the changing values in the doctor-patient relationship means that other systemwide problems receive less critical attention. Mechanisms responsible for organizational ethics need to identify which values must be given priority and how to rank competing values.

The ecology metaphor has limits, especially if it hides important differences. In the overall ecology of organizations, it is important for moral analysis to recognize the unique features of health care organizations. The variety of professionals inhabiting health care organizations (physicians, nurses, managers), the kinds of health care organization (hospitals, nursing homes, managed care providers), and the unique range of missions and goals require that moral analysis be clear about specific social features that characterize health care organizations and distinguish them from others. Otherwise the mechanism responsible for organizational ethics could perform an inadequate moral analysis of the context and ultimately fail to meet its mission.

Organizations

As is fully described in Chapter Two, theories of organization accentuate different characteristics. Classic studies characterize organizations by (1) noting division of labor; (2) focusing on mission, goals, or products; (3) observing how agents (employees) report to principals (managers or leaders); and (3) noting how goals are accomplished through rules and procedures. If an organization's mechanism analyzes ethics through the lens of formal characteristics of organizations, it reveals certain moral problems: mission lapse, the risks associated with unclear division of labor, the burden of too much or too little attention to policies and procedures. The business ethics literature often takes this perspective and offers a moral analysis related to agent-principal relationships—that is, to the moral problems that occur between an employee (agent) who reports to an employer (principal).

In contrast, contemporary sociological theories of organization focus on complementary issues—for example, the gap between an organization's formal policies and operations and the informal culture that animates it. Viewing ethics through the lens of an organization's informal cultural characteristics, we notice moral problems that are specific (if not unique) to that organization, such as the gap between policies and practice. Formal and informal theories of organizations examine issues across the organizational ecosystem. Thus, both are necessary for an adequate moral analysis. Also, an ethics mechanism must be self-conscious about which theory it uses and which it omits.

Health Care Organizations

Even though characterizing health care organizations seems nearly impossible, given the volatile, opportunistic managed care market, one can still highlight characteristics that distinguish health care organizations from others. Health care organizations possess a distinctive organizational ecology characterized by (1) their mission of health care service to alleviate pain and suffering and restore patients to health; (2) the complex, highly regulated environment—internal and external—under which they operate; (3) professional cultures (physicians, nurses, health care managers); and (4) the rapidly changing health care market.

One remarkable feature of today's health care organization is the move toward industrialization. Health care organizations in the first part of the twentieth century were physician-dominated, guild-like systems that depended upon diagnosis and treatment of the patient as an individual. In the course of that century, health care organizations almost imperceptibly moved toward an industrialized model relying on population-based, statistical evidence to organize and provide health care predictably. This shift highlights two characteristics of the ecosystem to which moral analysis must attend. One is a move from domination by a medical professional to direction by a managerial professional. Another closely associated characteristic is the ascendancy of statistical, population-focused, and evidence-based health care, used to ensure predictable health outcomes and costs.

These characteristics create the conditions for many organizational moral problems that health care institutions face. As they vest decision-making power in managerial professionals who use the industrial tool of population-based health care, multiple challenges arise. In the case of PHC and the development and execution of practice parameters, it is reasonable to ask: Did the managerial professional fully understand the consequences of her decision on patient care? Did the system offer adequate checks and balances to oversee the managerial professional's decision making? Do clear policies articulate which decisions have been vested in the managerial professional? Has too much discretion been given the managerial professional? How do managerial professionals collaborate with health care professionals? Do their values overlap? (See Cases Fifteen and Sixteen.)

Characteristic similarities among health care organizations should not blind those pursuing moral analysis to the distinctive features of the organizations that make up the rapidly changing health care ecosystem. When people think of health care organizations, they tend to picture an individual hospital like St. Somewhere, or in the era of managed care systems a network of hospitals like PHC. It must be noted that health care organizations are at differing stages of organizational development and complexity, especially with respect to the shift from medical to managerial professionalism. Also, imagining that PHC is a representative health care organization excludes important parts of the ecosystem for which this book is also designed. Take, for example, institutional purchasers of health services, such as self-insured employers that purchase health benefit plans, and others that not only manage but also provide health services to reduce health benefit costs. To the extent self-insured employers manage and offer services, they are part of the ecosystem that organizational ethics must address.

Vendors that support larger providers such as PHC but do not engage in direct patient care are also part of the health care ecosystem. These vendors may provide one service, such as management of information systems, or they may distribute medical equipment or lend support to direct providers of care, such as PHC. Whatever they sell, they are not merely external forces playing upon health care organizations, but rather part of the community for which close attention to organizational ethics might help in moral analysis. Organizational ethics in health care applies not simply to traditional health care organizations such as PHC but to all the organizations that populate the health care ecosystem.[1]

The Actors

Health care organizations are populated by a variety of professionals. Each group makes specific choices, thus confounding moral analysis. Among the potential players are trustees, stockholders of for-profit health care organizations, executive leaders, managers, employees, institutional purchasers (employers), individual patients, the community, institutional partners, and vendors. In other areas of applied ethics, the moral analysis often focuses on one actor (for example, the virtuous manager in business ethics) or a significant relationship (such as doctor-patient in clinical ethics). Yet in health care organizational ethics, the focus on a single actor or relationship obscures identification of ethical problems. For instance, focusing on the moral lives of leaders and managers who make up only a small number of actors in any organization might overlook the moral choices and risks the greater number of employees face.

Given that numerous actors in health care come from a variety of professions, an important moral challenge for health care organizational ethics analysis is to understand the organizational psychology and behavior of each professional group (see Chapter Two). The motivation and behavior of managers within the health care organization is illustrative. Typically, managers in a hierarchical organization report to a leader or executive, and their behavior is regulated by detailed policies and procedures to accomplish a mission. One risk that managers face is not having policies and procedures spelled out sufficiently. Consequently, managers can exceed the bounds of job discretion or—for a host of reasons— pursue a mission other than the organization's. In contrast, the organizational motivation and psychology of leaders suggest they are willing to take credit (even when it is not deserved) and shift blame to managers (even when the responsibility is theirs). Chapter Two examines in depth the implications of organizational psychology for organizational ethics. Ethical analysis of the health care organization requires that the ethics mechanism (which may be an ethics committee) pay attention to generic characteristics of actors (managers, CEOs, boards) and actually account for the particular moral psychology of the actors in an individual organization.[2]

The Focus of Organizational Ethics

If discussion of the nature of health care organizations and their moral inhabitants seems complex, the added layer of moral analysis is likely to daze even persons trained in moral theory. Before exploring how an ethics mechanism might tackle the problems occurring at PHC, it is important to be clear what this book assumes about ethics—and in particular about organizational ethics. If most of us think about ethics, we can identify choices, behaviors, or actions that we consider good and worth pursuing, or not good and worth avoiding. Yet we are often uncertain why a particular action is to be preferred, or what is to be gained by acting morally (or by reflecting on acting morally). At a minimum, some people construe ethical reasoning to be conflict resolution or compliance with the law.

Although ethical reflection might serve those interests, this understanding frames the meaning and purpose of such reflection quite narrowly. Ethics as a discipline is a systematic and critical reflection on all the components of moral choices. This reflection includes framing the questions, identifying relevant facts to answer the questions, clarifying concepts (such as conflict of interest), exploring the burdens and benefits of all alternatives, giving a reason for action, and deciding on a course of action that holds competing values in balance (see Exhibit 1.3 later in this chapter).

The terms *ethics* and *morality* are used interchangeably, but some theorists distinguish the two, defining *morality* as the lived experience of making choices and *ethics* as systematic reflection on that lived experience. Sometimes ethics and morality are construed to be the difference between secular and religious ethics respectively. This book is principally concerned with secular, nonreligious reflection on the moral problems endemic to an organization.

What is to be gained by systematic reflection on moral experience? No agreement exists about there being any one goal of moral philosophy. Most people who engage in moral reflection are not conscious about what goal they hope to attain (such as happiness or compliance with the law). Yet which goal is sought determines what does and does not count as a moral problem and solution. For example, if the goal of ethical reflection is simply conflict resolution, one can find cases of a lapse in organizational truth telling or promise keeping in which employees experience no conflict; therefore these lapses are not considered moral problems. Or if the goal is legal compliance, there are health care advertising practices that violate no laws, even though the advertisement might subtly coerce patients.

Still another popular goal of ethics is seen in the slogan "ethics is good business." This is an amalgam of goals, the views that moral organizations garner the support of customers; that organizations resolving a moral problem before it becomes a liability are better off; and that by addressing moral conflicts among employees, workforce friction can be reduced and outcomes improved. These pragmatic views sell ethical reflection on its immediate, tangible, even monetary benefits. They also appeal to organizational leaders, especially as they consider expending resources—including employee time—in pursuit of these goals. Yet there exist some goals of ethical reflection and behavior that do not necessarily appeal to self-interest and may be worth pursuing. This book assumes a long-standing view that ethical reflection and moral living promote integral human fulfillment, of individuals and communities. Ethical reflection and action pursue values that allow humans to flourish as individuals and communities. Later chapters of this book examine the values that encourage this outcome and explore complex cases to sort out whether choices promote or undercut such flourishing.

The case of billing irregularities at St. Somewhere highlights some of these threats to thriving. There could be many explanations for the irregularities, but suppose the reason was an employee's inaccurate, even untruthful, reporting (see Case Twenty). Society cherishes truth telling because it is the glue of human community—it is difficult to live and flourish in a community where everyone is unsure about who is telling the truth. Truth telling is a prerequisite for business and organizational operation. Without it, it is impossible to make verbal agreements and contracts. In this case, the value of truth telling is easy to identify for moral analysis, and the deleterious moral consequences for community thriving are obvious. But more often, throughout this book as in life, the values that promote flourishing are difficult to identify, and it is hard to know whether our choices concerning them help or inhibit individual and community growth.

If ethics is systematic reflection on moral life that brings integral human fulfillment to persons and communities, what part does organizational ethics play in that flourishing? To understand its role, one should examine the family resemblance between business ethics and organizational ethics. Discussion of business ethics predates the recent emergence of organizational ethics; the former has been chronicled, taught, and discussed for the past half century. One theoretical puzzle in the discussion is whether organizational ethics is a subset of business ethics or a larger umbrella. If it is simply a subset, then all the theoretical questions may have been resolved by business ethics and no new unanswered questions remain.

Similarity between these two areas of applied ethics can be seen in a workable definition of business ethics (by Laura Nash) as "the study of how personal moral norms apply to the activities and goals of a commercial enterprise. It is not a separate moral standard, but the study of how the business context poses its own unique problems for the moral person who acts as agent of this system."[3] This characterization makes clear what most people surely agree upon: that business ethics is not separate from other forms of ethics but rather focuses on the context of business. Similarly, organizational ethics as an area of applied ethics is not separate but focused on moral choices within organizations.

There is unlikely to be any disagreement that organizational ethics, at minimum, studies personal moral norms as they apply to the activities and goals of organizations. The most obvious family difference between business and organizational ethics is the latter's focus on the moral life of an organization. Some have argued that it is not simply a matter of projecting the moral life of individuals on organizations, but rather of ascribing moral responsibility to organizations. They cite as evidence the legal transformation of organizations from merely legal entities to ones that have civil rights (such as freedom of speech) and are held civilly and criminally liable. In ordinary language and perception, many people talk and think about an organization as more than a sum of individuals. An organization exists after its original members die, it has power to hire and fire, and it pursues missions that override any individual employee's desires. Moreover, the organization's actions are not reducible to the actions of its employees.

Some people infer from this evidence that an organization, like an individual, is a moral agent that can be praised, blamed, credited, or held morally accountable.[4] If this were the case, then the focus and goal of organizational ethics would be defined as the study of personal and organizational moral norms and choices as they contribute to the activities and goals of an organization and to the integral human fulfillment of persons and communities. Also, if this characterization were adequate, the difference between business and organizational ethics would be plain. Business ethics focuses on the choices of the individual *in* an organization, whereas organizational ethics focuses on the choices of the individual *and* the organization. Organizational ethics studies not only personal moral norms but also organizational moral norms as they apply to the activities and goals of an organization.

Moral norms can be glimpsed throughout the organization. Norms are manifest in an organization's formal structure, in its mission statement; policies and procedures; codes of professional conduct; strategic objectives; business plan; and contracts with employees, vendors, and purchasers. Organizational moral norms are less clearly seen, but no less palpable, in the organizational culture (which includes informal policies and procedures) and in the gap between what is formally expected and the ways things really get done. Throughout this book, we attempt to highlight organizational moral norms. Chapter Two offers a lens through which an ethics mechanism can begin to identify, study, and respond to such norms. We also argue the view that organizational ethics is not just new wine in the old wineskin of business ethics. Rather, organizational ethics proceeds on the view that organizational moral norms can be identified and morally evaluated. Although organizational moral norms may be difficult to disaggregate from personal moral norms, both sets of norms must be considered in an adequate analysis of organizational ethics.

What facets of organizational ethics are most important in this endeavor? As noted earlier, the field of health care organizational ethics remains underexplored compared to clinical health care ethics. Even so, the range of questions that should be considered is beginning to solidify (Exhibit 1.1). Not all the questions, however, are necessarily helpful in the day-to-day discussion carried out by an ethics committee or other mechanism responsible for identifying and resolving ethical dilemmas in the health care organization. One approach a mechanism might employ to identify the most important issues is to examine a laundry list of problems that have been found in most organizations (Exhibit 1.2).

After identifying the problems on the list in Exhibit 1.2 that are most prevalent and corrosive within some part of the organization, the ethics mechanism can then create a priority list to deal

**Exhibit 1.1. The Scope and Character
of Organizational Ethics.**

1. Theories of organizational ethics
   - What is the focus of organizational ethics?
   - How does it differ from other forms of applied ethics?
   - Is the organization a moral agent?
   - If an organization is a moral agent, what are the consequences for analysis and action?
   - What, if anything, distinguishes health care organizational ethics from organizational ethics?
2. What concepts, if any, apply to most organizations?
   - Conflict of interest
   - Discretion and control
   - Allocation of resources
   - Human relations
3. Are the concepts of autonomy, justice, and beneficence, or similar ones, useful for analysis of organizational ethics?
4. How do a professional code and job descriptions contribute to organizational ethics?
   - Ethics of leaders
   - Ethics of managers and administrators (competing interests among the board, the community, clinicians, and patients)
   - Employee ethics
5. What virtues contribute to organizational ethics?
   - Integrity
   - Honesty
   - Fairness
   - Respect for others
   - Promise keeping
   - Prudence
   - Trustworthiness
6. What formal structures contribute to organizational ethics?
7. What role do mission and values statements play in organizational ethics? What role should they play?

Exhibit 1.1. The Scope and Character of Organizational Ethics, Cont'd.

8. How do policies and procedures support—or undercut—organizational ethics? Who should participate? What values should be considered? What checks and balances exist?

9. What informal features of an organization promote or inhibit moral behavior?

10. What parts of organizational culture should organizational ethics attend to?

11. How does the ethics mechanism (for example, ethics committee) study the culture of the organization?

12. Which aspects of the external environment affect moral choice for the individual and the organization?

13. How do external forces affect organizational ethics?

14. What role can and should external regulation play in shaping organizational ethics?

15. What conflicts exist between personal moral and organizational norms as they apply to an organization?

16. What are the moral issues among health care organizations and other organizations?

17. What obligation of toleration and cooperation does the health care organization have with its partners, such as purchasers of health care, vendors, and other managed care organizations?

18. What challenges of organizational ethics, if any, are unique to a health care organization?

19. What part, if any, should religious values play in organizational ethics?

20. What mechanisms exist for organizational ethics? Which are optimal?

21. What is the scope of jurisdiction?

22. What authority should the mechanism possess?
    - Where should it be located within the organization?
    - How should it relate to the clinical ethics mechanism?

23. What is the relationship of the organization to corporate compliance?

24. What systemic supports promote ethical behavior?

Source: Adapted from Khushf, G. "Administrative and Organizational Ethics." *HEC Forum,* 1997, *9*(4), 299–309.

Exhibit 1.2. Common Problems Found in Organizations.

Greed

Cover-up and misrepresentation in procedures for reporting and control

Misleading product or service claims

Reneging or cheating on negotiated terms

Establishing policy that is likely to cause others to lie to get the job done; unarticulated, unclear, or inappropriate policy

Overconfidence in one's own judgment, with risk for the corporate entity

Disloyalty to the company as soon as times get rough

Poor quality—performance below expectation, apathy about goals

Humiliating people by stereotyping

Lockstep obedience to authority

Self-aggrandizement over corporate obligations

Favoritism; partiality, not meritocracy

Price fixing (choosing customary charges regardless of real cost)

Sacrificing the innocent and helpless to get things done (blaming subordinates)

Suppression of basic rights: freedom of speech (in other words, voice), choice, and association (in other words, union)

Failing to speak up when unethical practices occur (whistle-blowing)

Neglect of one's family or personal needs

Making a product decision that perpetuates a questionable safety decision (affecting practice parameters, resident and nursing duties, and so on)

Not putting back what one takes out of the environment or the community (for example, sale of a nonprofit to a for-profit entity)

Knowingly exaggerating the advantages of a plan in order to garner support

Failing to address probable areas of bigotry, sexism, or racism

Courting the business hierarchy, as opposed to doing a job well

Climbing the corporate ladder by stepping on others

Promoting the destructive go-getter who outruns his or her mistakes

**Exhibit 1.2. Common Problems
Found in Organizations, Cont'd.**

Failing to cooperate with other areas of the company (the enemy
   mentality)

Lying by omission for the sake of business (nondisclosure by leaders)

Cooperation or alliance with questionable partners, albeit for a good
   cause

Not taking responsibility for injurious practices (intentional or not)

Abusing (or just going along with) corporate perks that waste time and
   money

Corrupting the public political process through legal means

Goal substitution (for example, pursuing a mission—legitimate or
   not—other than the organization's)

Dithering

Obstruction, stalling

Inefficiency

Source: Adapted by permission of Harvard Business School Press. From *Good
Intentions Aside: A Manager's Guide to Resolving Ethical Problems* by L. Nash.
Boston, MA. 1990, pp. 8–10. Copyright 1990 by the President and Fellows of
Harvard College; all rights reserved.

with them. Another method is to select issues that cut across the
organization. For example, everyone within a health care organization makes choices about how to expend resources, including
use of time, medical appliances, drugs, and the like (see Chapters
Eight and Nine). Careful examination of resource expenditure
highlights use and abuse. Another issue that cuts across the organization is each employee's use of discretion, that is, exercising
judgment that is not specifically articulated in policies, procedures,
and professional codes (see Chapter Seven). Still another issue that
cuts across an organization is the problem of competing (and perhaps conflicting) interests on the part of employees, as between
professional and home life or between managerial and clinical
obligations (see Chapter Six).

   A final way to estimate the importance of issues is to focus on
a department or a function. Take, for example, the human resource function (see Chapter Five). Following the course of an em-

ployee's relation to an organization—being hired into it, being promoted through it, and leaving it—helps identify the range of problems and evaluate which of them are debilitating to an organization's mission and culture. In short, at this period in the emergence of health care organizational ethics, it is premature to establish once and for all which substantive moral problems are most critical. Those interested in, and responsible for, organizational ethics will want to look and listen carefully as members of the organization consider what the most potent problems are.

Organizational Ethics: A Method

During the past twenty years, those in health care who have engaged in moral reasoning in clinical dilemmas have often remarked that they feel inadequately prepared. They wish they had more training in ethics and substantive moral issues associated with end-of-life care and the like. In part, they have been comforted by the prodigious study and writing done by those in clinical ethics. In contrast, there is currently nothing like the same volume of material on substantive moral issues in organizational ethics. Consequently, those interested in organizational ethics need to devise methods for identifying, analyzing, and addressing moral issues. To facilitate developing such a method, it is helpful to consider three steps: understand your moral perspective, evaluate the strengths of the moral perspectives of others, and be clear about all the things that have to be considered.

Understanding Your Moral Perspective

Anyone approaching organizational value dilemmas brings, explicitly or implicitly, tools (in other words, theories) to evaluate value conflict. Some evaluate the situation with a moral tool that weighs the good and bad consequences accruing from personal or organizational moral choices. Others evaluate the situation according to whether the moral choice violates some norm ("do unto others") stemming from human reason or revelation. Still others evaluate the situation in terms of a moral theory; for example, in the ethics of clinical health care some people proceed with a version of "principlism," which evaluates a dilemma in light of core concepts of autonomy, justice, and beneficence. It is not the purpose of this book to evaluate these tools or theories. But it is imperative to remember that practical, irresolvable conflicts over organizational values may be rooted in fundamental differences among those who are discussing the dilemma. Therefore, one step in the method is to understand your moral perspective. Which theoretical tools do you employ—those based on consequences, or on rules, principles, or narratives?

Evaluate the Strengths of Other Moral Perspectives

Depending on the theory assumed for moral analysis, certain features of a case come to the foreground for discussion. With PHC, if one relies on principlism, certain features of the dispute over practice parameters come to the fore. The problem might be framed in terms of the doctor-patient relationship. The dispute is whether a patient should be given some choice in treatment even if the protocol does not allow choice, or whether physicians are morally obligated to set aside practice parameters if doing so is good for the patient. In contrast, if one relies on a theory examining the moral norms of the organization, the moral issues are framed differently, with other problems standing out.

The problem of practice parameters can be construed as the moral choice of a health care organization adopting policies that direct clinical practice. Other moral problems might surface, including what the motivation is for the rules (and whether that motivation is defensible) and what the limits are, if any, for an organization's directing health care. Each person participating in the discussion that an ethics mechanism carries out is likely to bring an individual moral perspective; each one inserts a valuable piece in the organizational ethics puzzle.

All Things Considered: A Case Workup

The moral story of PHC, as with most of life, seems complex and irresolvable. With its refractory, almost impenetrable problems, the case illustrated by PHC is reason enough to simply avoid taking up the questions in the first place. However, when parties are pitted against each other, some benefit can be gained by teasing apart the elements to understand the locus of disagreement.

There are many variants of case workup; by and large, they are attempts to ask as many questions as possible—all things considered—along the way. We employ a step-by-step method in this book (prominently in the case studies of Part Two). It includes (1) identifying questions, (2) gathering facts, (3) clarifying concepts, (4) sizing up alternatives and consequences, (5) finding justification for action, and (6) seeking integrity-preserving compromise (Exhibit 1.3).

Mechanisms for Addressing Organizational Ethics

During the rise of clinical health care ethics, health care institutions rushed to establish ethics mechanisms—most notably ethics committees—to deal with such substantive issues as decision making and termination of treatment. But in spite of all the staff goodwill and enthusiasm, the participants in the mechanism had difficulty in successfully organizing and sustaining enthusiasm. Committee members attributed the obstacles to lack of knowledge about substantive ethics issues; "If I only knew more about health care ethics, the committee would be successful" is a refrain often heard. Although an improved knowledge base could fortify ethics committee functioning, the movement has paid little attention to the fact that the *process* of addressing ethics issues might be as great an obstacle as the lack of substantive knowledge. What is the best process for addressing ethical issues? Who can best address them? What resistance does this process, and do these people, face? What is the scope of authority for this process? What are the expected outcomes of the process and the best ways to accomplish them?

In developing an ethics mechanism for organizational ethics, one encounters a formidable obstacle: identifying and addressing the unwieldy range of issues found throughout the organization. In contrast, clinical health care ethics faces a simpler process insofar as it focuses on the patient, and clinicians have familiar structures (such as clinical case conferences) that they can imitate and use to discuss clinical ethical problems. It is too early in the discussion of health care organizational ethics to know if the clinical model of an ethics committee is adequate to the task of organizational ethics. (More about this later.)

One frequently hears "Why do we even need a mechanism for organizational ethics?" If the clinical health care movement is any

**Exhibit 1.3. All Things Considered:
A Method of Moral Analysis.**

1. Question identification
   - What questions need to be answered?
   - Are there any priorities among the questions? For example, do some questions need to be asked and settled before others can be asked? Or are some questions necessary for the current problem while others can wait? Or are some questions so complex that they have historically resisted answers?

2. Fact gathering and assessing
   - Depending on the question to be explored, what facts are important for that question?
   - What facts are missing?
   - If certain facts are clear, will they sway the case one way or another?
   - Do you have enough factual understanding of the organization's mission, policies, procedures, and culture? Do you understand the context? Do you understand the moral psychology of the actors— for example, the professional motivation of leaders or managers?

3. Concept clarification
   - Suppose that when a question is framed, someone alleges that the problem involves a conflict of interest, or an abuse of discretion, and insubordination. What do those concepts mean? Is there any agreement about the characteristics of the concepts?
   - What facts are needed for the concept to be applicable in this case?
   - Is there a priority among concepts in this case? Sometimes a case raises several concepts. (For example, in health care advertising, it is alleged that the concepts of coercion and truth telling are relevant.)

4. Alternatives and consequences
   - Have you considered the case from the perspectives of all those who might have an interest in resolving it? Have you imagined the resolution of this case from the perspectives of all who have an interest?
   - What are the burdens and benefits of pursuing each alternative? Whose interests will suffer if a course of action is taken?
   - Have you examined short- and long-range consequences?

**Exhibit 1.3. All Things Considered:
A Method of Moral Analysis, Cont'd.**

- Which consequences are important? The economic ones? Health-related? Survival?

5. Justification

- What are the reasons to prefer one alternative over another?
- Does any rule of thumb apply? For example, would you do X in all cases—in a sense, universalize your actions? Would you apply the decision to yourself? Are equals treated equally? Has the decision-making process been fair and open to inspection? Would there be a moral hazard if the community knew about the decision?

6. Integrity-preserving compromise

- If a course of action is decided upon, is there a means to protect the values important to others in the dispute?

---

indication, those within an organization might see no need for a mechanism. The objection stems from several sources of resistance. One is "We don't have any moral problems around here—everything is just fine." The common notion that if it ain't broken, don't fix it is plausible, since health care organizational ethics is not front and center in the media or on the docket of trustees or administration. However, accrediting agencies and some clinical ethics committee members understand that adverse patient outcomes can be caused by problems on the organization's business side.

Another reason some see no need for an ethics mechanism is duplication. The corporate compliance committee, the ethics officers, internal audit, an ethics hotline, and the human resource department are identified as adequate mechanisms to deal with organizational ethics problems. The managerial rule of thumb to favor existing, functioning mechanisms demonstrates not only good stewardship but also the wisdom of avoiding turf conflicts. When a mechanism is established, therefore, it must be clear what it does and does not address if one is to ensure there is no overlap with other mechanisms. Even if other mechanisms (such as a corporate compliance program) exist, their membership, scope of authority, and focus tend to be restricted. Any mechanisms adequate to the task of identifying and addressing organizational ethics require having all things considered, as we have said, which includes multidisciplinary input.

Still another reason some think an ethics mechanism is unnecessary is the cost involved. In the competitive health care environment, time—that is, staff time—is money. If the clear concern is cost and not actual need for addressing organizational ethics, then creativity is in order. An organization may consider fortifying existing mechanisms, integrating them into the fabric of each department's operations, or collaborating with another health care organization. This book consciously avoids recommending that an organization establish one more committee or task force; instead, we simply recommend—as do the JCAHO requirements—that an organization have some mechanism in place to address organizational ethics.

As health care ethics committees developed, a common obstacle in the way of efficient functioning was turf warfare. A committee would encounter a roadblock when some people perceived that it had overstepped its bounds by interfering with the role and responsibility of existing authority. Part of the expressed concern was that the ethics committee would get out of control—stirring up all kinds of trouble that could be managed differently. What was overlooked was that the mechanism needed to be managed; it needed a clear scope of authority and accountability, which was often missing in a clinical ethics committee. Whatever mechanism an organization relies upon, there must be explicit discussion of who gives the authority to the mechanism, to whom the members of the mechanism report, what its functions are, and what goals it is held accountable for meeting. Too often, a clinical ethics committee was established with little thought to these issues, which can make or break a mechanism. Turf wars can be avoided with advanced planning of a mechanism's authority and accountability.

Misperceptions about the mission of the mechanism are also likely to cause it to falter. A common, lethal misconception about a mechanism is that it should have a police function within the organization. As we address several times in this book (see, for instance, Chapter Three), any connection between an ethics mechanism and guarding, patrolling, watching, reprimanding, and punishing undercuts its broader mission.

As noted earlier, organizations pursue ethical identification, analysis, and action for a variety of reasons. Even if the members of the mechanism pursue this activity only for legal liability, that pursuit will be stymied. Problems are likely to go unnoticed and unaddressed if the mere thought of them brings sanction. Issues that are identified as "organizational ethics dilemmas" might be moral problems with greater ambiguity than is first seen. Consequently, ambiguous problems rooted in numerous factors might be difficult to resolve though disciplinary measures. Equally important, if an organization is using the ethics mechanism to meet its mission or to improve employee and patient satisfaction, then using sanctions might undercut promoting the virtues the organization desires. Whatever mechanism is adopted to address organizational ethics, it should present a safe, confidential place to address potentially troubling issues. Creating a safe place for unsafe ideas encourages discussion of problems that might find no other place to be voiced.

Some misperceptions about the mechanism can be traced to confusion about its functions and its workload. Whatever form the ethics mechanism takes, an organization is likely to expect it to permit education, consultation, and policy conferral. If those in the mechanism group are unclear about its scope of authority and accountability, problems arise and conflicts can occur in providing such education and consultation. Consider the potential confusion related to consultation: Is it a true consulting function, or a mandating one? If an employee seeks information about an issue that is clear in the law (for example, accurate coding and billing), consultation on this matter might be perceived by the employee as mandating compliance. This in turn suggests a policing function, which the mechanism must avoid. Mandating compliance also usurps the power and authority of existing structures and occasions turf battles. Mandating sends the message that the mechanism is not a fair, confidential, safe venue for exploring moral issues. If clear lines of authority and accountability are established, however, the mechanism—should it identify a clear-cut moral and legal liability—is responsible to report the matter to the organizational structure that commissioned it. Appropriate reporting sends the message that the mechanism is not acting on its own, nor overstepping its bounds by duplicating existing organizational functions.

Given the number of pitfalls awaiting the organizational ethics mechanism, four pragmatic guideposts are worth highlighting. First, any hope of launching a mechanism requires support from the top down. A mechanism that starts at the grass roots is likely to flounder without the support of leaders who might perceive the movement as a threat. Influential leadership participation in the design and function of the mechanism contributes to its acceptance and successful operation.

Second, whoever commissions the mechanism should be realistic about its workload. Many clinical ethics committees have become disillusioned when unrealistic outcomes were placed on them. Realistic priorities and time lines should be set once a mechanism has mapped the moral ecology of an organization. Third, the mechanism can succeed with as little effort as appropriately advertising its existence. Take, for example, the use of the term *ethics,* which immediately connotes wrongdoing for some employees. Instead, using the word *values* might be less threatening, because it avoids association with policing or with flagrant problems that need little in the way of subtle moral consideration.

Fourth, adopting the committee structure that is found in a clinical ethics committee might obstruct the productivity of the mechanism. If the moral problems in health care organizational ethics are broader than doctor-patient relations, for example, it is ill-advised to create a committee that simply mimics the clinical ethics committee in its membership and moral analytical abilities.

Throughout this book, we make the case that the problems of health care organizational ethics require innovation and departure from doing things as usual. The discussion in the next chapter suggests that those interested in organizational ethics need a new way of seeing problems—and a new way of responding.

Notes
1. Moskowitz, E. H., and Nassef, D. T. "Integrating Medical and Business Values in Health Benefits Management." *California Management Review,* Fall 1997, *40*(1), 117–139.
2. Messick, D. M., and Bazerman, M. H. "Ethical Leadership and the Psychology of Decision Making." *Sloan Management Review,* Winter 1996, *37*(2), 9–22.
3. Nash, L. *Good Intentions Aside: A Manager's Guide to Resolving Ethical Problems.* Boston: Harvard Business School Press, 1990, pp. 8–10.
4. Goodpaster, K. E., and Matthews, J. B., Jr. "Can a Corporation Have a Conscience?" *Harvard Business Review,* 1982, *60*(1), 132–141.

Chapter Two

Organizational Theory, Culture, and Psychology
Tools for Organizational Ethics

Information gathering is at the center of organizational ethics. It is the second step of the method outlined in Chapter One (under the head "Organizational Ethics: A Method"). In traditional bioethics, the fact-gathering stage is relatively simple. The common practice is to observe a physician-patient relationship in which the ethical issues, decision-making process, alternatives, and consequences are relatively transparent or framed by some set of ethical principles, such as beneficence. In contrast, fact gathering in organizational ethics is much more complicated. The investigator faces a difficult challenge in identifying and understanding many sets of relationships, multiple organizational cultures, and numerous informal practices that often are hidden.

Fact gathering is an important part of ethical analysis for three reasons. First, the ethical problems of an organization fundamentally rest on the behaviors, decisions, policies, and structures of the organization. Thus investigators need to understand how an organization works, both on paper and in reality. Second, fact gathering unearths the raw material from which investigators can begin to answer their questions. For example, if the ethics mechanism at a hospital is charged with examining a problem of discretion related to billing irregularities, some first steps might be to identify how discretion is practiced in the billing department and the degree to which the practice conforms to the policy or more informal norms and practice. Third, it may encourage investigators to raise new or alternative questions, because the information collected reveals real or possible ethical problems related to the structure or practices of the organization.

To successfully complete the data-gathering phase of ethical analysis, the investigators need a set of tools that help them understand how an organization operates. This chapter reviews several explanations. In doing so, it introduces a set of diagnostic tools or alternative lenses capable of focusing attention on certain features of organizational life that may pose ethical problems.

Three Classic Approaches to the Study of Organizations

Most organizational theories start from the premise that the fundamental strategic and moral problem facing an organization is uncertainty. Organizational analysts offer a variety of theories to account for how organizations handle the uncertainties and ambiguities that arise from outside the organization (changes in the market or regulatory environment) and inside (coordinating tasks or setting goals). Two theories focus on internal problems: the *rational systems approach* examines the formal structures and processes that govern organizational behavior, while the *natural systems approach* looks at the role of informal structures. A third theory, the *open systems approach,* stresses external relationships and how an organization adapts to changes in the environment. Each theory highlights certain moral features of organizational life.

Rational Systems Approach

The rational systems approach grew from work done in the late nineteenth and early twentieth centuries on the emerging modern corporation. By focusing on organizations with bureaucratic forms of governance and those using assembly-line production techniques, early theorists defined the organization as a collectivity oriented to pursuing specific goals in which the activities and interactions of members are centrally coordinated to meet these goals. Means-and-ends thinking guides organizational behavior. Action is ordered in such a way as to realize some set of predetermined rules or goals with maximum efficiency.

The hallmark of the rational organization is a formal structure. It is characterized by explicit rules to govern behavior, division of labor with clearly defined relationships of authority, and job roles that are prescribed independently of the personal attributes of the individuals holding them.[1] Formalization may be viewed as an attempt to make behavior predictable by standardizing and regulating it. Thus, according to this perspective, an organization has (1) a visible set of hierarchical authority relations in which (2) work activities are governed by formal rules and clearly defined criteria for evaluation, relations that (3) are designed to pursue some set of goals.

Rational systems analysts focus on how the formal structure of an organization facilitates or hinders realization of goals. Historically, this approach has been used to study systems of authority and control and production processes. The strength of this approach is that it focuses attention on formal structures, official rules and policies, and employer-employee relations, allowing analysts to ask a pair of questions: How are relationships among health care workers in providing services such as surgery regulated by explicit rules, and how do these rules influence the quality of care? Do hierarchical or egalitarian authority systems make a hospital or clinical team efficient? This approach can be used profitably to study recent changes in health care—for example, how the ongoing shift from professional control (by physicians) to managerial control (HMOs) in health care is affecting patient care, billing efficiency, or system profitability.

This approach focuses attention on a range of ethical issues: violations of explicit rules, routinized procedures, organizational norms, and the negative and positive outcomes that result from strict adherence to rules. Key areas in which to look for problems are employee evaluation and discipline (How is rule breaking disciplined? Is promotion tied to meeting targeted goals or following company policy? How does the organization address a situation in which following the official rules harms the patient or compels the patient to switch to a competitor?) and authority and production systems (How does the shift from a paternalistic to a shared-governance nursing model affect patient care or employee morale?).

In the case of the billing and coding irregularities at Partnership Health Care described in Chapter One, a rational systems approach can be used to identify the degree to which explicitly defined rules for the practices are followed and formal relations of authority remain intact. Members of an ethics mechanism might ask: Are there explicit rules or policies that define who is or is not allowed to enter codes on patient charts? Are physicians prohibited, or are they allowed, to delegate coding responsibilities to subordinates? Are there disciplinary procedures established to correct coding or billing practices that violate the law or system policy?

Alternatively, the members might examine how work activities related to billing and coding are intended to operate so that they can discover if there are problems with the organization of work itself. They might look at clinicians' patient loads: Do physicians have too many patients under their care and not enough time to do the paperwork, and therefore delegate it to subordinates? In brief, the goal of this type of analysis is to discover whether the formal coding and billing structure is causing the irregularities or whether the official structure is sound but violations of policy and procedure are the source of the problem.

At the same time that a rational systems approach accomplishes this, it fails to see how informal processes, structures, and relationships shape the nature and identity of an organization. This approach assumes that the only goals are those that are formally defined, that an organization's culture is unified and shared, and that work tasks are accomplished according to official rules. It ignores the reality that most organizations are made up of multiple subcultures (physicians, nurses, and administrators all have their own, unique culture or set of values, beliefs, symbols, language, and rituals); that there is often a disparity between the official goals and those that are actually realized; and that how one is supposed to get work done is often not how work is really accomplished. The second theory, the natural systems approach, focuses attention on the informal or unofficial aspects of organizational life.

Natural Systems Approach

The natural systems approach starts with the assumption that examining official rules and policies, organizational charts, and goal statements tells only a partial story of how an organization operates. In any organization, an unofficial or informal set of goals, rules and norms, work procedures, and cultures run parallel to the official or formal set. Formal structures exist independently of the characteristics of individuals in particular roles, while informal structures are very much grounded in the personal characteristics or resources of specific individuals. Suppose an attending physician is vested with authority in a hospital unit, but everyone looks to one of the nurses for guidance on difficult cases. The question for an ethics mechanism in such a situation is, To what extent does the informal authority system create ethical problems related to patient care, evaluation, or staff morale?

Many natural systems analysts argue that the informal aspects of an organization are more important than the formal ones because they often undermine, replace, or transform them. This occurs, in part, because individuals enter an organization with existing ideas and expectations about work, and with values and interests that may be at odds with official values and goals; and in part because, as Richard Scott puts it, "formalization places heavy and often intolerable burdens on those responsible for the design and management of an organization." Attempts to program all behaviors in advance may stifle individual problem solving, discretion, initiative, and creativity and thus create an inefficient, apathetic, or alienated workforce.[2]

A comprehensive moral analysis of an organization attends to both formal and informal structures and goals. Heeding the informal requires the analyst first to identify the degree to which actual norms, rules, and practices differ from official or formal ones, and then to inquire into how the informal counterparts influence production outcomes, interpersonal relations, and goal attainment. This comparative method is an important tool for identifying the points at which formal and informal are in tension, and then for assessing the degree to which the tension between the formal and informal (or relying primarily on the informal) creates ethical problems for an organization.

One of the strengths of this approach is that it focuses on the politics of the workplace, since struggles over power, resources, status, and even survival often take place within the informal realm. A study of middle managers documents how promotions have little to do with actual job performance or formal goal attainment and more to do with attaching oneself to a rising star, *appearing* to be a team player, and participating in the social rituals that grease the wheels of patronage (discussing the news or sports by the water cooler).[3] As we have suggested, the informal aspects of organizational life pose different moral problems from those related to formal organizational structures and processes. Informal practices may undermine official or formal practices, as when friends or insiders are given preference in hiring or promotion despite official rules that prohibit this activity (see Chapter Five). Such practices make an organization's commitment to ethics appear superficial to both employees and outsiders.

Within a health care organization, the natural systems approach can be a useful tool for examining the clinical and professional cultures and work relationships. It may also be a lens by which to discern a breakdown between clinical and administrative units or to identify how and why official policies and rules are not followed.

For example, a natural systems approach might help an ethics mechanism uncover some of the causes of the billing and coding irregularities at St. Somewhere Hospital. Using this perspective leads members of the mechanism group to ask different questions from those raised in a rational systems analysis. Do physicians neglect their charting responsibilities because the culture of the clinic marginalizes administrative work and emphasizes hands-on patient care? Are certain clinical departments overworked and understaffed and therefore relying on ad hoc coding procedures because following the official guidelines takes too much time away from patients?

From the administrative side, the mechanism might inquire into the nature and level of training of individuals who maintain hospital records or handle the billing. Has the manager or the hospital provided ongoing education so employees are aware of changes in legal regulations or industry standards? What is the managerial style in the billing office? Has the manager given too much discretion to her employees or failed to exercise adequate oversight?

The natural systems approach alerts an analyst to examine how employees and managers act in their particular work environment and to identify workgroup cultures that might encourage unethical, illegal, or morally questionable behaviors. It also suggests that an ethics mechanism should consider the extent to which staff members resolve conflicting job demands or policies through informal measures.

Open Systems Approach

The first two approaches concentrate on internal issues, but the open systems approach focuses on external relationships. The emphasis is on seeing that an organization is embedded in a set of much larger organizations on which it is dependent for resources, personnel, and legitimacy. The environment, made up of customers, suppliers, competitors, allies, and regulatory bodies, is often unstable and highly variable. How easily an organization can adapt to an uncertain environment largely determines its survival and success. Moreover, these external relationships and the need to adapt shape the internal structures and practices of an organization. For example, the rise of JCAHO means that hospitals must create accreditation mechanisms and empower compliance officers (in other words, they must create structures, roles, and review practices) to survive; failure to do so results in loss of accreditation.

An open systems approach focuses on an organization's interdependent relations and efforts to span boundaries (that is, to create cooperative, interdependent relationships with other organizations). A new set of ethical problems arises in viewing an organization this way. Does adaptation to change in the market mean that mission and values must be sacrificed? How are external relationships created and maintained? What principles guide these relationships (caveat emptor, principle over profit)? If an organization allows subunits to enter into some contractual relations on their own—as in the case of Partnership Health Care, where each of the five hospitals was allowed to contract directly with medical suppliers—what kind of oversight does the system practice? Does subunit autonomy promote good stewardship?

Returning to the case of the billing irregularities at St. Somewhere, an open systems analysis sees the possibility that the problems may be caused, in part, by the hospital's relationships with insurers or regulators. An ethics mechanism might study the history of St. Somewhere's relationships with insurers to check for incidents or patterns of fraud or abuse. Similarly, the members might look into the hospital's relationships with regulators: Have recent outside reviews of the billing office been thorough? Have changes in regulations been effectively communicated to the hospital?

Ethics mechanisms relying on the open systems approach should also examine the strategies an organization uses to minimize environmental uncertainty. Merging with a similar organization is a common tactic because it eliminates competition, allows greater economies of scale, and may expand the range of services or products. However, it could also fundamentally change the mission or values of the organization or create new conflicts, because the merging partner having greater power (larger assets, larger share of the market) may create policies, allocate resources, or eliminate jobs that adversely affect the weaker partner.

In our case study, Jewish Health Care (JHC) was pushed into the merger with PHC largely because of declining revenues and growing debt. After the merger, the hospital was turned into an ambulatory care center, while acute care services were transferred to Suburban Hospital. JHC employees and leaders believed their facilities were being underused (a stewardship issue). In addition, its mission to serve an indigent population has been undermined because it cannot offer acute care. Yet its weak financial position leaves Jewish Health Care officials in a poor bargaining position. In this case, the demands of survival overrode preservation of the system's historic identity and mission.

Table 2.1 highlights the key features of each approach and identifies the health care arena in which each is most applicable.

The table also suggests that no one theoretical approach is complete. Each focuses attention on certain aspect of organizational life. Each may be used to reveal a host of ethical problems related to formal and informal structures, and internal and external relationships. Using all three requires a set of investigation strategies:

1. Examining organizational documents. These include operating rules and procedures; the employee handbook (which lists behavioral guidelines, performance evaluation criteria, grievance procedures, and so on); and statements of mission, values, or organizational philosophy. This is necessary to identify the formal structures and practices and should be the first step in investigating any issue. This creates a baseline from which to compare actual practices.

Table 2.1. Summary of Primary Approaches to Organizational Analysis.

Approach	Key Problems	Analytic Focus	Applicability	Ethical Issues
Rational systems	Integration, control, goal attainment	Formal rules, procedures, structures	Hierarchical or bureaucratic organization; administration and management units within health care organization	Violation of formal rules, practices, norms; negative outcomes of following rules
Natural systems	Integration, control, goal attainment	Informal rules, procedures, structures, workplace politics	Hierarchical or bureaucratic organization; professional units within health care organization	Discrepancies between formal and informal structures; power politics
Open systems	Adaptation, resources, boundary spanning	Organization-environment relationship	Integrated delivery system, health care alliance	Boundary spanning; niche marketing

2. Observing people doing their work. This strategy allows the analyst to uncover the informal rules, communication network, relations of power, and goals, as well as compare the informal and formal structures. This might entail attending staff meetings and disciplinary hearings and listening carefully during unit meetings and social rituals.

3. Interviewing an organization's leaders and employees. The members of the ethics mechanism ask about the mission, values, and goals of the organization and how they are implemented in practice, to identify how formal and informal structures operate and reveal how closely the two fit.

All three strategies also are useful for examining an organization's external relationships. Interviewing employees who deal directly with outside agents and with leaders who can explain adaptation strategies may be the most effective approach. These suggested investigative techniques do not conform to the familiar case-study method used in traditional bioethics, nor are they commonly used by managers in leading and running their departments. However, the complexity and breadth of organizational ethics problems demands investigative strategies (such as those we have outlined) that help the members of the ethics mechanisms fully understand how their organization works and why ethical problems occur.

Organizational Culture

A great deal of research in the 1980s and 1990s emphasized the importance of culture in understanding how an organization works. Every organization has a culture—most likely several. *Culture* refers to a set of *beliefs* (opinions about how things are) and *values* (statements about how things ought to be), which over time are validated by the organization and transformed into shared *underlying assumptions about the world*. These last beliefs are now based on experience and thus no longer need to be tested and can be taken for granted. All of these values or beliefs are manifested by a variety of symbolic devices, such as *myths* and *stories* (for instance, how the organization was founded), *rituals* (weekly after-work happy hour), *specialized language* (gallows humor), or *ideology* (a set of ideas about how the world is or ought to be).

Culture serves to integrate people into an organization because the set of shared values, beliefs, and meaning creates a sense of identity and belonging, encourages loyalty and consensus, and presents a rationale for appropriate and inappropriate workplace behavior. At the same time, culture differentiates subunits within an organization from one another and from the official culture. Many organizations consist of numerous subcultures, each of which, as we have suggested, holds a specific set of values, beliefs, rituals, specialized languages, and symbols. Some cultures simply differ from the official one, while others are created in self-conscious opposition to it.

A moral analysis of an organization is not complete until the analyst understands its culture or cultures. Because culture constitutes the orienting and motivating values and beliefs that guide organizational behavior, it has the potential to do great good or great harm. Table 2.2 identifies seven key dimensions of organizational culture.

How an organization answers the questions in the table reveals a great deal about its ethical standing and helps the inquirer target a moral analysis. For example, if an organization has an aggressive, profit-driven identity, does this influence how it interacts with competitors and regulators? How does a short-term, present-day time horizon shape organizational decisions and behaviors regarding resource allocation, pollution, worker safety, or profit seeking? What are the consequences for employees if the organizational culture regards individuals as mere cogs in the machine?

The ethical problems that arise as organizational cultures collide are illustrated in the creation of Partnership Health Care. As part of the merger, some clinical services and their personnel at St. Somewhere were shifted to Suburban Hospital. Integrating St. Somewhere's staff with Suburban's clinical teams has been difficult. The problems stem from competing philosophies of patient care: St. Somewhere favors a low-tech, compassionate approach, while Suburban favors a high-tech approach that does not encourage creation of staff-patient relationships. As a result, the new staffs spend a lot of time arguing about use of expensive tests and invasive procedures. Patient care has been compromised on a number of occasions because of constant change in the care regimen. An ethics mechanism might be able to resolve the conflict first by helping both sides understand how their particular culture

**Table 2.2. Underlying Dimensions
of Organizational Culture.**

Dimension	Questions
1. Relationship to Environment	At the organizational level, do key members view the organization's relationship to its environment as dominant, submissive, or harmonious?
2. The Nature of Reality and Truth	How do members of the organization define what is true and what is not, what is a "fact," and how truth is to be determined?
3. The Nature of Human Nature	What does it mean to be "human"? Is human nature basically good, evil, or neutral? Are humans perfectible or not?
4. The Nature of Human Activity	What is the "right" thing for human beings to do, on the basis of the stated assumptions about reality, the environment, and human nature: to be active, passive, self-developmental, or fatalistic?
5. The Nature of Human Relationships	What is the "right" way for people to relate to each other, to distribute power and resources? Is life cooperative or competitive; individualistic, collaborative, or communal; based on traditional lineal authority or participatory? Does the organization value diversity or homogeneity? What are the basic assumptions about how conflict should be resolved, and how decisions should be made?

Source: Schein, E. H. *Organizational Culture and Leadership.* (2nd ed.) San Francisco: Jossey-Bass, 1991, pp. 95–96. Adapted with permission of Jossey-Bass, Inc., a subsidiary of John Wiley & Sons.

of care bestows privilege on certain practices and discourages others; second, by highlighting the features of each culture that enhance patient care and that can serve as points of agreement and hence cooperation; and third, by identifying practice parameters that define the conditions under which high-tech or low-tech care procedures are to be implemented.

Researchers have identified a variety of organizational cultures, as outlined in Table 2.3.

Each culture creates the conditions for particular moral problems. For example, a clinical culture may be a power culture in which physicians exercise professional authority and create an atmosphere of frustration, resentment, and perhaps fear among nurses. Nurses' concerns about patient care may go unheeded if their medical authority is unrecognized or subordinated to that of physicians. This may result in poor care.[4] Generally, some organizational cultures foster "moral silence" (that is, failure to verbalize and act on one's moral convictions) among employees. Moral discussion and behavior tend to be muted or prevented in an organization whose culture emphasizes these features:

- Business is seen as morally neutral; the only ethical obligation is to turn a profit for shareholders.
- Loyalty to the team or to one's boss outweighs voicing concern about ethically questionable practices, especially if speaking out or whistle-blowing carries negative consequences (losing one's job, being ostracized).
- Efficiency and pragmatism are so highly valued that considering the ethical implications of organizational policy or practice is seen as interfering with getting the job done; discussion of ethics or moral issues is defined as naïve, idealistic, or utopian.[5]

Assessing Organizational Culture

Evaluating an organization's culture is a difficult task. Even identifying the key characteristics of a culture is problematic. Deeply held values and assumptions are often taken for granted and rarely articulated. The most important investigative strategies are simply to ask questions and listen. Researchers have developed three general strategies to identify and assess organizational cultures: gather stories, identify problems, and "learn the language."

Table 2.3. Types of Organizational Culture.

Type	Main Characteristics
Power	Centralization of power Emphasis on individual rather than group decision making Fundamentally autocratic; suppresses challenges from below Individual members motivated to act by a sense of loyalty to their superior (patriarchal power) or fear of punishment (autocratic power) Implicit rules rather than explicit rules Key values: control, stability, loyalty
Role or bureaucratic	Hierarchical structure Emphasis on formal procedures and written rules to guide work behavior Clearly defined role requirements and boundaries of authority Risk minimized Impersonal and predictable work environment Individuals as cogs in the machine; position more important than the person Key values: efficiency, predictability, production, control
Achievement, innovative	Emphasis on team and strong belief in the organization's mission Work organized according to task requirements High degree of worker autonomy and flexibility Decision making pushed downward Workers acquire cross-functional knowledge and skills Key values: creativity, adaptability, risk taking, teamwork
Support	Emphasis on egalitarianism Functions to nurture personal growth and development of members Tends to be found in nonprofit rather than commercial organizations Workplace is safe, nonpoliticized Key values: commitment, consensus, growth

Source: Adapted from Cartwright, S., and Cooper, C. L. "The Role of Culture Compatibility in Successful Organizational Marriage." *Academy of Management Executive,* 1993, 7(2), 62; and Zammuto, R. F., and Krakower, J. Y. "Quantitative and Qualitative Studies of Organizational Culture." *Research in Organizational Change and Development,* vol. 5. Greenwich, Conn.: JAI Press, 1991, p. 86.

Gathering Stories

One of the best ways to learn about an organization's core values and identity is to ask members to relate stories about its founding, legendary figures, and notable successes and failures. Stories reveal what an organization and its people consider to be the distinctive and ideal characteristics of the place. They are also a central means by which the organization transmits messages about obeying authority and power, following rules, or enacting the mission. The organizational story commonly focuses on three themes: equality and inequality, security and insecurity, control and lack of control.[6] Identifying which term in each pair is emphasized in a story reveals important clues about how it treats employees or what values and principles guide the mission. Additionally, this practice exposes disjunction between the ideals of an organization and its lived practice.

Identifying Problems

Another strategy to uncover values is to ask employees of an organization what they consider to be the tough problems and how the organization, or their particular subunit, addresses them. The areas that health care workers identify as problems (say, patient satisfaction, or malpractice) indicate what people consider to be important. Uncovering how they resolve problems (for example, settling a malpractice suit out of court to avoid public admission of guilt) reveals what kind of moral message an organization sends to its employees, customers, and the general public. Observing organizational rituals or following employee evaluation and promotion procedures helps an analyst assess how closely values match practice.

Learning the Language

Attending to language is crucial for understanding organizational culture. One scholar notes that "labels, metaphors and platitudes are building blocks" for the worldview and philosophy that an organization uses to motivate or control behavior.[7] Informal norms and rules are often buried in the complaints that subunits have regarding one another. A direct way to assess dominant and alternative cultures within an organization is to ask a variety of people (from the CEO to the administrative assistant) to rank a set of statements that best describe their organization (see Exhibit 2.1).

This exercise is also a useful tool to identify differences between how management and labor, professionals and administrators understand their organization's mission, values, and identity. It helps identify which aspects of an organization's culture are commonly agreed upon and considered important and which are in dispute and considered less important. Comparison of groups at different levels in the hierarchy (professionals, administrators, and so on) and within subunits (physicians, nurses) strengthen the analysis.

Organizational Psychology

Organizational psychology is concerned with understanding the motivations underlying workplace behavior and explaining how and why employees process information, interpret policy, and make decisions. In particular, the decision-making arena presents a potential ethical minefield. The organization strives to make the decision-making process rational, relying on cost-benefit analysis or comparable evaluation of how well a decision meets goals. Staff members, from the CEO to the nurses, rely on a variety of practices to reduce uncertainty and simplify and rationalize decision making. In practice, however, rationality often fails. An uncertain or ambiguous environment, the sheer complexity of decisions, and human foibles conspire to reduce rationality. A strategy to enhance rationality or simplify decisions may create moral problems.

One tool often used to facilitate this process is routinization. Here, decisions are defined according to categories—in other words, this is a resource allocation or a personnel decision—each of which has a set of rules to follow. Problems arise if a particular decision falls into multiple categories or if it poses an exception to the rules. One common rule allows individuals to look for a satisfactory solution to a problem rather than the optimal one. This practice expedites the decision-making process and helps the organization or subunit reach a particular goal, but it may also create ethical problems and expose an organization (especially one in the field of health care) to litigation. In an effort to save money, Partnership Health Care has cut nursing staff by 15 percent at all five hospitals and replaced the nurses with less skilled, but less

Exhibit 2.1. Diagnosing Corporate Culture.

Please rank this set of statements describing features of an organization according to how closely they resemble your organization or work unit.
1 = most closely resembles your organization
4 = least like your organization

Dominant Characteristics

_____ Organization A is a personal place. It is like an extended family. People seem to share a lot of themselves.

_____ Organization B is a dynamic and entrepreneurial place. People are willing to stick their necks out and take risks.

_____ Organization C is a formalized and structured place. Bureaucratic procedures generally govern what people do.

_____ Organization D is competitive in orientation. A major concern is with getting the job done. People are very production- and achievement-oriented.

Organizational Glue

_____ The glue that holds organization A together is loyalty and commitment. Cohesion and teamwork are characteristic of the organization.

_____ The glue that holds organization B together is a focus on innovation and development. The emphasis is on being at the cutting edge.

_____ The glue that holds organization C together is formal procedures, rules, and policies. Maintaining a smooth-running organization is important.

_____ The glue that holds organization D together is emphasis on production and goal accomplishment. Being aggressive in the marketplace is a common theme.

Organizational Climate

_____ The climate in organization A is participative and comfortable. High trust and openness exist.

_____ The climate in organization B emphasizes high energy and readiness to meet new challenges. Trying new things and trial-and-error learning are common.

_____ The climate in organization C emphasizes permanence and stability. Expectations regarding procedures are clear and enforced.

_____ The climate in organization D is competitive and confrontational. The emphasis is on beating the competition.

Source: Quinn, R. E. *Beyond Rational Management: Mastering the Paradoxes and Competing Demands of High Performance.* San Francisco: Jossey-Bass, 1988, pp. 142–143. Adapted with permission of Jossey-Bass, Inc., a subsidiary of John Wiley & Sons.

costly, nurse's aides. Such a move is consistent with what other health care systems are doing, and it allows PHC to avoid cutting other programs or staff. In the short run, PHC realizes substantial savings in labor costs, but the long-term costs may make this decision damaging in terms of employee morale, reputation, and finances. If the level of care declines, PHC loses customers. If having less skilled caregivers harms patients, then PHC faces malpractice suits.

As the ethics mechanism identifies the rules that guide decision making and its rationale, the members should ask a number of questions: Which organizational practices and structures constrain how decisions are made? How do they influence what decisions are actually made? Do individuals use organizational structures and procedures to escape responsibility for decisions? How are decisions routinely made, and how is conflict over applying rules resolved? Answers to these questions speak loudly about the ethical nature of an organization.

Another simplifying tool that executives use to guide their decision making is a set of general assumptions about the world and people.[8] These assumptions are based on beliefs about how the world operates, about the causes and consequences of action in the world, and about the characteristics and expected behaviors of groups of people. This last set of beliefs serves as a means to divide the world into *us* and *them.*

Assumptions of this sort minimize the complexity of an organization's environment and the context of decision making and thus render both environment and context predictable. As a result, executives tend to rely on a number of simplifying assumptions or theories to make decisions, as shown in Exhibit 2.2).

For example, some executives tend to give little weight to, or even ignore, possible consequences of an organizational action or policy whose risk have low probability. This is related not only to the near-sacred quality of the means-and-ends rationality that dominates organizational thinking but also to the sheer pragmatic imperative of getting things done (having to consider every imaginable consequence and cost can paralyze the decision-making process). Giving little weight to the consequences of a decision also relates to one's assumptions about others; an executive may be likely to ignore the consequences of an organizational action if those most

Exhibit 2.2. Strategies Executives Use to Simplify the Decision-Making Process.

Assumptions About the World

1   *Ignoring possible outcomes or consequences.* Ethical decisions must be based on accurate information about the world, which means that decision makers must consider the full range of consequences of any decision. Ethical problems may arise if executives commit any of the following decision errors:

1.1   Underestimating the importance of risk (tendency is to emphasize the benefits of a new policy or activity and ignore risks that have low probability)

1.2   Ignoring the consequences for stakeholders, especially if they belong to relatively powerless groups (women, children, minorities) or diffuse groups (the public)

1.3   Pretending the public or stakeholders won't find out about the decision and why it was made

1.4   Discounting the future; overvaluing short-term costs and benefits

1.5   Treating collective costs as "externalities" or as not ethically relevant

2   *Judging risk.* Ethical decisions rest on accurate evaluation of the risks associated with the consequences of any decision. Ethical problems may arise if executives commit the following errors of risk assessment:

2.1   Denying uncertainty; pretending that the world is stable and predictable

2.2   Pretending that events in the world are not ruled by chance but can be explained according to a favorite reason or cause (for example, success comes to those who work hard)

2.3   Expecting perfect evidence; for example, ignoring strong statistical evidence that smoking leads to negative health outcomes such as cancer because the evidence is not foolproof (not true that in 100 percent of cases, smokers contract cancer)

2.4   Defining or framing risk in negative terms (for example, losing a job or closing a hospital); affects how difficult trade-off decisions are made, with executives tending to avoid risk associated with perceived loss

3   *Perceiving cause.* Ethical decisions also rest on accurate understanding of the causes of problems associated with any

**Exhibit 2.2. Strategies Executives Use to
Simplify the Decision-Making Process, Cont'd.**

decision. Ethical problems may arise if executives commit the
following errors of causal misperception:

3.1 Blame the person rather than systemic causes or organizational
structures (authority systems, technology)

3.2 Sin of omission; failing to take action is not seen as causal; used
as a way to shield individuals and organizations from moral
responsibility

Assumptions About Others

1 *Ethnocentrism.* Judging other groups as inferior or abnormal
because they are different from one's own group

2 *Stereotyping.* General beliefs about the traits, behaviors, skills, and
so forth of particular groups that may not hold for any one
member of the group in question

3 *In-group favoritism.* Special preference is given to preferred
groups

Source: Adapted from Messick, D. M., and Bazerman, M. H. "Ethical Leadership
and the Psychology of Decision Making." *Sloan Management Review,* 1996, *37*(2),
9–22.

affected are not stakeholders (for instance, the public) or belong
to a negatively valued group (indigents).

These decision-making problems have the potential for great
harm to individuals or groups and to the organization. Consider
the shift of clinical services in St. Somewhere's merger with others
to form Partnership Health Care. After the merger, the leadership
of PHC decided to consolidate reproductive health services at Deaconess Hospital and one of the suburban hospitals. This decision
reflected the system's well-intentioned effort to reduce costs. However, it left the inner-city clients of St. Somewhere without local reproductive health services, a problem compounded by the facts
that many of these patients lack private transportation and there
is no public transportation to the four suburban sites. Is it ethical
for a health care organization to reduce or eliminate services for
some populations to meet broader systems goals? Would exhaus-

tive analysis of the possible consequences of such a decision create ethical alternatives (such as providing free transportation from St. Somewhere to one of the other hospitals)? An ethics mechanism can use the list of simplifying assumptions in Exhibit 2.2 to evaluate decisions and the decision-making process at all levels of the organization. The list may be a particularly valuable tool if the mechanism evaluates decision making as it unfolds, rather than after the fact.

Decisions within an organization are guided by more than routine procedure and simplifying assumptions. Some scholars argue that informal practice and structure, as well as the varied cultures of an organization, are often powerful influences on decision making; according to James March and Johan Olsen, "[Sometimes] the decision-making process is not strongly related to the organizational action, in other words, the policy selected, the price set, the man hired. Rather it is connected to the definition of truth and virtue in the organization, to the allocation of status, to the maintenance or change of friendship, goodwill, loyalty, and legitimacy, and to the definition and redefinition of 'group interest.'"[9]

In such a case, self-interest, emotion, group bias, and organizational culture influence how decisions are made and who makes them. A study of how middle managers make decisions in an engineering firm demonstrates that loyalty to one's superior, opportunism, and office politics often govern decision making. In many organizations with pyramidal authority structures, decisions often are made not to fulfill a particular set of goals or stay true to the mission and values of the organization, but rather to protect one's superior and hence oneself. Robert Jackall observes that "fealty to the boss" becomes the overarching decision rule as success and promotion come to those who follow the rule, while blame for problems and "nonpromotability" befall those who deviate (even when they act to meet official goals). Concern about authority relations and the security of one's place in an organization may blind individuals to the ethical consequences of their decisions.[10]

The members of an ethics mechanism would be wise to attend to both the formal and routine procedures that are intended to guide decision making, as well as the informal politics, interpersonal motivation, and group pressure that can turn a decision into ethical liability (see Exhibit 2.3).

**Exhibit 2.3.   Steps to Identify How
and Why Decisions Are Made.**

1. Observe the behavior of decision makers. Attend staff meetings and clinical conferences, and observe organizational members in situations where they routinely make decisions. How do relationships of power and authority influence the decisions made by subordinates and superordinates? What are the operative decision rules? Do they systematically lead to ethically questionable outcomes?

2. Interview organizational members. Ask members how and why they make decisions, especially those involving trade-offs. Ask members what motivates decision making. Ask how pressure from the top influences what and how decisions are made.

3. Examine organizational documents that articulate operating procedures or decision rules, and then examine a variety of decision episodes to determine how closely action matches policy.

Source: Adapted from March, J. G., and Simon, H. A. *Organizations.* New York: Wiley, 1958. Reprinted in Grusky, O., and Miller, G. A. (eds.). *The Sociology of Organizations.* New York: Free Press, 1981, p. 140.

The theories reviewed in this chapter are tools for individuals and groups interested in conducting a moral analysis of an organization. Alone, they do not yield ethical insight or moral diagnosis, but they should help the investigator frame questions and discern features of organizational structure and behavior in which potential ethical problems reside.

Notes

1. Scott, R. C. *Organizations: Rational, Natural, and Open Systems.* (2nd ed.) Upper Saddle River, N.J.: Prentice Hall, 1987.
2. Scott (1987), p. 55.
3. Jackall, R. *"Moral Mazes: Bureaucracy and Managerial Work."* In T. Donaldson and P. H. Werhane (eds.), *Ethical Issues in Business.* (5th ed.) Upper Saddle River, N.J.: Prentice Hall, 1996 [1983].
4. On the competing cultures of nurses and physicians, see Chambliss, D. F. *Beyond Caring: Hospitals, Nurses and the Social Organization of Ethics.* Chicago: University of Chicago, 1996.
5. Bird, F. B., and Waters, J. A. "The Moral Muteness of Managers." In Donaldson and Werhane (1996).

6. Martin, J., Feldman, M. S., Hatch, M. J., and Sitkin, S. B. "The Uniqueness Paradox in Organizational Stories." *Administrative Science Quarterly,* 1983, *28,* 438–453.

7. Czarniawska-Joerges, B. "Merchants of Meaning: Management Consulting in the Swedish Public Sector." In B. A. Turner (ed.), *Organizational Symbolism.* Berlin: De Gruyter, 1990, p. 139.

8. Messick, D. M., and Bazerman, M. H. "Ethical Leadership and the Psychology of Decision Making." *Sloan Management Review,* 1996, *37*(2), 9–22.

9. March, J. G., and Olsen, J. P. "Organizational Choice Under Ambiguity." In J. G. March and J. P. Olsen (eds.), *Ambiguity and Choice in Organizations.* Bergen, Norway: Universitetsforlaget, 1976, p. 16.

10. Jackall, R. "Moral Mazes: Bureaucracy and Managerial Work." In Donaldson and Werhane (1996).

Chapter Three

Organizational Support for Ethical Behavior

The medieval theologian Thomas Aquinas summarized human moral obligation in this way: "Good is to be done and promoted, and evil is to be avoided."[1] With the possible exception of Catholic health care providers, it is unlikely that people in modern health care organizations or those who lead them would turn to St. Thomas for counsel on organizational ethics. From an organizational perspective, however, his formulation is noteworthy because it highlights the need to *support* the good. Good is to be not only done but *promoted*. By this reckoning, a health care organization should act to support the staff in doing good on its behalf. It also seems that the organization should act to discourage employees from conduct that is wrong.

One can read Thomas's dictum as a reminder that the organization has an obligation to promote health-related goods in its external relationships, especially in the community it serves. Elaborating other external obligations certainly warrants attention as an aspect of organizational ethics. However, an organization's obligation to promote good is not limited to external relationships and activities. It extends to *all* the organization's activities, internal as well as external, and entails promoting good conduct and actively discouraging wrongdoing on the part of all who work for the organization or otherwise represent it.

At the same time, asserting a need to support right action begs the question of what constitutes "moral support." What can a health care organization do so that staff experience moral support?

The analysis offered in the previous chapter suggests that the answer must encompass the formal and informal cultures of the organization. Employees participate in and are influenced by both cultures and also by various subcultures, such as the one (or more) in their department or professional group.

The challenge to any organizational ethics initiative is to find ways to influence these cultures and the staff who work within them. A variety of misconceptions and related missteps can undermine a beginning ethics initiative; the first section of this chapter discusses some of these potential pitfalls. But there are also many ways to support ethical behavior. The concluding portion of the chapter identifies a number of those means and resources and suggests how they function as ingredients in a program extending moral support to the staff.

Promoting Good Conduct Within the Organization

Devoting attention to organizational ethics is itself a significant way to promote ethical consciousness and conduct among the staff. By disseminating the message that ethics is important, promulgating an organizational ethics statement or code of conduct, and providing education in recognizing and responding to ethical issues, a health care organization both signals concern for ethical behavior and offers a measure of support to employees concerned about conducting their activities ethically. (See "Moral Commitments Guiding Organizational Conduct" in Appendix Two.)

By and large, these components of a basic ethics initiative seek to raise consciousness and impart essential information about ethics, and perhaps furnish basic training in ethical problem solving. A code of conduct may also aim to discourage wrongdoing by threatening sanctions for violation of or noncompliance with specific dictates of the code of ethical conduct, which may in fact function largely as a code of legal compliance. Important as such measures are, however, they are only a beginning for the organization that genuinely desires to support good conduct among those who act on its behalf. There are significant moral realities within any health care organization that such efforts barely touch—or miss completely. Insufficient recognition of these realities can block or delay the progress of an ethics program.

The Problem of Consistency

For one thing, elements of the organization's moral culture may be—or be perceived as—inconsistent with one another. The inconsistencies may involve formal and informal cultures among or within those cultures. Thus, for example, the lived moral experience of those working in the organization may contradict the values espoused in the ethics program—even if those values are implicit in the organization's mission statement. People may cite instances in which their desires or actual efforts to do the right thing have been frustrated by some feature of the organization's policy, prevailing practice, or moral climate. Far from supporting its staff in doing the good they are ostensibly employed to perform, the organization may be perceived as actually hindering people in their efforts to carry out its mission and implement its values.

Clinical staff dedicated to competent, compassionate care and the healing of sick people may feel that hospital procedures, financial pressures, or staffing patterns actually serve as barriers to the very care they are called to give. Or human resource personnel who take seriously their organization's stated commitment to diversity in recruitment may find that actual hiring practices favor insiders or (particularly at the executive level) those in an old-boy network, effectively circumventing the diversity that a recruiter seeks to incorporate in submitting a candidate list to a hiring manager.

Some might object that such examples reflect sour grapes on the part of people who refuse to accept change or who simply don't get their way. Complaints about staffing patterns, for example, may be attributed to, or written off as, classic labor-management differences of opinion, part of the inevitable tension that accompanies the inequality of power in this relationship. There is often more than a grain of truth in such an objection. But there may also be legitimate reasons for people's moral distress, which in any case does not go away by being ignored or dismissed.

At the least, the situations just described reflect failure to achieve ethical *alignment* in the organization's implementation of its espoused values, a failure not uncommon in complex organizations confronting rapid change in the economy and in the health care environment. Such situations are a profound reminder that multiple forces are constantly at play in shaping an organization's ethical climate and its formal and informal cultures, forces that rarely achieve complete harmony with one another. Thus an organization's formal organizational ethics program may sometimes run afoul of other, often hidden, forces that influence staff to act in ways that are questionable, or simply out of line if weighed against the program's espoused values.

Whether this phenomenon is labeled an "alignment" problem or a "corporate integrity" problem,[2] from the employee's perspective one result is that the organization appears to apply its own values inconsistently. Staff people then feel unsupported in pursuing the good they believe they should pursue; some may even report that the organization discourages them from doing the right thing. An additional side effect is the advent or deepening of moral cynicism and dampening of morale, especially among those who have high ethical expectations and aspire to work for an organization in which they can take pride.[3]

It does not do simply to object that those with moral qualms about their organization's activities, or about what they feel constrained to do, have a duty to speak up and seek to bring about change. Although it is true that individuals bear responsibility for their own actions[4] and may sometimes be obligated to take a stand even at some risk to their own position in the organization,[5] the health care organization cannot expect its associates to be moral heroes on a regular basis. The reality of power relationships, and many staff members' perceptions of power and its possible use against them, mitigates against the likelihood that most employees will take courageous positions or even raise uncomfortable questions. Moreover, most human beings are not likely to assume the role of prophet or act as a rugged individual in the face of cultural or leadership opposition within an organization. Pressures to conform are too great, and most individuals are not prepared—or perhaps politically savvy enough—to call for ethical change without evidence that some external support for their effort is available.

"Knowledge" Problems and "Doing" Problems

A second shortcoming of some organizational ethics initiatives is a tendency to proceed as if the common denominator among ethics problems is essentially a knowledge deficit: people don't *know* what constitutes an ethical problem or don't *know* how to respond if they do identify an ethical conflict. The evident remedy for such an underlying problem is information and education about ethics and compliance. To be sure, disseminating information, and perhaps developing a process for ethical decision making, surely helps people recognize and categorize ethical and legal pitfalls and perhaps sort out at least some ethical problems. Enhanced knowledge can, in turn, relieve the anxiety or moral distress that accompanies uncertainty about what to do or how to think a problem through. If knowledge is in some sense power, it can also be a source of security.

But are all ethical problems in the health care organization primarily attributable to lack of ethical knowledge? Does the availability of additional information by itself enhance the ethical conduct of organizational associates? The implicit assumption that knowledge is *the* answer overlooks other problem scenarios. For one thing, and perhaps most obviously, even offering basic ethics education and training in problem solving does not help employees know how to proceed ethically in all situations. There are still hard cases in which additional consultation with someone (perhaps an ethics officer or consultant) or some group (an ethics committee) is necessary to help an employee think through complex or novel problems. That is, having consultative resource people available may be an indispensable supplement to the foundational knowledge imparted by an elementary ethics training program.

Less obviously, even when people more or less know the answer to a problem—that is, when education and training have worked, cognitively speaking—sometimes they are still hesitant to *act* on what they know. Perhaps they harbor residual doubt or lack confidence in their still-fresh knowledge and skills. In such an instance, the staff may need more than information and a decisional formula; they may need to talk things through with an experienced person or persons before they can feel confident enough to act on what they know. Clinical ethicists and health care ethics committees have long encountered similar phenomena in the clinical arena. A physician, for example, may recognize intellectually that it is ethically preferable to discontinue life-sustaining treatment in appropriate circumstances, but if such a situation actually arises, the physician may be uncomfortable with the decision (or be plagued by legal fears) and seek ethics committee consultation.

Such a request may conceal a covert, even unconscious, wish for the committee to confirm a course of action the physician has already thought through. If the committee finds itself readily concurring with the doctor's ethical reasoning or wondering what the "issue" or "conflict" is, members may wonder why the case came to the committee at all. Far from being a pointless exercise, however, such consultation may prove critical to optimal management of the case. Without the opportunity to consult with others face-to-face, in a dialogical fashion, the physician might shrink from following the course that he or she recognizes intellectually is best—with results that are detrimental to the patient and the family, not to mention staff morale. In such a case, the doctor's ethical need is not only for information but also for other forms of moral support, at least in part because deciding and acting on what one knows often requires courage, a virtue that may need relational support to help it take hold in guiding one's actions.

Mere Compliance Versus Excellence

A third problem in some introductory ethics programs, especially those focusing largely on corporate compliance (see Chapter Four), is a tendency to stress accurate knowledge of ethical and legal pitfalls on the one hand, while strongly reminding associates of the legal sanctions or institutional discipline they face if they fail to avoid those pitfalls. The tacit assumption of this approach is that Thomas's promotion of the good and avoidance of evil are best achieved if associates are made vividly aware of the negative consequences that can befall them or the organization, which might in turn pass on the pain, if they "screw up" through some form of noncompliance (whether intentional or inadvertent).

There are a number of problems with this approach. For one thing, by stressing legal and regulatory issues it can, albeit unintentionally, contribute to a mentality that says "If it's legal, it's ethical." For another, focusing on the negative—which, in many cases, can include a compliance hot line that invites anonymous reporting of possible wrongdoing—threatens to turn ethics into a policing mechanism, at least in the minds of personnel.[6] This use of an ethics program distorts the meaning of ethics itself; it also undermines the climate of trust that, as noted in Chapter One, is a cornerstone of any comprehensive ethics initiative, and indeed of any real possibility of transforming organizational moral culture.

Even the explicit threat of penalty or disciplinary action may not be sufficient to counteract other organizational forces (for example, fear of not meeting productivity goals) that lead employees to compliance violations,[7] intentionally or unintentionally. Moreover, fear of negative sanctions, such as peer disapproval or retaliation, may be strong enough to prevent those who know of violations from telling on others who have committed them.

A deeper criticism of such an approach is that the negative focus of a compliance-centered program is unlikely to help an organization achieve genuine ethical excellence. By its very nature, the law establishes minimal standards and tends to support little more than "moral mediocrity."[8] The legal emphasis is on avoiding violation, not on promoting good as Thomas urges. As a result, a program that concentrates on imparting knowledge of ethical and (mostly) legal pitfalls, while stressing the various sanctions that can follow a lapse, is unlikely to elicit the ethical best from an organization's staff. It does not promote alertness to opportunity for ethical improvement or reflection on their practice in serving the organization.[9]

Moreover, many professionals and paraprofessionals in health care organizations are motivated daily in their work by deep commitment to care and serve, and to do so in the most competent way possible. The idealism that led employees into the health care field in the first place is often very much alive within them. It constitutes a moral resource that can be marshaled by the organization and by leaders with vision and idealism of their own. Any organizational ethics program worth its salt seeks ways to support and positively elicit the energy inherent in such motivation and ideals. For this reason (and for others to be discussed), an organizational ethics program does well to seek to understand the moral psychology both of organizations and of the individuals who constitute and lead them (see the discussion of organizational psychology in Chapter Two).

Means for Assessing the Needs

If the leaders of an organization recognize that their employees need ethics education and other forms of organizational moral support, how do they go about addressing this need? A fitting approach is to begin with some form of assessment using tools such as those described in Chapter Two. One way to start is simply to ask, Where is the support wanted or needed? To ask this question is, in large measure, to inquire after the moral experience of staff throughout the organization. Observing the staff and receiving oral reports can be an initial diagnostic resource. What have those responsible for the organizational ethics program heard in the hallways, or otherwise been told, about the ethical condition of the organization? Even at second and third hand, there is something to be learned from the word on the street about ethical perceptions of the organization.

If, however, the aim is truly to engage the range and depth of associates' moral experience in all sectors and at all levels of the organization, it is imperative to solicit their firsthand reports—their own stories of moral experience—whether through formal interview or informal conversation. In particular, what are the ethical conflicts (those they consider ethical) that staff in various areas encounter in their work? There are a number of ways to frame such a question since for some people the term *ethical* may seem rarefied or unclear, while for others it needlessly confines thinking. It may be more productive to ask something like, "What kind of problem do you encounter that makes your insides churn or keeps you awake at night?"

In addition, or alternatively, those charged with proposing or enhancing the range of organizational supports for ethical conduct may seek to develop a priority list of target audiences whose voices they especially want to hear. The list includes those whose ethical experience of the organization seems essential to understanding and addressing the existing need for moral support. Which areas, and which personnel, are especially likely to experience significant ethical conflict? What group or individual conduct or decision making seems most important to the success of the overall effort in organizational ethics? What are the decisional pressure points where ethical conflict arises, where a moral misstep seems especially possible,[10] or where a moral lapse is particularly detrimental? Such questions may rightly lead to a focus on executives and their decision making (see Chapter Two) or on middle managers and the day-to-day choices they make. The tendency to concentrate attention on positions of formal authority, however, needs to be balanced by recognition that daily decisions and the actions of line staff are often prime areas for investigation.

Hence it is important that those responsible for the ethics initiative identify clearly what they hope will result from enhanced moral support. Do they, for example, want to influence the decision making—including policy decisions at the senior management level—and the actions that they discern are the most ethically sensitive? Do they wish also (or instead) to modify the culture and moral ecology of the organization by altering employees' attitudes and dispositions (their "readiness or tendencies to act in certain ways"[11]), and thus to touch "the way we do things around here" at a level deeper than that of individual decisions and their implementation?

The answers to these questions are likely to vary with the organization. The primary focus might be on spotting and addressing some or all of the thirty-odd problems listed in Exhibit 1.2 of Chapter One. Others might develop a priority list of broad issues or cultural themes that seem to pervade the organization. Still others might seek to identify (or they might already know) one crucial problem that requires focused attention. How potential themes for attention are formulated informs not only the choice of assessment modalities to be used and the questions to be asked of the staff but also the selection of the target groups to be surveyed or interviewed, as already noted.

Ethics information gathering with selected individuals and constituencies can proceed in various ways; using a combination of approaches may work best. A written survey asking for an individual's perception of the ethical climate and identification of problem areas is one way to gather information. A series of ethics-centered meetings, forums, and focus groups with selected groups at various levels is another. Individual interviews with selected leaders and key people in various areas, especially those where pivotal decisions are made, are an additional option.

Another, partially overlapping perspective on people's need for support can emerge from identifying the impact that the organization's culture has on their decision making and other aspects of their daily practice. As Chapter Two indicates, organizational culture is a highly complex phenomenon. One strategy for evaluating its effect is to compare the content of such formal elements as mission and values statements, policies and procedures, and employee handbooks with empirical observation of how things are actually done from day to day and with findings from the surveys, interviews, and other conversations suggested earlier. (See Chapter Two for other potential tools of analysis.)

Identifying Existing Supports

In the assessment process, it is important not only to identify the negatives—the problem areas in which support is needed yet inadequate—but also to look for the positives—those features of organizational life that are already experienced as moral support or demonstrate the potential to function in this way. The results of such an inquiry may vary widely, with their range surprising and even encouraging. Possible forms of support might include the most general and abstract: the statement of mission and core values, an organizational ethics statement or broadly formulated code of behavior, or the reigning ideology that brings together values and a descriptive picture of how things work to shape habits of thinking and pragmatic values.[12] Concrete or specifically focused features of organizational life that people experience as support might include the clear direction afforded by a corporate compliance program, the counsel of managers and supervisors, guidance received from supportive risk managers and legal departments, day-to-day peer support, an ongoing ethics education program, consultation with an ethics office or committee when needed, the shelter afforded vulnerable employees through the chain of command, a policy and practical protection available to the whistle-blower, and inclusion of ethical conduct and ethics leadership as recognized factors in job performance and performance evaluation.

Having discerned both the need for support and existing supportive resources, those responsible for organizational ethics are in a position to identify and select the means of support that seem best suited to particular needs. As they begin this process, however, they should also consider the nature of the human beings who are the target audience for the various supportive mechanisms.

Human Nature: Recognizing Diverse Needs and Motivations

Efforts to support the staff in recognizing and addressing the organization's ethical concerns can benefit from awareness of the diverse needs and motivations that people bring to their involvement with the health care organization. Psychologist Abraham Maslow contended that all human beings share basic needs for safety, belonging, love, respect, and self-esteem, which must be met before they feel free to attend to higher needs and the motivations those needs create.[13] Even so, everyday observation suggests that individuals display quite varied needs (and intensity of need) and proclivities, variety that might be attributable to such diverse influences as culture, education, family, economics, religion, and the accidents of biology. Several schemes that classify individual tendencies by personality "type" have evolved; whatever their validity, at least they serve as a reminder that people are not all wired in the same way, that people learn differently and respond to innumerable stimuli.

Moreover, in a health care organization, employees are variously situated, have diverse responsibilities, and are to some extent creatures of the power relationships within which they function. Further, individuals within an organization vary in their susceptibility to and dependence on feedback and influence from those around them, whether peers, superiors, or subordinates (whose influence on—indeed, whose power in relation to—those above them may be underestimated). All these factors also affect motivation and inclination; they deserve to be taken into account by those seeking to design appropriate forms of moral support for diverse and diversely situated people in their organizations.

But how are such considerations actually relevant to selecting and developing support systems for ethical conduct? At the least, they suggest that when it comes to need and motivation, one size does not fit all. No single formula for support, no one form of it, is likely to be effective for everyone in the organization. Yet there appears to be enough commonality among human beings generally— a commonality that may be reinforced within an organization by its culture—to permit some forms of support to reach and influence many, if not all, associates.

Thus moral motivation, or motivation to do the right thing, may come from many sources and take many forms. Some people may be left cold, untouched at their moral center, by references to the lofty but abstract language of an organizational mission statement. They may find the statement insufficiently concrete, or by virtue of their previous experiences it may arouse in them cynicism rather than moral inspiration. Other staff, however, may derive greater commitment to the mission from the very language that turns off their colleagues.

Conversely, some find the strongest support—and perhaps for them the *only* relevant support—in the directness with which a corporate compliance program guides them away from unlawful conduct and indeed threatens punishment if they fail to comply with its directives. What for the idealistic seems only a minimal and negative form of moral guidance, couched in the terminology of fraud and abuse and threatening penalty and discipline for violations, may serve as ample motivation to be ethical, as these people are inclined to understand the term. Still others may be moved by exhortations that insinuate (or, better, show data to demonstrate[14]) that their organization can minimize risk to its reputation,[15] or even gain a competitive edge in a crowded health care market,[16] by cultivating ethical business conduct. It has, for example, been argued persuasively that diversity initiatives are unlikely to achieve long-term success unless organizational leaders and hiring managers see clearly that affirming diversity and managing it well not only meets a social and moral responsibility but clearly makes good business sense.[17]

As a general rule, those designing the support program are probably best advised to draw on as many motivational resources as are available to them. One reason is simply that, in enhancing an organization's ethical character, we need all the help we can get. From the concrete to the abstract; from legal requirements *cum* punishment to rules of thumb; from pragmatic motives to idealistic reasons for being moral; from fears of discharge, fine, or jail to the promise of superior financial performance . . . any number of rationales, motivations, and incentives might conceivably be brought into play at one time or another, with one group or individual or another.

Of course, as suggested previously, some forms of support and the motivational appeal they make do not engender a favorable response in all members of the staff. Some motivational tactics can even precipitate negative reactions, as when clinicians are urged to act ethically because it's "good business" to do so. Motivations that allude to the patient-centered values inherent in the clinician's professional discipline are more likely to strike a responsive chord in clinical staff members and demonstrate that the organization supports them. Appeals to what sound like financial considerations often sound callous or simply beside the point, even given the enhanced financial consciousness of the managed care era.

It is important to consider the potential fit between the rationale or motivation and the group to which the ostensible support should be tailored. Sensitivity to the particular groups whose ethical conduct the organization wants to support can inform a corresponding selectivity about the supportive tools to be used with those groups and in the organization generally. Such sensitivity and selectivity entail having a sense of what people in the organization value, of how they think. This familiarity with the people is indispensable to the success of the motivational aspects of any organizational ethics program. It is most likely to be acquired through developing positive relationships, which are essential to the success of such a program because they create trust and convey integrity on the part of those leading the program.[18]

Developing and Using Ethically Supportive Resources

The remainder of this chapter is devoted to considering features of organizational life that can serve as resources or tools for moral support of health care employees. Many of these features exist already in most organizations, whether or not they have previously been identified as resources for an ethics initiative. Some may be well known in another guise, for example, as a function of an existing ethics committee that is primarily concerned with clinical issues. Other resources discussed here may not yet exist but could be developed in many organizations. The very process of selecting, developing, and using the range of resources available to a given organization presents an additional opportunity to reflect on just what the organization hopes to accomplish in its distinctive ethics effort. It also promotes creativity and innovation, both in choosing resources and in tailoring them to the organization's unique needs.

The suggestions here are meant as a representative sampling rather than an exhaustive list. They may well spur readers to generate additional ideas. These examples span formal and informal cultures. Some are abstract or indirect, insofar as they function at a high level of generality or address the context in which ethical action occurs. Others are concrete or direct, addressing specific issues or likely to function as tools for a particular purpose. The examples begin with those that may already be well known in an organization that has formal ethics mechanisms, such as an ethics committee that addresses issues arising in clinical care. Subsequent examples suggest possible development of new resources or involve adapting and using resources not typically thought of as support for the organization's ethics endeavor.

Ethics Mechanisms and Their Roles

The ethics committee already functions as an important mechanism and resource in many health care settings. As Chapter One notes, it has typically served three functions: education, consultation, and policy review or development. By carrying out these functions, and perhaps expanding them to accommodate an organizational focus (see Chapter One), an ethics mechanism can extend substantial moral support for ethical conduct in organizational activities generally as well as in clinical activities.

One caution to heed in this process is the reminder that the role and effectiveness of the ethics committee can easily be jeopardized by any hint that it is functioning as the ethics police. Although members sometimes lament the committee's lack of genuine clout or enforcement power, in general the capacity for moral support is best secured by arrangements that preserve the committee's role as an optional resource rather than a mandatory one. This approach seems the best insurance that a committee can be—and be perceived as—a safe and confidential place in which fair and impartial exploration of issues can occur.

Policy

From a rational systems perspective, written policies and procedures are indispensable formal means of guiding and supporting employees in ethically desirable behavior. As the natural systems and open systems approaches make clear, policy by itself cannot create and promote ethical conduct. Even if it is not sufficient for this task, however, policy is surely necessary to it. A given policy or set of policies, such as those governing human resource questions, can function as a solid basis and a source of baseline criteria for moral alignment throughout the organization and within particular areas or departments (see as examples Chapter Five and "Protecting the Whistle-Blower and Other Dissenters" later in this chapter). From the perspective of informal culture, both the quasi-legal function that policies fulfill and the message that policies send provide substantive moral support.

Policy signals to the employee what the organization values in fairly specific circumstances; given a reasonable effort by leaders to implement and enforce it, policy can be an effective guide to acceptable conduct in those circumstances. In its messaging function, policy can also set a tone and create an aura of expectation, and even aspiration, that extends beyond specific provisions addressed to the matter at hand.

The potential for policy to contribute to the ethics effort suggests that policy-making and policy-reviewing processes merit a different sort of attention than they have typically received. Policy is often treated as an instrument to be written in the simplest, most straightforward terms, in order to get the job done. Policy writing has also been viewed as a necessary evil, to be endured for the sake of bureaucratic mandate or accreditation requirements.

When policy making is informed solely by such quasi-legal and pragmatic considerations, the question of ethical rationale or connection to organizational mission and values tends to fall by the wayside. It may even be seen as fluff that adds little to—or even detracts from—the instrumental function that policies primarily serve. This pragmatic perspective makes an important point (policy is not, after all, a sermon), but it may overlook the importance of the messaging function of policy and procedure. In those policies dealing with issues that have evident ethical implications, a concisely written rationale that addresses ethical concerns or organizational values can simultaneously make the ethical connection explicit and signal to users of the policy that the organization takes the ethical dimension seriously. A by-product of writing such a rationale is that it invites those who draft and approve policy to reflect on the ethical implications of the issue at hand and the possible need to align the policy with other aspects of the organization's ethics program.

Educational Programs

It hardly needs to be said that some program of education in organizational ethics is critical in developing a strong ethical climate and ethical consciousness among the staff. One way in which an educational initiative functions as an actual *support* for ethical conduct is that even basic ethics education facilitates recognizing problems. Clarity about what constitutes a problem leads people to attend carefully to choosing the best course of action in the problematic situation. Support also comes from the fact that, as indicated earlier, increased knowledge (both as information and as methods for problem solving) tends to reduce anxiety. Lessened anxiety, in turn, counteracts the tendency to ignore problems because people feel ill-equipped to address them. It also heightens people's ability to be inclusive and creative in their moral thinking, whereas excessive anxiety may constrict deliberation.

Process and Audiences

In practice, supportive educational programs can and do take many forms. At the beginning of an ethics initiative, for example, there may be a multifaceted blitz of introductory educational resources:

- Well-designed brochures
- Informative articles in an associate newsletter or other venue
- An introductory ethics orientation or series of training sessions for all associates
- Modules for new-associate and new-manager orientation programs
- Other modules tailored to the needs of particular sectors of the organization (for example, billing, marketing, human resources, and physicians and other clinicians)
- Additional pertinent written materials, including case discussions and a basic schema for case analysis

After the initial educational offerings, there can be multiple forms of continuing ethics education, such as an "ethics for lunch" or "ethics brown-bag" program, either in a specific department or as a housewide offering. These programs often feature reflection on difficult cases, but they may also focus on particular ethical

concepts or policy matters. Most people in health care organizations do not need (or want) to be deluged with theoretical material about ethics in this or any sort of educational venture; they are
likely to want only enough theory to help them recognize issues
and select a way to approach them. In designing organizational
ethics education, the institution (especially if it is a hospital) will
likely have a track record of education that grew out of the clinical bioethics movement and formation of the institutional ethics
committee. Some of the same formats that have proven useful in
clinical ethics education can be adapted and translated into the
framework of organizational ethics issues and concepts.

Specific Content

Simply to discuss an educational plan, its potential audiences, and
program formats is not yet to specify what the content of such programming should be. Even to say that some programs focus on specific cases begs the question of what kinds of issues are considered
and what value framework is used to examine them. The issues, values, and case-consideration processes outlined in Chapter One
pose many possibilities for program content. Organizing and
adapting this material to distinctive circumstances is part of the
challenge any health care organization faces in turning the material into effective educational programming.

At the outset, the organization may wish to prioritize content
issues according to very basic criteria. It may want first, and perhaps even exclusively, to make associates aware of the "evil" that is,
in St. Thomas's words, "to be avoided." In that event, special educational attention to the so-called negatives, to the ethical and legal
pitfalls that compliance programs address, is in order (see Chapter Four and also "Corporate Compliance" later in this chapter).

However, ethics education should go well beyond the essentials of compliance education to enter the realm of some or all of
the issues addressed throughout this book. In the process, an educational program ought to pay special attention not only to issues but also to the values framework used to address them: the
values and virtues associated with health care and their relationship to other values associated with business and the life of organizations. Thus such well-known values and virtues as respect for
autonomy, beneficence, fidelity, avoidance of harm, compassion,
and justice may be discussed in relation to other values and virtues:

utility, stewardship, quality, pragmatism, integrity, cooperation, and tough-mindedness.[19]

Clinical staff members and those involved with the financial side of health care may learn from values and virtues that are not native to their own disciplines and training. Clinical staff members, particularly, may discover that exposure to concepts of business ethics—even if they are leery of business connotations in connection with their work—helps them understand issues and appreciate the perspectives of those who might otherwise be seen as the enemy. Exposure to a well-crafted summary of business ethics theories[20] may prove particularly interesting and instructive in this regard.

Senior Leaders and Trustees

A particular, and frequently overlooked, venue and focus for education is the organization's executive group or senior leadership team. Senior management and the governing body should by no means be overlooked in the educational picture, nor should they exempt themselves from it by claiming lack of need or irrelevance to their function. Indeed, it may be wise to design educational modules and materials that address these leaders' distinctive role and responsibility (Exhibit 3.1), for they too are likely to need both guidance and encouragement in fulfilling their fiduciary role as *moral* trustees of the organization.

If the needs assessment for organizational ethics education and support incorporates interviews with senior leaders and a structural analysis that identifies the pressure points where significant decisions are made,[21] the assessment can be the basis for educational programs that target leaders who face particular difficulties and opportunities. Here the fruits of research on the psychology of executive decision making and the contextual factors influencing decision making may prove relevant insofar as the research suggests that decisions are not always as rational as they appear or purport to be (see Chapter Two). In this light, usable moral support for executives might address the ethical principles and values that they consider in decision making, educate them about the psychology of decision making, and invite examination of their habitual way of seeing situations and context. As factors that affect decision making, these considerations are relevant, ethically speaking, to the virtue of prudence.[22]

**Exhibit 3.1. Creating an Ethical Environment for
Employees (Ethical Policy Statement of the
American College of Healthcare Executives).**

The number and magnitude of challenges facing health care
organizations are unprecedented. Growing financial pressures, rising
public and payer expectations, and the increasing number of
consolidations have placed hospitals, health networks, managed care
plans, and other health care organizations under greater stress—thus
potentially intensifying ethical dilemmas.

Now, more than ever, the health care organization must be managed
with consistently high professional and ethical standards. This means
that the executive, acting with other responsible parties, must support
an environment conducive [that not only is conducive] to providing
high-quality, cost-effective health care but [. . .] also encourages
individual ethical development.

The ability of an organization to achieve its full potential will remain
dependent upon the motivation and skills of its staff. Thus, the
executive has an obligation to accomplish the organization's mission in
a manner that respects the values of individuals and maximizes their
contributions.

March 1992 (revised August 1995)

Policy Position

The American College of Healthcare Executives believes that all health
care executives have an ethical and professional obligation to
employees of the organizations they manage to create a working
environment that supports, but is not limited to:

- Responsible employee ethical conduct and behavior
- Free expression of ethical concerns and mechanisms for discussing
  and addressing such concerns without retribution
- Freedom from all harassment, coercion, and discrimination
- Appropriate utilization of an employee's skills and abilities
- A safe work environment

These responsibilities can best be implemented in an environment
where all employees are encouraged to develop the highest standards
of ethics. This should be done with attention to other features of the
Code of Ethics, particularly those that stress the moral character of the
executive and the organization itself.

Note: Formerly titled "Responsibility to Employees."

Source: Adapted with permission of the American College of Healthcare
Executives, copyright 1995.

Other research suggests that through the choices and behavior of its leaders an organization often arrives at a decision about strategy and tactics on the basis of a "rational myth," essentially a cultural assumption about the world and what works in growing or maintaining the organization.[23] In addition, the choice of strategic direction may reflect a need to demonstrate to various stakeholders that the organization is adopting widely accepted best practices (for example, reengineering) in an effort to improve or at least maintain its competitive position.[24]

Those interested in extending moral support in the form of education to executives and other managerial decision makers should not ignore such environmental influences and the related psychology of decision making. Consideration of these dimensions of morality or the moral climate, sometimes called "descriptive ethics,"[25] is a legitimate focus of ethical interest and concern. Thus it is important to persuade the organization's senior leadership that education on these aspects of decision making belongs within a program of concerted moral support for ethical behavior.

Administrative Case Rounds

Another potential means of education that involves executives as teachers as well as learners is holding administrative case rounds. In such a session, senior leaders discuss situations and experiences in which policy alternatives and the need to make decisions have raised significant issues,[26] including managerial or leadership issues and ethical concerns. In the process of sharing experiences and administrative ways of thinking about issues, leaders have the opportunity to reflect on and learn from that experience while offering it as a learning opportunity to others.

For the attendees, in turn, such rounds illustrate how senior leaders integrate the practical and the ethical in their effort to be faithful to the institutional mission and their vision of ethics while fulfilling a fiduciary responsibility for the organization's well-being (see Chapter Ten). In the process, middle managers and other staff might enhance their appreciation for the difficulty—and the art—of making complex decisions under fire, and quite possibly their appreciation for the integrity that executives show in the midst of crisis (Exhibit 3.2).

One might ask, at least theoretically, whether such rounds, concerned as they would be with the practicalities of administration,

Exhibit 3.2. Educational Training in Ethics for Health Care Executives (Ethical Policy Statement of the American College of Healthcare Executives).

Statement of the Issue

Increasingly, managers of hospitals and other health care institutions are facing situations involving serious ethical and bioethical conflicts. A number of factors have contributed to this increased tension: pressures to lower costs, scarcer financial resources, advances in medical technology, decisions near the end of life, and increased patient demands, to name just a few. Health care executives must take a leadership role as facilitators and advocates in articulating and upholding the values of their respective institutions; specifically, they must act to safeguard the rights of patients and promote a full and fair discussion of the issues.

Simply stated, ethics can be defined as the application of a person's values in decision-making situations. These values are derived from a number of sources—family background, religious training, social interaction, education, and employment experiences. In addition, an individual's ethics are often impacted by societal boundaries such as state and federal laws and business practices. And, of course, any value system is always subject to change.

Policy Position

The American College of Healthcare Executives supports the development of defined programs and courses on ethics (1) in undergraduate and graduate programs in hospital and health care administration; (2) in the College's membership criteria (Board of Governors Examination in Healthcare Management and Executive Skill Builders, formerly known as Professional Assessment programs); and (3) as part of the curriculum of professional organizations (including the College) which offer continuing education courses to health care executives.

It is imperative that hospital and health care executives receive specialized and ongoing training in the area of biomedical and managerial ethics so that they can approach institutional ethical and moral decisions with a firm background and knowledge of the issues. This training should be part of a lifetime commitment to high ethical conduct, both personally and professionally. It should be included as part of a formalized educational process, beginning with the preparation for entry into the profession, continuing through graduate training, and ongoing throughout the manager's professional career.

The American College of Healthcare Executives supports current educational efforts for hospital and health care executives in the areas of ethics and biomedical ethics, and it stresses a continued emphasis on these efforts.

(Approved by the Board of Governors of the American College of Healthcare Executives, Aug. 6, 1993)

Source: Reprinted with permission of the American College of Healthcare Executives, copyright 1993.

are also in any recognizable sense ethical. One reply is that, if at least some of the analyses made and arguments offered can be labeled ethical[27]—even as they are also and unquestionably practical and administrative. Indeed, it is the confluence of these ways of categorizing the problems that lends relevance and interest to such rounds and renders them potentially a genuine form of moral support for executives because the educational opportunity appears at precisely the decisional pressure points noted earlier in this chapter.

Consultative Mechanisms

Consultative resources such as those described in Chapter One may be the most evident example of systemic moral support that a health care organization can make available to associates. It is not necessary here to reiterate the functions and general benefits of the consultative function of an ethics mechanism, but something further may be said about the nature of the moral support it can offer. Those who experience an ethical problem may feel that the problem is theirs to puzzle over, solve, lament, wait out, or perhaps avoid. A clearly identified, readily available consultative mechanism may prove a true lifeline to associates floundering in a moral slough of despond.

Of these mechanisms, the ethics committee is probably the best known and best prepared to serve as a support to associates in the organizational ethics arena. If the mechanism is an ethics office (sometimes staffed or led by a designated ethics officer), its advantage is typically that it has some clout: the appearance, and often the reality, of having teeth can exact compliance or press for examination and possible change in an ethically questionable situation. The existence of an ethics hotline (often associated primarily with a corporate compliance program) that affords a caller anonymity can heighten the utility of the ethics office for anyone reluctant to invoke the administrative hierarchy for one reason or another.

But it is precisely at this point that a potentially unique contribution of an ethics committee comes into play. Even if another administrative channel (such as an ethics officer) is available to address a perceived problem, staff may feel reluctant to invoke the hierarchy, fear being blamed themselves if they report a problem, or be reluctant to tell on others—whether superiors or peers—lest they suffer interpersonal or career-jeopardizing repercussions. (This last fear may be a factor even if the organization has a policy of protecting the whistle-blower.) A mechanism that is not part of the chain of command, whose use is optional, and whose process is confidential may offer a welcome alternative that at least some morally distressed employees will use.

Moreover, the availability of consultation from either of these sources, or in some instances from external consultants, can help a staff person withstand the moral anxiety caused by lack of knowledge; the uncertainty that persists despite one's knowledge of issues and problem-solving strategies; or the uneasy feeling of hanging out there alone, however much one knows. By fostering moral community as well as the assurance of at least a measure of expertise with ethical issues, the ethics committee or ethics officer and staff can allay fears while providing valuable education when issues are hot, as well as promote a kind of learning that is likely to last because it is grounded in the moment's existential urgency.

Mission Statements and Core Values

An organization's mission statement (or, in some cases, a mission and values statement) can, if properly employed, serve as a significant resource for the organizational ethics endeavor and the moral support of staff. Unfortunately, the potential of a mission statement to serve in this capacity is easily missed. Often enough, an organization's mission statement is viewed as a nice document and little more. This perception sometimes arises because the mission statement expresses the organization's purpose and values at a high level of generality. In other instances, the document may appear to be an afterthought, one that every organization has to have rather than one grounded in *this* organization's deeply held values.

A mission statement's generality, however, need not prevent it from serving as a supportive foundation or shaping significant context for the organization's ethics effort. The mission statement can set a tone for the organization's informal culture, particularly if leaders make a concerted effort to incorporate it as an ingredient in specific activities. Most health care mission statements profess a commitment to health as a good for humanity and for the organization's community. Thus they assert explicitly or implicitly that values beyond survival and financial success are the driving force behind the organization's activities.

At the same time, mission statements often take financial realities into account; thus, to those who attend carefully to them, they acknowledge that any tension between maintaining solvency and delivering quality health services must be negotiated in some way. Even more important, a mission statement that incorporates this tension expresses a tacit confidence that the organization accepts and can accommodate the tension. Staff people who work every day within this tension may find it important, and a source of moral support, to discover that the mission statement does not gloss over the tension but recognizes it, even if the statement alone cannot solve it.

Even at a relatively high level of generality, a mission statement can include (or be accompanied by) a statement of the organization's core values. If they are widely communicated in the organization and frequently acknowledged as a point of reference, these values can serve as an ethical touchstone for many activities. That is, core commitment to such frequently highlighted values as equality, respect, quality, and stewardship can gradually become internalized in the minds (and hearts) of those who carry out activities. This internalization is particularly likely in a health care organization since the high aspirations typically found in a mission statement likely cohere with health care values at the heart of practicing professions such as medicine and nursing.

Even though the values may not give specific guidance about how to handle a particular situation or a hard case, they almost always present some fundamental criteria against which particular decisions and actions can be weighed. It is usually possible to ask, for instance, whether a particular decision demonstrates respect for the parties involved and affected, or whether stewardship is a value that has been adequately considered in deploying human and financial resources.

Optimal use of the statement of mission and core values may require a certain amount of interpretation or translation in order for associates to make the mission their own, or for the values to come alive as usable reminders and guides. A concerted effort to familiarize all associates with the mission, and sometimes an effort to modernize or shorten it, may be required. Education as to its meaning and implications may need to include case examples or suggest ways to interpret the applicability of the core values in a particular situation. Perhaps especially in an organization with a religiously grounded heritage and mission, telling the story of the organization's history and the dedicated service of the founders often enlivens the mission and inspires present-day employees with a similar spirit.

One criticism of mission statements and statements of core values is that they are subject to multiple interpretations.[28] As a result, the ability of the mission statement to support ethical conduct may be compromised, as when people in different sectors or layers of the organization hold varying definitions of stewardship, or when they prioritize the values differently. To focus on the stewardship example, the interpretations that leaders in finance and those in human resources give to stewardship may differ greatly. For the so-called money people, stewardship may concern the need to manage financial resources cautiously, while for the HR function stewardship encompasses both appropriate deployment of personnel and ongoing development of staff. For still others in the organization, stewardship may be a correlate of, or even a handmaid to, quality, so that part of quality is using resources to obtain optimal outcomes for those served. Again, others may cast stewardship primarily as a limiting value, a continual reminder that an organization dare not outspend capabilities and compromise future ability to deliver the services its mission promises. Where such differences of perspective exist, they should be recognized and addressed rather than ignored.

One other way in which a well-disseminated and widely internalized mission statement can function as a genuine moral support to the organizational ethics effort is through its very nature as a public declaration. That is, the organization that seeks to take its mission and values seriously and successfully conveys this commitment to the staff tacitly invites employees to evaluate the organization continuously in light of its faithfulness to the mission. Those associated with the organization (and even members of the public at large) are in a position to ask whether it is treating people (either external or internal) in accord with the values it professes.[29]

In effect, these constituents now have a promissory note with which to call the organization itself to account, even as they are accountable under the mission statement for their own actions. The very willingness of the organization to expose itself to such ethical scrutiny may serve as a positive model, inspiring the individuals it employs to greater commitment to ethical conduct. In the process, this approach may also heighten the loyalty of associates who are pleased to be part of an organization with high ethical standards.

Of course, organizational accountability has its risks as well. It is probably inevitable that, at some point, employees catch the organization professing values it does not implement consistently—failing, that is, to "walk the talk." If this exposure is not met with corrective action, or if employees keep their perceptions of the incongruency to themselves, the result may be moral disenchantment and cynicism. Thus care must be taken not to deny or cover up the flaws that do emerge in the organization's conduct of its business, perhaps especially in its treatment of employees. The organization that is not straight with its employees has a hard time selling organizational ethics to them, again because trust is so crucial in associates' acceptance of such programs (see Chapter Seven). But the organization that openly acknowledges ethically questionable decisions or activities, and then moves promptly to correct the problems or make amends, may ultimately gain greater ethical commitment from its employees.

A quite different risk may arise from attributing organizational accountability if the staff judge that the organization has failed to meet its mission commitments but base their judgment on partial or inaccurate information. In such an instance, the fact that there is a labor-management dynamic in any employment relationship renders it possible that some employees will accuse the organization of mission shortfall when they are actually (or also) disgruntled about their inability to control decisions that do not go their way. An organization cannot protect itself against every potential ethical criticism, even unfair ones. The organization that generally acts with integrity in its dealings and whose leaders have a reputation for embodying such integrity is more likely to weather any storm of misplaced criticism than one lacking such a history and reputation.[30]

Meeting Accreditation Standards: Ethics Statements and Codes of Ethical Behavior

In 1995 JCAHO added the first standards for "organization [*sic*] ethics" to existing standards on patient rights in accreditable health care settings. The central requirement of the new standards was development of a "code of ethical behavior" for the organization.[31] The code was specifically to address practices in four areas: billing; marketing; admission, discharge, and transfer; and relationships with other health care providers, educational institutions, and payers. As a practical matter, an organization was not initially required to have an actual code of behavior; it could meet this standard through an equivalent set of policies and practices in the four requisite areas. By 1998, JCAHO materials seemed to imply that a specific code of ethical behavior should exist, although some room for exceptions remained.

Some health care organizations, especially those in Catholic health care, already had codes of ethics or ethics statements (see Exhibit 3.1). Some viewed them as a natural outgrowth of mission and values commitments; others apparently followed the lead of the many non–health care organizations adopting such statements. Among those that had not yet developed such statements, many viewed this requirement of the standards more as a burden than an opportunity. From an organizational ethics perspective, however, the imposed need to formulate a code of ethical behavior may eventually yield an additional form of support for ethical conduct on the part of associates. As with a compliance program (discussed briefly in this chapter and again in Chapter Four), a perceived requirement may be a blessing in disguise if it is reframed as an opportunity and seized as such. The anxiety-laden motivation and energy typically generated by the external requirements of accreditation can be harnessed to support the ethics effort in several ways.

For the most part, a statement that conforms to JCAHO standards must address only a limited range of concerns (the four practice areas just listed). Further, the stated intent of these standards shows that they are not meant to be ambitious; the organization is to ensure simply that activity in these four sectors of "business and patient care" is "honest, decent, and proper."[32] Far from setting the bar too high, the standards themselves stop well short of exacting a standard of behavior that constitutes a burden for most health care organizations. The advent in 1998 of a standard requiring organizations to insulate clinical decision making against undue influence by financial incentives and other financial arrangements with providers appears to mark an initial and salutary turn by JCAHO toward a more rigorous approach to organizational ethics.

Nevertheless, from the perspective of support for ethical conduct, even the minimal accreditation standards may give aid and comfort to internal forces seeking to promote organizational ethics. The code of behavior or organizational ethics statement need not, for example, be limited automatically to the four areas listed (plus, perhaps, the clinical decision-making arena). Other areas, such as allocation of resources, or policy matters in patient care other than admission, transfer, or discharge concerns, may also be addressed. In addition, an ethics statement may seize the moment by referring not only (or even principally) to JCAHO standards as its ethical beacon, but rather to the organization's own mission and values, or the values inherent in the practice of health care. It might, for example, correlate the tenets of the code of behavior with the organization's core values. (See the "Advocate Health Care Ethics Statement" in Appendix Two.)

Moreover, the very process of developing the ethics statement may be viewed as an opportunity to enhance ethical awareness among employees, particularly those who work in the areas addressed by the statement. Not only managers and supervisors but especially those from the grass roots in these areas may be enlisted to help craft the portion of the statement that pertains especially to their own activities. Thus those who are closest to the action may have voice, and perhaps even vote, in creating the statement serving as a criterion for ethically evaluating their own function in the future.[33] Such involvement is empowering, and it also yields personal investment in (and enhanced buy-in for) the completed statement.

The process itself can be a step toward creating a reflective, committed moral community among those working with the areas addressed in the statement. Indeed, it is quite likely that these associates will display ethical insight into the areas of moral risk in their activity that others, even ethics "experts," can miss. Participation in drafting the statement may also lead them to consider deeply the interplay between the organization's mission or core values and their daily activities. In the process, they may discover that their organization is indeed ethically concerned, seeks to support them in acting morally, and has committed itself not only to creating an ethics statement but as well to supporting their development as moral agents in the workplace.

Of course, merely creating an organizational ethics statement, whether it remains within or extends beyond the parameters of the JCAHO mandate, is no guarantee that all employees will act ethically or even find the statement relevant to their activities. A genuine effort to make employees and other associates of the organization aware of the statement and its content, followed by additional reminders and efforts to connect it to specific issues and practices, can expand a statement's usefulness. The organization may enhance staff ownership of the statement by recognizing that the initial version of its statement is not likely to be definitive. (After all, these statements often suffer from a process of hurried creation if their composition coincides with preparation for a JCAHO survey.) Even the first published edition of a statement might best be viewed and presented as a work in progress, on which personnel are always invited to comment.

Corporate Compliance

As discussed in Chapter Four, a corporate compliance program seeks primarily to educate employees about legal pitfalls (which usually prove to be ethical pitfalls as well), induce them to avoid these pitfalls, and guide them to seek consultation on any potentially problematic situation involving themselves or others in the organization. Although further consideration of the particulars of a compliance initiative appears in Chapter Four, here it is worth observing that a compliance program may yield more than useful ethical information. For some staff, the program may supply needed motivation not just to act ethically in matters where they already know the issues but also to attend to ethical concerns that they might otherwise ignore. Fear-based motivation that appeals to legal penalty, an intraorganizational discipline process, or potential damage to organizational reputation may work effectively with some individuals in a way that other motivations do not.

Cultivating a Climate for Moral Learning

Merely providing education and educational resources does not guarantee that genuine moral learning takes place. In recent years, many health care organizations, like other corporations around them, have emphasized the need to become "learning organizations." For educational programs and resources truly to offer optimal moral support, an organizational climate that supports learning should exist, and intentional efforts to integrate the spirit of that climate with ethics education should be made.

In particular, an environment that values and supports honest inquiry and permits authority to be questioned is likely to foster an ethical climate in which not mere conformity with established norms but active, creative reflection on moral conduct can take place. In addition, an environment that views mistakes as a potential path toward learning—one in which hesitancy and lack of certitude are not devalued as weakness or lack of confidence—can permit genuine ethical exploration and development among the staff. As Robyn Golden and Sallie Sonneborn put it, "Organizations should have a learning and supervisory process that allows for feelings of uncertainty and professional vulnerability"[34] if they wish to "grow" ethically conscious and conscientious staff members. Such a context can also facilitate employees' own self-examination, a process that is another important but often overlooked dimension of moral development. The nonpunitive approach to and encouragement of associates' ethical self-assessment and self-disclosure can become one more form of moral support for the organization that seeks to construct a comprehensive framework of support.

Recognition of Ethical Conduct and Ethics Activities

Finding ways to recognize ethical behavior and ethics involvement can become a significant means of promoting ethical conduct and offering systemic support to individuals engaged in promoting such conduct.

Recognition and Awards

Recognition of contribution to the ethical climate can be formal or informal. Many organizations already give awards to employees who exemplify organizational values. Besides recognizing alignment with the mission or core values, these awards can, if properly framed, constitute another form of moral support in the ethics enterprise.

Supervisory recognition of employees' ethical conduct or contributions to the ethics program might have an informal impact equal to or even greater than the formal awards process if the recognition is timely and conveys the leader's genuine appreciation. Such recognition can reinforce employee commitment to ethics because ethics becomes deeply associated with relationships that matter and with moral community in a personal way.

Performance Assessment and Compensation

Another opportunity to demonstrate institutional support for ethical conduct and involvement concretely is the individual performance assessment or review process. Historically, the performance review has not stressed ethics or even used ethics language; ethics as an explicit focus has been unlikely to enter the evaluation process unless an employee commits a significant ethical lapse, in which case the employee is subject to the disciplinary process.

In reality, however, ethical behavior and the attitudes, knowledge, and skills that support it are implicit in any review process. Attempting to make this ethical dimension explicit is one way to integrate ethics fully into day-to-day consciousness and operations and to enhance ethical alignment throughout the organization.

Integrating an ethics focus into the review process can enlist a variety of means. On the one hand, an employee can be rewarded for going above and beyond minimally required forms of participation in the ethics effort, as by attending a nonmandatory, ethics-related in-service or by serving on the institutional ethics committee. In this model, ethics participation is, so to speak, gravy; it is presumably rewarded with higher scores on some portion of the performance review.

Some organizations now incorporate into employee evaluation criteria for performance or behavior that draw their content from the mission or core values. In this model, the employees may indeed be rewarded for doing well in relation to the criteria, but they are also at risk should they score poorly in relation to these values or ethics measures. Doing well or poorly in turn affects the pocketbook, and even a career path, for good or ill by contributing to the employment track record. Here an organization might give careful thought to just what criteria are used, how they are scored, and whether the way this portion of the review is structured can assure basic fairness to all who undergo it.

Another possible use of the review process to promote ethics in the organization is through restructuring the compensation package of those who occupy an upper management or senior leadership position. It is common for the incumbent in this position to receive a portion of compensation in the form of executive incentives or a similarly titled "benefit" whose amount (if any) in a given year depends on the organization's or upper management's collective annual performance in some preselected areas of activity. Such incentives can be structured to reward performance against one or more criteria that correlate with ethical criteria, for example, appropriate stewardship of resources or patient survey data affirming the presence of compassionate care. Again, such incentives require attentive structuring, particularly if part of the goal is to recognize management's key leadership role in ethics without unduly separating recognition of the leader's activity from appropriate recognition of ethical behavior by the associates in the trenches.

Enlisting the Scruples of the Silent Majority

One impetus for the growth of organizational ethics has been research suggesting that, although individuals are accountable for their own misconduct, such conduct often depends in some way on the tacit support or complicity of other individuals in the organization.[35] A permissive context often involves the sin of omission on the part of those around a culprit who know, or suspect, that something is amiss but do not act on their misgivings.[36] The organization would be wise to consider how it can encourage associates to act on their scruples rather than remain silent while wrongdoing is contemplated or occurring.

Protecting the Whistle-Blower and Other Dissenters

It is at last widely acknowledged that an organization needs to support employees who know of possible misconduct but have fears about the consequences of reporting what they know. Protection of the whistle-blower has become a staple of some approaches to organizational ethics, particularly those that closely identify organizational ethics with corporate compliance.

It should be noted that whistle-blowing in the world of business and governmental affairs outside of health care has typically referred to instances of truly serious wrongdoing in which somebody goes over the head of the immediate superior and reports the problem higher up in the organization (internal whistle-blowing) or, in well-known cases, discloses the situation to parties outside the organization (external whistle-blowing).[37] By contrast, in a health care setting the term is often used loosely to refer to problems of lesser magnitude for which reporting is most likely to be internal. Perhaps the word *dissent*[38] would sometimes be more appropriate in this setting, insofar as it may connote honest disagreement about the ethical acceptability of a course of action rather than the question of appropriate response to obvious and flagrant violation.

In any event, there is both practical wisdom in and ethical justification for protecting the person who sees or suspects misconduct but fears the repercussions of telling. Practically speaking, as Emily Friedman concludes, "if those who expose ethical problems and wrongs are ignored, hushed up, or worse yet, punished, the obvious lesson will spread rapidly through the organization: We claim to have ethics, but we do not use them."[39] Ethically, the reluctance to report wrongdoing often reflects a power differential between parties involved, with the potential whistle-blower fearing that another's power will cause her professional harm if she reports what she knows. This disparity has long affected clinical relationships, such as those between physicians and nurses. It can be especially difficult when the actual or potential unethical conduct emanates from, say, a manager or supervisor to whom the whistle-blower reports. It is a requirement of justice that the organization protect the less powerful party in this situation, even as such support promotes the aims of the organization's ethics program.

Implementing policies that promise protection to those who report ethically problematic behavior can thus be a significant component of an ethics program generally as well as a corporate compliance program specifically. The promise of protection should, however, follow careful deliberation about what it actually takes to provide the needed protection in *this* organization's specific context. Mere statements that those reporting wrongdoing are to be exempt from reprisal may not be convincing to employees who have learned (perhaps with good reason) to avoid provoking any in their circle of relationships who might do them some harm in return. Policies that promise protection may be perceived as mere words on paper unless a plausible protective mechanism exists, one that over time becomes known in the organization's culture as effective and therefore trustworthy.

A whistle-blowing mechanism that allows anonymous reporting to a hotline number (a common feature of compliance-oriented programs) may offer a form of protection that is necessary before some staff members will come forward. As part of a policy to encourage such reporting, there may be a need to affirm good-faith reporting of situations about which an employee has qualms, and thereby to invite reports that later prove unfounded. Such errant reports sometimes rest on suspicion without much evidence, involve errors of fact or misinterpretation of a situation, or reflect reliance on secondhand reports (perhaps even the rumor mill).

These considerations are a reminder that mistaken allegations might have unwelcome consequences for all involved, not the least for implicated parties who are at risk of unwarranted damage to reputation. The potential for such mischief suggests it may be advisable to define the threshold of "appropriate" reporting, to serve as a caveat to would-be whistle-blowers. The recognition that some reporting might be driven by dubious motives or ill-considered judgments should, however, be balanced by the recollection that, historically, whistle-blowers have often been subject to crushing retaliation, with little or no protection.[40] Due process protections are available to those accused of wrongdoing; this is a kind and degree of protection that whistle-blowers and other dissenters simply did not have in the past (and sometimes still lack). At the same time, whistle-blowing policies might wisely suggest using (and exhausting) other appropriate channels before turning to this option as a last resort.

Sins of Omission

It may take more than mechanisms protecting whistle-blowing to extend optimal support to people whose better impulses prompt them to intervene if they perceive that unethical behavior is afoot.

The impetus for reporting ethically problematic conduct is likely to stem from the dual sense that an important norm is being violated *and that it is important to do something about the behavior involved.* That is, there is a need to develop and cultivate within the culture the idea that one is responsible for more than merely keeping one's nose clean—a consciousness that there really are sins of omission and that these may be as culpable as the sins of commission that they tacitly permit and protect. "It is an old adage," organizational psychologists Donald Messick and Michael Bazerman write, "that evil prevails when good people fail to act, but we rarely hold the 'good' people responsible for the evil."[41] Those who do not report their misgivings to someone or to some office in a position to intervene, or who fail to confront colleagues they believe are acting inappropriately, place themselves in the position of moral accomplice. Finding ways to instill this awareness and helping people accept the inevitable measure of interpersonal risk that responding to misconduct entails are two of the challenges for the organization that wants to go beyond the first (admittedly important) step of protecting the whistle-blower.

Other Forms of Administrative Support

It may seem obvious that any effort to infuse an organization's culture—and thereby to "infect" individual associates—with a belief that ethical conduct is important, and with a willingness to act accordingly, depends not only on the avowed support of leadership but also on evidence that the leaders are taking steps to implement the espoused values in the upper echelons as well as at the staff level.

Executive Behavior and Modeling

Whenever such administrative initiatives as an ethics program are rolled out, many employees wait in the psychological wings to see whether or not executive leadership seems truly to support and to live out the espoused attitudes and behaviors. The importance of administrative modeling behaviors, of walking the talk, can hardly be overestimated. Leaders who demonstrate commitment to the values they claim to support (for example, by exemplifying and rewarding the ethical behavior that they call for) build loyalty among the troops to that behavior and associated attitudes. In the process, the leader who demonstrates such integrity builds trust[42] and can even inaugurate what some have called a mutual "transformational" process, as Dawn Carlson and Pamela Perrewe describe it, "in which leaders and followers actually raise one another to higher levels of morality and motivation."[43]

Consistency and Alignment

A sincere and thoroughgoing administrative effort to align policy and practice with avowed values in all the organization's dealings can go a long way toward creating a culture in which people recognize ethical integrity and are willing to contribute to it. In a health care organization, employees are frequently individuals with high ideals, and they are often quite alert to incongruence between their organization's expressed values and those displayed in practice. Those who have witnessed such incongruence in the past often develop a protective veneer of cynicism and may need to be convinced of the sincerity, effectiveness, and long-haul character of any ethics initiative. Leadership that can pass the "cynicism test" has a far better chance of rekindling and evoking the latent idealism of people who, beneath the veneer, are often looking for moral leadership worth following.

Treatment of Employees: A Special Test

A highly visible proving ground for an ethics initiative is the organization's attitude toward and treatment of its employees. Phyllis Mitzen puts it simply: "Ethical behavior of an organization begins with ethical behavior toward its own employees."[44] The organization that communicates consistently and unambiguously to employees that it values them, even if it cannot guarantee them permanent employment,[45] has already gone a long way toward creating a climate supporting ethical attitudes and conduct.

In health care, especially, the organization that esteems employees and treats them well displays consistency between the values driving its externally focused health care mission and the values that govern its internal activities.[46] Employees are, in turn, likely to believe that the organization truly supports their efforts to act in alignment with its mission and values, and with the principles espoused in ethics initiatives (see also Chapter Five).

Resources and Tools

Supplying staff members with resources and tools designed to facilitate their integration of organizational values or implement particular aspects of the ethics program can be an important ingredient
in moral support. What should characterize such resources is ready
availability ("It's there when you need it") and usability. Tailoring
resources to specific needs and activities, packaging them in a convenient and concise format, and presenting information or guidance in the clearest terms possible are some of the ways that such
resources can meet the objective of usability.

Portable Mission and Values Statements

Some organizations have reduced their mission statement or statement of core values to a compact form. Reduction may still retain
the whole mission statement in small print or abridge it in some
way, perhaps by restating it in simpler language or highlighting selected tenets that amount to a mission within the mission. Wallet-
sized cards may be especially useful if they feature—and even
better, explain briefly—the central values inherent in the mission.
Staff may find it convenient and helpful to refer to a card for a
brief refresher on the values, and even on their possible meaning
in a difficult situation.

   As an adjunct to the bare bones of a mission statement, some
organizations have designed a pocket- or wallet-sized card that
seeks not merely to restate but to interpret the mission's relevance
for the day-to-day attitude and activity of staff personnel. In distributing such a resource, an organization demonstrates a desire
to have the mission (and by implication ethics as well) infuse its
culture and the consciousness of its staff. Thus it displays the commitment to an enhanced moral ecology that is at the heart of an
effective organizational ethics effort.

Checklists

An example of a task-focused tool is a checklist of possible ethical
questions to ask and procedures to follow in various decision-making
situations. It can be a relatively generic list of questions for assessing whether an ethical problem actually exists in the situation (see
Exhibit 1.2 in Chapter One), or questions and procedures in-

tended to help people make moral choices in the unique circumstances of their work in a particular organization. The checklist can be included in, or appended to, a code of ethics or ethics statement. Other checklists, adapted to the health care setting, have appeared in the health care management literature.[47] Still others have been developed specifically to assist staff in meeting the requirements of a corporate compliance program or JCAHO accreditation standards.

Some checklists aim to link decision making explicitly with the organization's mission and values. They may identify a set of questions to be asked sequentially in reaching a decision,[48] thus being especially suitable for use in a deliberative group process of collective decision making. Or a checklist can identify considerations that the individual decision-making manager or supervisor should take into account. Such tools may also attempt to correlate those considerations with specific organizational values (equality, stewardship, compassion, collaboration, quality, and the like; see Exhibit 3.3).

Another possible variation on the checklist theme incorporates recent research on the psychology of managerial decision making and addresses common blind spots in such decision making (see Chapter Two). This sort of checklist could, for example, include questions that invite recognition of the full range of potential consequences and risks (both short-term and long-term) as well as the stakeholders affected by these consequences. The checklist might also prompt managers to assess the possibility of egocentric and ethnocentric bias and of self-deceit in their decision-making instincts.

Not least, it might raise the critical follow-up issue of postdecision communication: Is the preference for disclosure, characterized by honesty and openness; for a high degree of secrecy or concealment; or perhaps for measured disclosure, marked by a certain spin on controversial realities? Here the communication checklist might note prospective use of the sunshine test (Would a decision maker want her decision and rationale to appear on the front page of the *New York Times*?) as a last check to run *before* the decision is finalized.[49] Introducing a managerial checklist might prove especially useful as a practical sequel to an educational program that explores the psychology of decision making and the ethical issues arising from that psychology.

**Exhibit 3.3. Sample Decision Checklist,
Developed as Part of a Cultural Transformation
Initiative Within Advocate Health Care.**

When making decisions, ask ourselves if our actions and decisions are
consistent with our values

√	*Compassion*
_____	Have I evaluated the total impact of this decision on patients, employees, and physicians?
_____	Have I developed a communication plan to ensure proper communication of the issue so that all can fully understand it?
_____	Have I made myself or others available to counsel those affected by this decision?

√	*Equality*
_____	Does this decision ensure respect to those whom it affects?
_____	If this decision initiates change, have I anticipated the impact and needs of those affected?
_____	Have I anticipated the impact on organizational diversity in this decision?

√	*Excellence*
_____	Is this decision the result of listening to the needs of those affected?
_____	Have I anticipated the impact and outcomes to this decision, and do I have a plan to address them?
_____	Have I tried to communicate a "half full" rather than "half empty" attitude toward the outcomes of this decision?

√	*Partnership*
_____	Have I communicated with all parties that may be affected or even concerned about this decision?
_____	Does this decision take into consideration the need to team with others in order to best implement?
_____	Have I anticipated barriers that may make implementation difficult?
_____	Have I been fair, and my thoughts free of turf issues, in coming to this decision?

**Exhibit 3.3. Sample Decision Checklist,
Developed as Part of a Cultural Transformation
Initiative Within Advocate Health Care, Cont'd.**

√	*Stewardship*
_____	Does this decision make the best use of our resources?
_____	Does this decision augment our desire to provide the best possible service while being sensitive to the financial impact?
_____	Can I personally assume responsibility for this decision?

Source: Adapted with permission of Advocate Health Care. Copyright 1996 Advocate Health Care.

A Few Maxims for Ethics Activists

Once an organizational ethics program is up and running, those who aim to make it a source of moral support for staff members may find these additional suggestions helpful.

First, *build on the moral resources that already exist.* It is possible for an ethics initiative, especially one heavily focused on compliance issues, to start with the negative and continue to emphasize it. Perhaps inadvertently, installing a compliance or ethics hotline may reinforce the message that people are all too likely to "screw up"— or, worse, to act with wanton disregard for the law, for patients, or for the organization's interests.

All things considered, it is preferable to assume (and the assumption is normally valid) that organizational staff already act ethically in the great majority of instances and that they *want* to act ethically in what they do. This approach builds on a natural human inclination to do good and right things; it also draws on and encourages the idealism and associated motivations that typically drive the behavior of those who work in health care. People whose vocation entails providing care and resources for healing to vulnerable people already approach their work with a strong internalized sense of morality; the health care organization can only benefit from publicly recognizing and cultivating this moral sense.

Second, *recognize that all ethics programs have growing pains and meet resistance.* Any concerted effort to develop an organizational ethics program and extend moral support to staff in taking ethics seriously has its struggles and encounters obstacles. Moreover, those struggles are likely to seem particularly difficult and unwelcome to ethics officers, members of an organizational ethics committee, and others who champion the initiative or lead it. If high expectations are not met, there can be a sense of failure even though gradual progress is being made. The inevitable fact that at least a few people, including some in management positions, balk at aspects of the program or even engage in passive sabotage can undermine morale further.

If such circumstances and experiences arise, it may be a good idea to benchmark initial experience against that of others in a more mature ethics program, preferably one with a good reputation. It is quite probable that the benchmarking conferees will report their own periods of struggle and encounters with pockets of resistance (perhaps even large ones), even as they report significant progress overall. Such a report from a respected quarter may ease some of the self-generated pressure to make the ethics program meet its objectives all at once.

It is also probably good to remember that an organizational ethics initiative, like any other management-supported initiative or program, is likely in some measure to participate in the labor-management dynamic of the organization. Some criticisms of the ethics program may derive from the perception that even the ethics initiative is "only" another management ploy to increase administrative control. Moreover, some staff are surely aware of—and not silent about—perceived ethical shortfalls on the part of the administration. Managers, in turn, may note the recalcitrance of workers who fail either to "get it" or to fall in line with the new initiative. None of these dynamics need prove fatal or severely damaging to the organizational ethics program, but awareness that they are a predictable part of the landscape may help those leading the program to retain perspective in times of rough sledding.

Third, *set the bar high—and keep it there.* Though struggle and resistance are inevitable, it is nonetheless important to establish and maintain high standards, and even stretch goals. Disappointment over unmet expectations may reflect an unrealistic sense of how long it takes to achieve the goals, but unmet temporal expectations should not translate into lowering the bar itself. In the biblical story of Israel's relationship with its God, Israel ever and again falls short of the divine expectations (indeed, of covenantal standards to which the people agree). God grieves over these failures even as he repeatedly forgives Israel—but God never relaxes the standards (commandments and laws) against which Israel's performance is assessed.[50] In organizations, easing the standards may ease the pain of unmet expectations, but lowering aspirations also undermines the impetus for continuing ethical improvement.

Fourth, *encourage ethical alertness by cultivating conscience and spiritual awareness.* People in health care organizations need moral support if they are to live out a high vision of ethics that goes beyond compliance and doing the more or less obviously right thing. Organizations must show that they value ethics as a process of continuing reflection, one that involves asking new, often hard questions about organizational activities. If ethics education includes acknowledging the associate's role as the ethical eyes and ears of the organization, and explicitly affirming the need for alert and questioning conscience as well as conformity with the rules, then the organization can only gain from the added attention to issues that results.

Conscience itself may be nourished by organizational efforts to respect and cultivate spiritual awareness, which for some is the wellspring of conscience as reflective moral awareness.[51] Religiously sponsored organizations may seem to have better, more established resources for undertaking this task, but it is also true today that spirituality is less often construed as the handmaid, let alone the special possession, of particular religious traditions. As attention to that which gives meaning, purpose, and direction to life and work, spirituality can take nonreligious forms and be cultivated within any organization. As such, it is a potential ally and support, both to an organization's mission and to its ethics initiative.

Notes

1. Thomas Aquinas, *Summa Theologica* I-II, Q. 91., Art. 2. (Dominican Friars of the English Province, trans.; T. Gilbey, ed.). Cambridge: Blackfriars, vol. 28, 1966. Cited in Veatch, R. *A Theory of Medical Ethics.* New York: Basic Books, 1980, p. 36.
2. Tuohey, J. F. "Covenant Model of Corporate Compliance: 'Corporate Integrity' Program Meets Mission, Not Just Legal, Requirements." *Health Progress,* 1998, 79(4), 72.
3. Maslach, C., and Leiter, M. P. *The Truth About Burn-Out: How Organizations Cause Personal Stress and What to Do About It.* San Francisco: Jossey-Bass, 1997.

4. Potter, V. R. "Individuals Bear Responsibility." *Bioethics Forum*, 1996, *12*(2), 27.
5. Friedman, E. "Ethics and Corporate Culture: Finding a Fit." In E. Friedman (ed.), *Choices and Conflict: Explorations in Health Care Ethics*. Chicago: American Hospital Association, 1992.
6. Brown, M. T. *Working Ethics: Strategies for Decision Making and Organizational Responsibility*. San Francisco: Jossey-Bass, 1990.
7. Paine, L. S. "Managing for Organizational Integrity." *Harvard Business Review*, 1994, *72*(2), 106.
8. Paine (1994), p. 111.
9. Goodpaster, K. E. "Conscience and Its Counterfeits in Organizational Life." (Public lecture.) DePaul University, Chicago, Oct. 28, 1998.
10. Messick, D. M., and Bazerman, M. H. "Ethical Leadership and the Psychology of Decision Making." *Sloan Management Review*, 1996, *37*(2), 10.
11. Gustafson, J. M. *Theology and Christian Ethics*. Philadelphia: United Church Press, 1974, p. 153.
12. Goodpaster, K. E. "Business Ethics, Ideology, and the Naturalistic Fallacy." *Journal of Business Ethics*, 1985, *4*, 228–229.
13. Maslow, A. H. *Toward a Psychology of Being*. (2nd ed.) New York: Van Nostrand Reinhold, 1968, p. 25.
14. Verschoor, C. C. "A Study of the Link Between a Corporation's Financial Performance and Its Commitment of [*sic*] Ethics." *Journal of Business Ethics*, 1998, *17*(13), 1509–1516.
15. Petrick, J. A., and Manning, G. E. "Developing an Ethical Climate for Excellence." *Journal of Quality and Participation*, Mar. 1990, p. 84.
16. Pastin, M. *The Hard Problems of Management: Gaining the Ethics Edge*. San Francisco: Jossey-Bass, 1986.
17. Thomas, R. R., Jr. "From Affirmative Action to Affirming Diversity." *Harvard Business Review*, 1990, *68*(2), 113.
18. Hinderer, D. "Hospital Downsizing: Ethics and Employees." *Journal of Nursing Administration*, 1997, *27*(4), 11.
19. Nash, L. L. *Good Intentions Aside: A Manager's Guide to Solving Ethical Problems*. Boston: Harvard Business School Press, 1990; Solomon, R. C. *Ethics and Excellence: Cooperation and Integrity in Business*. (Ruffin Series in Business Ethics.) New York: Oxford University Press, 1992.
20. Hasnas, J. "The Normative Theories of Business Ethics: A Guide for the Perplexed." *Business Ethics Quarterly*, 1998, *8*(1), 19–42.
21. Potter, R. L. "From Clinical Ethics to Organizational Ethics: The Second Stage of the Evolution of Bioethics." *Bioethics Forum*, 1996, *12*(2), 8.

22. Pieper, J. *The Four Cardinal Virtues: Prudence, Justice, Fortitude, Temperance*. Notre Dame, Ind.: University of Notre Dame Press, 1966.
23. Mohr, R. A. "An Institutional Perspective on Rational Myths and Organizational Change in Health Care." *Medical Care Review*, 1992, *49*(2), 242–244.
24. Arndt, M., and Bigelow, B. "Reengineering: Deja Vu All Over Again." *Health Care Management Review*, 1998, *23*(3), 64.
25. Beauchamp, T. L., and Childress, J. F. *Principles of Biomedical Ethics.* (4th ed.) New York: Oxford University Press, 1994, p. 4.
26. Reiser, S. J. "Administrative Case Rounds: Institutional Policies and Leaders Cast in a Different Light." *Journal of the American Medical Association*, 1991, *266*(15), 2127.
27. Goodpaster, K. E., and Matthews, J. B., Jr. "Can a Corporation Have a Conscience?" *Harvard Business Review*, 1982, *60*(1), 138.
28. Maslach and Leiter (1997).
29. Reiser, S. J. "The Ethical Life of Health Care Organizations." *Hastings Center Report*, 1994, *24*(6), 28–29.
30. Hinderer (1997).
31. Joint Commission on Accreditation of Healthcare Organizations. *Comprehensive Accreditation Manual for Hospitals.* Oakbrook Terrace, Ill.: JCAHO, 1998.
32. Schyve, P. M. "Patient Rights and Organization Ethics: The Joint Commission Perspective." *Bioethics Forum*, 1996, *12*(2), 16.
33. Schneider-O'Connell, A., and McCurdy, D. B. "Translating Values into Operational Standards: A Case in Health Care." In *From the University to the Marketplace: The Business Ethics Journey.* (Second of three diskettes.) Niagara Falls, N.Y.: Vincentian Universities of the United States, 1996.
34. Golden, R. L., and Sonneborn, S. "Ethics in Clinical Practice with Older Adults: Recognizing Biases and Respecting Boundaries." *Generations*, 1998, *22*(3), 86.
35. Paine (1994).
36. Messick and Bazerman (1996).
37. James, G. G. "In Defense of Whistle Blowing." In J. C. Callahan (ed.), *Ethical Issues in Professional Life.* New York: Oxford University Press, 1988.
38. Bok, S. "Whistle Blowing and Professional Responsibilities." In Callahan (1988).
39. Friedman (1992), p. 111.
40. Glazer, M. "Ten Whistleblowers and How They Fared." In Callahan (1988).
41. Messick and Bazerman (1996), p. 15.

42. Hinderer (1997).
43. Carlson, D. S., and Perrewe, P. L. "Institutionalization of Organizational Ethics Through Transformational Leadership." *Journal of Business Ethics,* 1995, *14,* 832.
44. Mitzen, P. "Organizational Ethics in a Nonprofit Agency: Changing Practice, Enduring Values." *Generations,* 1998, *22*(3), 104.
45. Noer, D. M. *Healing the Wounds: Overcoming the Trauma of Layoffs and Revitalizing Downsized Organizations.* San Francisco: Jossey-Bass, 1993.
46. Reiser (1994).
47. Curtin, L. L. "Creating an Ethical Organization." *Nursing Management,* 1995, *26*(9), 96–99.
48. Meyer, B. W. "Ensuring Accountability in Decision Making." *Health Progress,* 1997, *78*(3), 31.
49. Messick and Bazerman (1996).
50. Herman, S. W. *Durable Goods: A Covenantal Ethic for Management and Employees.* Notre Dame, Ind.: University of Notre Dame Press, 1997.
51. Goodpaster (1998).

Chapter Four

Corporate Compliance and Integrity Programs
The Uneasy Alliance Between Law and Ethics

It is not easy to establish an organizational ethics program that truly incorporates systemic resources to support ethical conduct and discourage unethical conduct. Senior organizational leaders and line managers need to be convinced not only that the goal is important but also that it is urgent enough to devote adequate resources to the means of implementation. Making the case in sufficiently clear and concrete terms can be problematic, because ethics sounds to many like philosophy, and thus impractical. Even suggesting that organizational ethics can help fulfill the organization's mission seems abstract to some—pie in the sky for which the organization does not have time or money in light of so many other immediately pressing concerns.

Given such difficulties, an organization may find that adopting a corporate compliance program presents an attractive alternative. Indeed, it appears that corporate compliance programs instituted in some health care organizations have become either explicit or de facto substitutes for (or competitors with) other ethics programs. It is clear, however, that organizational ethics is more than corporate compliance, as this chapter shows. At the same time, and despite the clear distinctions between them, corporate compliance and organizational ethics need not be adversarial. Thus this chapter also considers the prospects for a constructive relationship between them, as well as some possible pitfalls that may mark that relationship.

A Case

Fran works in the accounts payable office of Suburban Hospital. She has just gotten off the phone after a lengthy discussion with a health plan representative about a billing question. She takes a minute to catch her breath and then picks up the phone and pages Dale, a physical therapist. She tells him that the health plan is refusing to pay for most of the services provided to a patient because only one day of services was documented—even though the patient had actually received five days of physical therapy. Fran asks Dale if he can come to her office and initial the corrected medical record because "today is the last day that they will accept any changes." Dale responds, regretfully, that he is at an off-campus location and cannot return to the main campus for two days. "But that shouldn't be a problem," he adds. "Just initial it for me. You know nobody will question it."

This fictional incident raises concerns that differ from the standard ethical questions arising in clinical care. Here the problem is not the quality or the moral nature of the care itself but rather the conduct of those engaged in the business and operational activities that accompany the care. Moreover, the risks are not only ethical but also legal and financial, since for a health care organization inaccurate or incomplete charting may be a source of problems even if the mistakes are unintentional. In addition, what Dale urges Fran to do in this case would be considered fraudulent because he is actually asking her to forge his signature. If the payer were Medicare or Medicaid rather than a private health plan, discovery of fraud could subject the medical center to severe penalties. In recent years, some health care organizations and their employees have learned painful and expensive lessons about the cost of such behavior—the cost of failure in the area known today as corporate compliance.

Background

Responding to burgeoning federal health care budgets, the Department of Justice (DOJ) and Health and Human Services (HHS) regulators began targeting the health care industry in the early 1990s for investigation and prosecution of fraud and abuse cases. According to investigators with the DOJ, fraud and abuse have siphoned billions of dollars from health care programs.[1] During the period from 1995 to 1997, criminal investigations and prosecutions increased approximately 15 percent each year, while civil investigations increased almost 100 percent annually. Civil judgments and settlements in fraud and abuse cases for the 1997 fiscal year totaled $1.2 billion. Meanwhile, under a program entitled Operation Restore Trust, as of 1998 the HHS Office of the Inspector General targeted 4,660 hospitals to audit for overbilling.[2]

Fraud and abuse is a loaded and potentially misleading term (Exhibit 4.1). The types of practice being targeted in these enforcement efforts include

- Billing for service not rendered
- Billing for service not medically necessary
- Double billing for services provided
- Upcoding (billing for a service or product more highly reimbursed than the one provided)
- Unbundling (billing separately in order to get a higher reimbursement for a group of laboratory tests performed—and billed—together)
- Billing for nonreimbursable expenses
- Violation of the seventy-two-hour window (billing patients for outpatient services rendered within seventy-two hours of their admission to inpatient care)[3]

It is easy to see how these practices could represent efforts to defraud the government. However, to anyone familiar with the complexity of the law and the realities of the health care billing office, the potential for *accidental* violation of the law is equally apparent.

In many of the cases reported by the DOJ, particularly in criminal cases where intent is an element of the crime, the actions being prosecuted do involve criminal conspiracy to defraud the government. However, according to many observers (and as suggested in two 1999 reports criticizing the DOJ Medicare fraud and abuse initiatives),[4] in civil action government prosecutors routinely label *any* violation of the law in these areas as fraud, even those arising from clerical error or other mistakes. Because the penalties for violation of the law are so severe (including damages of up to 100 percent or more of the amount of money in question and—even worse—denial of the institution's right to participate in Medicaid and Medicare programs), the pressure to settle a civil suit is enormous.

Exhibit 4.1. A Simple Guide to Fraud and Abuse.

Although Medicare and Medicaid laws are complex, there are some red flags for clearly illegal deals. Most of these relate to federal law against paying for patient referrals. A deal is questionable if, when dealing with physicians or others who can refer patients to you:

1. You are making any payment back to the referral source that is based on the number of patients referred.
2. You are making any payment back to the referral source that is based on amount of dollars billed caring for the referred patients.
3. You are providing any services or goods to the referral source at a cost below fair market value: subsidized office rent, free office personnel, and so on.
4. You are buying or renting anything from the referral source at an above-market rate: paying $500 to a doctor's office to rent a square foot of counter space for lab samples, and the like.
5. You are paying for services you do not get: if you pay $100,000 a year for a doctor to provide services, you had better be able to prove the doctor worked enough hours in your facility or on your specific projects, including work product, to justify the pay.
6. You are waiving deductibles for Medicare patients.

These criminal and civil enforcement efforts are, however, only the most visible part of the government's war on fraud and abuse. Equally important, Congress and government regulators have sought to encourage corporate citizenship and to enlist the assistance of health care organizations as self-policing, proactive entities in this struggle, through creating corporate compliance programs. A corporate compliance program is a systematic effort by an organization to prevent violation of law by its employees and agents, and to detect and report such violation if it does occur.

Although at present much of the effort in health care is to address issues related to the government's war on fraud and abuse, corporate compliance can and should address violation of any law. The concerns of a compliance program encompass a case like this one:

Regina is a clinical nurse specialist at Suburban Hospital, a subsidiary of Partnership Health Care (PHC). She often works with Dr. Stone, a gastroenterologist who admits many patients to Suburban. She has noticed that when patients need GI lab testing, Stone often refers them to a particular non-PHC facility even though Suburban has its own well-run GI lab. Then she hears through the grapevine that Stone is a part owner of the other facility. She suspects a legal or ethical problem and wonders whether she should tell anyone in authority of her concerns.

Here the presenting issue is not the possibility of fraud but rather the potential for improper referrals. A set of laws[5] commonly known as the "Stark antireferral legislation" and implementing regulations (named for sponsor Rep. Peter Stark, enacted in 1989 and amended and broadened in 1993 and 2000) strictly regulate the business arrangements that physicians may enter into whenever it is possible that the physician could profit from his or her referral decision (a practice known as self-referral). The Stark legislation is complex, and its regulations do make certain exceptions. Regina should not assume that Dr. Stone is acting illegally, but she would be wise to discuss her concerns with Suburban's corporate compliance office or legal department.

The 1991 federal Guidelines for the Sentencing of Organizations, which are applicable to any malfeasance, explicitly affirm that one objective is to create "incentives for organizations to maintain internal mechanisms for preventing, detecting, and reporting criminal conduct."[6] These incentives explicitly include the potential to reduce fines for violations by up to 95 percent. Equally important, voluntary establishment of a corporate compliance program avoids the risk of government imposing a particular corporate compliance program (which could cost a large institution hundreds of thousands of dollars a year) as part of a voluntary settlement if fraud is discovered. Government investigators commonly demand creation of such a program in the absence of a voluntarily initiated "effective" one.

To be deemed effective, a voluntary corporate compliance program must be reasonably designed, implemented, and enforced so that it is generally effective in preventing and detecting criminal conduct (though failure to detect in a given instance does not prove that the program was ineffective). The program must satisfy seven conditions:

1. The organization must have established compliance standards and procedures to be followed by its employees and agents.
2. The program must be administered or overseen by "high level" personnel within the organization, such as a "corporate compliance committee" of the board of directors, together with a corporate compliance officer (usually not the general counsel) drawn from the executive staff.
3. The program ensures that substantial discretionary authority is not delegated to employees having a propensity toward criminal conduct (which may be discovered through an employee background check).
4. Steps must be taken to communicate these standards and procedures to all employees and agents (most obviously through mandatory training, although the guidelines do not stipulate means to be used).
5. Monitoring and auditing procedures must be implemented and publicized; as a key element, a reporting system must be implemented whereby employees can report wrongdoing without fear of retribution (for example, through an employee hot line or a toll-free phone number).
6. If a violation is found, standards must be consistently enforced through established disciplinary mechanisms.
7. After an offense is detected, all reasonable steps to respond and prevent further offenses must be taken.

The program is to be a systemwide, comprehensive effort to avoid and detect illegal behavior.

Across the nation, health care organizations are scrambling to develop and implement corporate compliance programs. The dangers of accidentally violating the law and the penalties for failing to develop such a program are far too significant to be ignored.

Moving Beyond Compliance

The relationship between corporate compliance and the incentives provided by the 1991 sentencing guidelines is clear: the latter serve as a direct inducement for the former. As a result, the corporate

compliance plan adopted by a health care organization can be—
and often is—designed simply to meet the legal requirement that
the organization and all of its employees and agents abide by the
law. However, on a deeper level, corporate compliance represents
a shift in thinking that corresponds to an emerging understanding
of bioethics and the role of an institution's mission in its delivery
of health care. This confluence of thinking has pushed many
health care institutions to move beyond a simple effort at corporate compliance to one directed toward corporate *integrity*—an attempt to merge ethics, mission, and law in one coordinated effort
(see Exhibit 3.1 in Chapter Three).

A corporate compliance program represents a shift in thinking
about the nature of corporations and corporate liability that began
in the defense industry in the 1980s and spread to health care in
the 1990s. It reflects an emerging view of corporate responsibility,
as distinct from the responsibility of individual employees. The 1991
sentencing guidelines reflect the new understanding that a corporate entity can be held legally responsible for its actions and not
just vicariously responsible for the actions of its employees. The
corporation's own actions (in the form of systemic procedures and
policies) can mitigate or exacerbate its culpability in the event of
employee malfeasance.

During roughly the same period, a somewhat similar shift began
in the realm of bioethics. From its beginnings in the late 1960s,
bioethics focused attention on the behavior of individuals and the
relationships between patients and their doctors.[7] But in the early
1990s, both the law and bioethics took more seriously the role of
the institution in patient care, particularly the institution's role
in educating and supporting patients in exercising their rights. The
federal Patient Self-Determination Act (effective Dec. 1, 1991) was
one legislative expression of this expanded approach. The emergence of managed care and the growth of for-profit health care institutions heightened concern about the institution's role. Ethicists
were compelled to consider how the organization, through its formal policies and its informal culture, affected patient care.[8]

As a response to this changing environment, in 1995 the
JCAHO promulgated a new set of standards in "organization
ethics" for accredited hospitals and health care providers. These
standards, plus additional standards issued subsequently, demand

that to be accredited an organization develop policies and procedures to address a variety of organizational ethical concerns (primarily related to billing, marketing, and potential conflict of
interest).[9] Here again, the organization is recognized as having
moral status separable from the acts of individual employees or
agents. It is the organization's responsibility to develop systems and
procedures to address these moral concerns, not just the responsibility of identified professionals within the organization.

The changing marketplace of health care has also provoked
many leaders of mission-driven (and, often, faith-based) institutions
to reflect about what it means to be mission-driven in a competitive
market. What is it that distinguishes these institutions from their
for-profit competitors? If the mission statement is to have meaning,
how is it to be made manifest within the organization? Again, these
questions suggest that an organization has *moral* standing—in other
words, the organization has certain values it seeks to realize—and
that it acts ethically by developing systemic ways of guiding its employees and agents to live up to the organization's ethical standards
(Exhibit 4.2).

At a practical level, an interrelationship among these three
areas of concern in organizational behavior clearly exists. For example, fraudulent billing practices such as those contemplated in
the first case above violate both the law and ethical norms of honesty. Questionable referrals like those made by Dr. Stone may or
may not violate the Stark legislation, but in either case they run the
moral risk of appearance of a conflict of interest. That is, they create a situation in which it appears that decisions about patient care
and the appropriate location of that care are influenced by personal or professional self-interest (see also Case Six in Part Two of
this book). Ordering unnecessary medical tests, which violates
Medicaid law, equally violates an organization's mission commitment to provide its patients with excellent health care services.
Nonetheless, efforts to control organizational behavior through
coordinated appeals to all three areas of concern have been
fraught with difficulty.

Problems in the Effort to Integrate

Among these three ways of approaching organizational behavior
(compliance, ethics, and mission), corporate compliance stands in

Exhibit 4.2. Example of "Business Conduct: Doing the Right Thing . . . for the Right Reasons."

Mission, Values, Philosophy, and Reputation

What's the value of a name? When it's your name—or ours—it's priceless. Protect our reputation—and yours—by complying with the law and representing our mission, values, and philosophy to patients, colleagues, and the public.

What is Advocate doing to ensure that we're doing the right thing? Because we've earned a reputation as a trustworthy and ethical organization, Advocate aims to be a leader among health care organizations in helping associates live out our values and understand how to comply with the law. To accomplish that, Advocate has created a business conduct program.

What are the advantages of a business conduct program? Caring for the patient, treating one another with respect, and conducting business properly are at the heart of successful health care companies. An effective business conduct program will help reinforce Advocate's heritage, reputation, and commitment to our patients, associates, and the community. It will also help us ensure compliance with the complex laws facing health care institutions and employees. Violations of the law could result in substantial fines and/or litigation liability for Advocate Health Care and jeopardize our tax-exempt status. Having an effective business conduct program will reduce our risks and penalties significantly. It also lessens an associate's chances of unintentionally violating regulations and thus incurring personal criminal or civil liability.

What does Advocate's business conduct program cover? The business conduct program applies to our interactions with patients and families; each other; vendors; and payors, both public and private. The program is designed to ensure that we act honestly and fairly. It has special emphasis on these key areas:

- Patient confidentiality
- Discrimination
- Sexual harassment
- Workers' compensation, safety, and OSHA
- Tax-exemption principles
- Medicare and Medicaid fraud and abuse
- Stark antireferral legislation
- Coding and billing procedures

**Exhibit 4.2. Example of "Business Conduct: Doing
the Right Thing . . . for the Right Reasons," Cont'd.**

What happens if an associate violates the law? Possible violations will be
reviewed thoroughly by Advocate's business conduct/corporate
compliance officer and may be referred to a systemwide corporate
compliance committee. Appropriate disciplinary action will be taken if
illegal, unethical, or improper activities are found to exist. No action
will be taken if associates are working to conform their practices to the
law and the business conduct program.

Source: Reprinted with permission of Advocate Health Care. Copyright 1999
Advocate Health Care.

a uniquely favorable position. The business justification for underwriting and supporting a corporate compliance program is obvious and compelling. The program is directed at a clear and
measurable goal: legal compliance. The very structure of the program is laid out, both in the law and in interpretive guidelines
disseminated by the Office of the Inspector General in the Department of Health and Human Services Office (HHS-OIG).[10]

In contrast, the justification for attention to ethics and mission
is often less clearly understood and appreciated. Despite many
claims that adhering to mission and high ethical standards is "good
business,"[11] the relationship between the two is not self-evident.
Moreover, any effort to link them tightly risks making attention to
ethics a business practice that can be cast aside whenever it does
not prove to be good business. From another perspective, those
whose primary charge is ensuring that the compliance program
minimizes violation of law may fear creating a program that tries
to do too much. If their underlying aim is to minimize the risk of
legal liability, any proposed alteration of the compliance program
that appears to weaken its focus on legal compliance may, under-
standably, not be entirely welcome. Their response might be to rel-
egate the "softer" concerns of mission and ethics to the margins of
the program. Then the mission and ethics focus, though present,
might appear to be tacked on to a program that essentially stresses
legal compliance.

Failure to integrate ethics and mission adequately into a corporate integrity program represents a lost opportunity to advance

ethical and mission concerns.[12] It may, however, also result in actual harm to the ethics and mission programs. Excessive focus on meeting the requirements of the law breeds cynicism among employees[13] in two regards. First, they may begin to perceive ethics and mission simply as nice-sounding words on pretty paper. Second, appeals to legal risk may prove unconvincing; writing in the *Business Ethics Quarterly*, Metzger, Dalton, and Hill assert that employees "are unlikely to see [legalistic] admonitions [about harm to the organization] as very compelling in situations where the perceived odds that their wrongdoing will be detected are slim."[14]

Excessive concern with legal compliance may actually detract from corporate efforts to avoid legal liability. One study found a higher incidence of legal violation in companies that stressed avoiding negative consequences to the corporation as the rationale for proper behavior.[15] Paradoxically, an organization narrowly focused on legal risks may lose the capacity to anticipate changes in the law. Law is fluid and subject to change. Behavior that is legal at one time (such as using asbestos as insulation, or silicone breast implants in reconstructive surgery) may at a later date threaten legal liability. In contrast, an integrity program that consistently seeks to envision the highest ethical standards and proactively directs the organization toward them may also anticipate future problems. Such an approach at least serves as mitigating evidence against accusation of corporate irresponsibility or moral failure to care for the people the organization serves.

Ironically, those responsible for ethics or mission leadership within an organization may themselves resist participating in a corporate integrity program. Leaders of an institution's effort in clinical ethics may hesitate to join the corporate integrity ethics initiative because they feel they are inadequately trained to do so, or because they fear that such participation will distract them from meeting the needs of individual patients.[16] They may also fear being seen as members of a new order of ethics police. In a clinical setting, it is not unusual for doctors or other professionals with little exposure to bioethics to be suspicious of any effort to address ethical issues. They may fear that the clinical ethics consultant will ride in with the intent of allocating blame. This suspicion may be exacerbated if the ethicist becomes deeply engaged in a corporate integrity program, one aspect of which is addressing legal liability issues and presumably determining responsibility or blame for illegal conduct.

A mission leader, too, may fear being, or appearing to be, an agent of legal enforcement. Leaders may also worry that linking the corporate compliance emphasis on legal concerns with organizational mission implementation tarnishes the image of the mission and compromises efforts to implement it by causing mission implementation to be seen, in reductionistic terms, as little different from the compliance program.

Moving Forward

The benefits of creating a corporate integrity program are considerable, in spite of the risks we have identified. Indeed, many find the need for an integrity program compelling. The leader of one Catholic health care organization put it very simply: "It's not enough that we weren't indicted today." The preceding survey of problems and risks in developing an integrity program suggests some possible ways to create a workable program, one that can avoid or counteract those risks.

First, the values of ethics and mission should be blended into the integrity program, not simply grafted onto the legal elements of the compliance program. At a fundamental level, the challenge is to make the goals and objectives of mission and ethics as concrete and practical as possible. Here the specificity of the program's legal requirements may serve as a benchmark. It is not enough to exhort employees to be honest or act with compassion. These admonitions must be given meaning within the day-to-day life of the organization. Employees need clear guidance about how they are to behave in their professional interaction with others— guidance that realistic examples and case discussions can offer (see Case Eighteen for an example).

Second, even with optimal effort to achieve clarity and concreteness, educating employees about ethics and mission is more difficult than the simpler process of educating them about legal obligations. Ethics and mission cannot be summarized in a simple listing of dos and don'ts. Employees need to be taught to think creatively if they are to confront the many and inevitable gray areas of ethics.[17] This type of training takes time and careful preparation.

On the other hand, it prepares employees to meet ethical and mission demands, while simultaneously helping them confront ambiguous or emerging areas of law.

Third, the organization might assess how systems and procedures support or hinder implementation of ethical and mission-based values, at the same time and in the same way that it evaluates those systems and procedures for their impact on legal compliance (see also Chapter Three). Support for legal conduct requires structural change and continual reinforcement no less than encouraging and changing ethical or mission-based behavior does.[18]

Fourth, a key feature of a corporate compliance program is engagement of employees in identifying and reporting improper behavior. This aspect of the program generally arouses mixed feelings because it is readily associated with witch-hunting, spying, or tattling on colleagues. If, however, the emphasis is not on reporting people and their questionable conduct but instead on identifying and recognizing specific behavior, this aspect of the program can play a positive role in the area of mission and ethics. It can begin with trying to develop specific understanding or pictures of what appropriate and inappropriate conduct actually look like.

Such a process has several benefits. It actively engages staff in thinking about the meaning of mission and ethics in organizational operations. In addition, it gives them permission and a reason to talk about any situations they find troubling, especially since the focus is not on catching evildoers or lawbreakers but on clarifying what conduct is appropriate to the organization's mission and values, and what is not. As a result, with this feature of the program ethical concerns and problems that might otherwise go undetected can surface. Unlike the requirements of law, which are set out in a statute or body of regulations, it may be that the daily requirements of mission and ethics are best recognized in communal reflection on lived experience.

Fifth, an integrity program should have buy-in at all levels of management throughout the organization. Just as a compliance program targets a senior administrator as a necessary leader for the program, an integrity program should be linked to senior management as well. Many organizational ethicists assert (correctly) that ethical behavior starts at the top[19] (see Exhibit 3.2 in Chapter Three). At the same time, common sense suggests that it cannot stop there; it must permeate all levels of management. An individual employee rarely works with or receives an evaluation from senior management. It is the front-line manager, and his or her behaviors and values, that most influence the employee.

Finally, adherence to ethical or mission values should have identifiable consequences for everyone. This suggests that adherence should be rewarded and nonadherence reasonably sanctioned. Otherwise, employees may be encouraged to think of the ethical and mission values as irrelevant to real life in the organization and their daily role within it.[20] However, rewards and sanctions should be carefully and creatively devised, lest they lead staff to see the program as one driven primarily by financial or career advancement incentives rather than by the moral aspirations that hold its deepest promise.

A corporate integrity program offers the organizational leader a powerful tool for implementing change and cultivating mission and ethical values. The decision to initiate such a program creates a unique opportunity. Yet the opportunity comes with significant risk, which a poorly conceived or implemented program may turn into reality. The challenge is substantial, but it can be met, as an increasing number of health care organizations are demonstrating by the progress they have made.

Notes

1. "Department of Justice Health Care Fraud Report Fiscal Year 1997." Available on-line at www.usdoj.gov.
2. Tuohey, J. F. "Covenant Model of Corporate Compliance: 'Corporate Integrity' Program Meets Mission, Not Just Legal, Requirements." *Health Progress*, 1998, *79*(4), 70.
3. "Fraud Report FY 1997." [http://www.usdoj.gov/01whatsnew/heffraud2.html]
4. GAO/HEHS-99-42R, Feb. 1, 1999; and HEH-99-170, Aug. 6, 1999.
5. 42 USC Section 1395nn.
6. 56 Fed. Reg. 21,762 (16 May 1991) at 22787.
7. See, for example, Jonsen, A. *The Birth of Bioethics.* New York: Oxford University, 1998.
8. Spencer, E. M. "A New Role for Institutional Ethics Committees: Organizational Ethics." *Journal of Clinical Ethics*, 1997, *8*(4), 372–376.
9. JCAHO. *Comprehensive Manual for Hospitals*, 1998. RI.4–RI.4.4.
10. OIG. "The Office of Inspector General's Compliance Program

Guidance for Hospitals"; OIG. "The Office of Inspector General's Compliance Program Guidance for Home Health Agencies"; OIG. "The Office of Inspector General's Compliance Program Guidance for Clinical Laboratories." Available at DHHS website [www. dhhs.gov/proorg/oig].

11. See, for example, Tuohey (1998), 70–71.
12. Giblin, M. J., and Meaney, M. E. "Corporate Compliance Is Not Enough: Catholic Healthcare Organizations Should Aim at the Development of Ethical Cultures." *Health Progress,* 1998, *79*(5), 30–31.
13. Giblin and Meaney (1998).
14. Metzger, M., Dalton, D. R., and Hill, J. W. "The Organization of Ethics and the Ethics of Organizations: The Case for Expanded Organizational Ethics Audits." *Business Ethics Quarterly,* 1993, *3*(1), 29.
15. Mathews, M. C. "Codes of Ethics: Organizational Behavior and Misbehavior." *Research in Corporate Social Performance and Policy,* 1997, *9,* 107–130. Cited in Metzger, Dalton, and Hill (1993), 29.
16. Spencer (1997).
17. Giblin and Meaney (1998), 31.
18. Metzger, Dalton, and Hill (1993).
19. See, for example, Nash, L. *Good Intentions Aside: A Manager's Guide to Resolving Ethical Problems.* Cambridge, Mass.: Harvard Business School, 1993.
20. Tuohey (1998).

Chapter Five

Managing Human Resources

The need to manage human resources is a central concern of every health care organization, and many ethical problems and opportunities arise in the course of dealing with employees. Human resource management thus offers a rich opportunity to explore a range of ethical issues that touch every area of the organization. Moreover, these concerns may surface at any point in an employee's involvement with the organization, starting with recruitment and hiring, continuing through the vicissitudes of a long or short period of employment, to eventual separation from the organization.

Thus, examining human resource management as a concern of organizational ethics permits latitudinal and longitudinal consideration of issues that can arise in a critical area of organizational activity. In the process, this examination can use rational systems and natural systems perspectives to understand employment issues in their formal and informal aspects. From an open systems perspective, it can also take into account the external factors that impinge on the organization's management of human resources.

Human resource issues may come readily to the attention of the ethics mechanism. Staff may approach the ethics committee with concerns they have, and committee members themselves may recognize that actual or potential issues exist in the human resource arena. It may be, however, that ethical concerns arising in human resource management do not reach the ethics mechanism, or that the committee is not perceived as an appropriate venue for these concerns. The legal considerations involved in human resource management, as well as issues of privacy and confidentiality, may mitigate against significant committee involvement with these matters. Thus in at least some organizations these issues are most likely to be addressed by those who encounter them in the course of their work, that is, by human resource professionals, by managers and supervisors, and by employees themselves—the actual "human resources" in question. It may be especially important for human resource professionals, and for managers and supervisors throughout the organization, to become familiar with the ethical issues that can arise in human resource management and with some ways of thinking them through.

Overarching Perspectives

If management is the art of getting things done through people, the contemporary shift from the language of "personnel management" to that of "human resource management" makes considerable sense. People remain the primary means of achieving organizational goals, in health care as in other enterprises, and like other resources people require management if they are to contribute optimally to those goals. Ethically, human resource management (which includes but is not limited to an organization's human resources function) is rightly concerned with deploying and directing employees in ways that promote the organization's purposes. In health care, this means furthering a mission devoted in some way to health and healing.

At the same time, human resources—both as an organizational concern and as a specific organizational function—has also signified organizational interest in and support for the well-being of employees themselves. Through compensation and benefit programs, intraorganizational programs of employee education and personal and professional development, and organizationally sponsored recreational activities, organizations have signaled to their human resources that they are valued as *humans*, not merely as resources. Therefore, from an ethical perspective health care organizations have also conducted their human resource activities in accord with the dictum that people should be treated as ends in themselves and not merely as means to serve others' ends. This is true whether those others are management, patients and their families, the board, stockholders, physicians and other clinicians, or staff employees. The inescapable corollary that treating employees in this way tends to increase employee satisfaction, build loyalty to the organization, and thereby benefit the organization itself is not incompatible with the claim that the organization is expressing genuine concern for employees' well-being in the process.

Some view the ethics of managing human resources as a set of issues that arise in administering the standard concerns of the human resource function or department: staffing needs; employment (recruitment, selection, and hiring); avoidance of discrimination; compensation; benefits; confidentiality and privacy; employee and labor relations,[1] including grievance procedures[2]; and discipline and discharge, including management of downsizing. This chapter considers the issues that arise in administering these relatively discrete concerns within the larger framework of human resource activity.

At the same time, the attention of the whole organization should be devoted to employees and how they are managed. Human resources is neither the domain of a specific department (HR) within the organization nor the purview only of line managers and administrators who must implement human resource policies every day. From the perspective of organizational ethics, human resource concerns pervade the organization's activities and suffuse its culture. How an organization approaches its human resources is critical to implementing that mission. Consequently, this chapter considers human resource concerns in light of organizational mission as well as the law, accreditation standards, and ethical principles and virtues.

Staffing Needs

In view of St. Somewhere Hospital's looming financial crisis, it is almost certain that in trying to find savings wherever possible the administration will reassess the hospital's staffing needs. In doing so, administrators might wisely consider staffing needs, or levels, in two senses. First, and perhaps most obviously, staffing level is the sheer number of staff needed to do the work in various areas, given the present configuration of the hospital's structure and current way of doing things. Reassessment might disclose that fewer nurses can reasonably provide care in some clinical areas or on some shifts.

Second, staffing level can refer to the number of staff with specific competencies needed to provide a particular service, or to the ratio of supervisory personnel to line staff in various models of reorganization. A reorganization might, for example, lead to a shift in the skill mix of the employees who provide care to patients in a given clinical area. Care that does not seem to require a nurse's training, license, and salary might be given by certified nursing assistants (CNAs) or patient care technicians. A smaller number of nurses would supervise all the work of the paraprofessionals and would still carry out those aspects of care requiring the greatest knowledge and skill.

What ethical considerations are relevant to issues of staffing level? In particular, what are the moral pitfalls of reduced number or competency level among staff? Many nurses, and others concerned about patient care, contend that such reductions threaten the quality of patient care along with patient safety. In reply, administrators often argue that if properly redesigned, care processes can create efficiencies without compromising the real essentials of care, in its technical and psychosocial aspects. Some would also argue (with questionable ethical validity) that JCAHO human resource standards for care are still being met. They might add that achieving efficiency without significant loss of quality depends on the understanding and cooperation of staff, that the need to set priorities in the context of limited numbers and time is really nothing new, and that failure to set task priorities is more likely to detract from the quality or safety of care than staff changes are.

Disputes of this sort ultimately turn on the definition of *quality* and *safety*, on devising ways to measure the goals implied in these terms, and on identifying data that can indicate trends in achieving those goals. The organization has to decide whether quality should refer to a high standard of excellence or to a more modest floor, a minimal threshold that should always be exceeded. Decisions about whether to define quality in objective terms such as patient outcomes or subjective terms such as patient satisfaction are also required. Further, what level of risk, if any, of failing to achieve safety norms is the organization willing to accept?

Clearly, the fundamental medical-ethical norm of avoiding harm to patients should be the preeminent value in the safety discussion. But its centrality does not imply that the administration should simply capitulate to demands for higher staffing levels based on claims of compromised safety without at least some data to support the alleged danger. Even in the absence of data, however, prudence suggests that administrators make commonsense judgments about a staffing situation that might conceivably result in a "sentinel event" (a singular catastrophic occurrence, such as death caused by medication error, or a public-image nightmare). Legal exposure may be the first consideration triggering alertness, but the real *ethical* challenge to the organization is the incongruity between such an event and the norm of doing everything reasonably possible to avoid harming the patient—not to mention the painful incongruity between the occurrence of a sentinel event and the health care organization's mission, its very reason for being.

Employment

Even at a hospital like St. Somewhere, where hiring activity may well decrease in the near future, the need to fill vacant positions—perhaps even to create some new ones—continues. Many issues, often interrelated, arise in meeting the ongoing need to recruit, select, and hire employees. The discussion here considers a representative sampling of these issues.

Rating Positions

Ethical questions can arise even before a position is advertised if an existing position description and compensation range must be reviewed. What aims should inform this process? Does the organization set compensation at a relatively low level because its reputation readily draws solid applicants? Or does it exceed the job market's compensation level to make the organization attractive in competing for strong candidates? Should it, as a matter of principle, meet some norm of fairness in compensation? Or should it, on pragmatic grounds, set compensation at a level that is likely to result in retaining satisfied employees once they have been hired? Again, for guidance in charting its course the ethical organization may look to its mission, to such virtues as prudence and justice, and to the principle of treating persons as ends and not means only.

Job Postings

It is no secret that the recruitment and selection landscape is dotted with legal minefields, but the ethical hazards along the way are too often unnoticed. For example, the hiring manager may know early on of an internal candidate she wishes to select for a position. In this case, mandatory internal posting of the position may become only a formality, and others within the organization who are interested in the position may in good faith apply for a position that is not truly open. Ironically, the very process intended to ensure that all qualified candidates have an equal chance at the job becomes a vehicle of organizational deception, one in which the hiring manager and the human resource recruiter may tacitly collude.

In part, this irony can arise because a position announcement is often the pro forma means of fulfilling legal requirements that those involved in the selection process have not also internalized as *ethical* requirements. In part, too, it may stem from fear—not unjustified—that to be open with nonpreferred applicants about their actual chance of being accepted for the position exposes the organization or manager to litigation. Such a fear does not, however, justify misleading use of the posting process.

Testing

Another possible pitfall in the selection process is using (or misusing) various kinds of testing as a screening mechanism. The common practice of requiring an applicant (especially a candidate for a senior management position) to take certain psychological tests raises significant questions of invasion of privacy[3] and even coercion. Those who must make these hiring decisions might reply that the weighty responsibilities involved in these positions—as well as the substantial compensation, benefits, and other rewards that the successful candidate receives—justify such an invasion (which, they might add, the candidate is free to decline, along with further pursuit of the job itself). In any case, a sound principle for an organization to follow might be to pursue the least invasive course needed to obtain information deemed critical to a hiring decision.

Other kinds of testing in the selection process can raise issues:

At St. Somewhere, all applicants for paraprofessional clinical care positions are required to take a "patient care test" before they are invited to interview. The test is primarily intended to evaluate an applicant's readiness to step into the increasingly demanding clinical paraprofessional role at St. Some- where. The test also attempts to assess the applicant's ability to actualize St. Somewhere's stated mission and values in the care process. The experience of recruitment staff and line managers who conduct posttest interviews, however, is that those who score well on the test often do not interview well, while those who score low in the passing range generally interview more strongly. This dynamic seems especially prominent among candidates for whom English is a second language. Moreover, because candidates must pass the test to be granted an interview, both recruiters and clinical managers believe that they and the organization have passed over applicants who were better qualified than some who were hired.

Assuming the possible validity of the anecdotal reports, this case presents an instance in which a well-intentioned assessment tool—one that seeks, laudably, to integrate the organization's dis- tinct values into the employment process—may function as a ve- hicle of unintended discrimination. Unfortunately, using the test to screen out all applicants who fail it effectively rules out the ap- plicant who has previously done excellent clinical work, or who has had solid clinical preparation in a training program, but scores poorly on the test. By ruling out the recruiter's or manager's dis- cretion in using the results, the test process ensures—as perhaps it was meant to do—that individual perspective on some aspects of a candidate's suitability does not result in an uneven selection– rejection process before the interview. The test's screening func- tion may also be intended to create efficiency by eliminating the need for some busy recruiters and managers to conduct time- consuming interviews. Regrettably, it appears to present an in- stance in which an organizational hoop through which applicants must pass ultimately achieves the opposite of its intended effect.

The result is evident injustice to would-be employees, as well as apparent loss for the organization itself. Once diagnosed and, one hopes, remedied at St. Somewhere, perhaps this unfortunate instance will serve to remind the administration and HR leadership that such an untoward outcome can occur despite the best of intentions. It may also suggest that giving the recruitment function a measure of discretion in using test results may be a prudent course, especially if the test's effectiveness at identifying and assessing what it is meant to evaluate has not yet been validated. If such discretion is reintroduced into the selection process, of course, other mechanisms to guard against misusing discretion may also need to be considered.

Interviewing

Other selection issues emerge in the interview process itself. The most obvious may appear to be legal problems that can arise when an interviewer asks a candidate questions that are inappropriate because federal law or regulations deem the requested information irrelevant to the requirements of the job at hand. The ethical issue is not solely, or even primarily, the pragmatic consequence that the organization is exposed legally; it is also the risk of discriminating or appearing to discriminate unjustly against a potentially deserving candidate. Such injustice may, in turn, be a product of the vice of sloth: in this instance, failure to think through and reach sufficient clarity about the real aims of the interview process, namely, to recruit a candidate for a particular position who can contribute to the goals of the organization. No doubt questions deemed inappropriate sometimes surface information about the *person* who would be the employee, information that proves relevant to the hiring decision. The subsequent question that must be answered, however, is whether there are other, less dubious ways— whose identification may require creativity—to discover the human information that is truly relevant to the requirements of the job itself.

Achieving such an outcome may well require not only carefully thinking through the interview process but also carefully preparing and coaching those who conduct interviews. In a day when many organizations have chosen, for good reason, to democratize the interview process by permitting others besides managers and supervisors to participate in a candidate interview, the process of guarding against inappropriate interview questions and techniques has become more complex. If the benefit to the organization and to the candidate is deemed to be worth the risk of an open interview process, however, it is incumbent on the organization to find creative ways of overcoming the obstacles.

References

As recruiters and managers interview candidates, at some point they want to check the references supplied by the candidates of greatest interest. In today's litigious climate, many organizations caution staff personnel named as references to say as little as possible about ex-employees, often nothing beyond "confirmation of employment." This approach, sometimes known as the "no comment reference," means that would-be employers fail to hear of an applicant's poor performance history and that those who know of such history must live with the moral distress created by withholding relevant information.[4]

As a result of this widespread practice, those who are desperate for reference information tend to seek it from whatever sources, and to pursue it in whatever ways, they find available. They may, for example, turn to known contacts in the candidate's former organization for an informal word about the performance of the candidate. Experienced recruiters and managers often learn to listen for the code—the message between the lines—from the candidate's former manager or from the former employer's human resource personnel. Even an answer whose words merely confirm employment dates may be voiced in a tone that communicates an attitude toward the candidate and insinuates a performance history without articulating one.

This dynamic exemplifies one of those moral situations in which two wrongs do not make a right, even though certain goals are achieved; the practice of withholding reference information provokes a recruitment end run that obtains a more-or-less crude approximation of a reference. It can be argued that, whatever an organization's legal affairs office may advise,[5] across-the-board withholding of performance information is an ethically dubious practice. It deprives the requesting organization of what it needs to make a sound hiring judgment, and it also contributes to a fear-driven recruitment atmosphere and fosters proliferation of questionable information-gathering practices in the recruitment process. Candidates themselves may be harmed by the comments of ill-informed informal contacts, by the misinterpreted meta-communication of reticent HR personnel, or by incomplete communication from references who would speak favorably of a candidate if they felt free to do so.

However unintentionally, such practice also reflects on the character of the organization. As Ellen Harshman and Denise Chachere argue, a no-comment policy signals to staff that their organization "is more concerned about its bottom line (in other words, guaranteeing that no one would have reason to file a lawsuit about a reference) than with the welfare of its good and loyal employees who depend on the reference of the employer for career mobility."[6] Such a policy also intimates something to outside observers: "An organization that will duck a candid reference for a troublesome, unproductive, or dangerous employee . . . will take the path of least resistance when the hard decisions need to be made."

In short, it makes ethical and pragmatic sense for a health care organization to value and promote freer exchange of reference information than is the norm in current practice. Obtaining and disseminating accurate information about the law and about the history of legal action over references may be one way to lessen the tendency to overreact to the specter of litigation. It is likely that many organizations have exaggerated the threat of litigation over allegedly defamatory references, and it may be that legally well-informed instruction about appropriate reference practices can diminish the actual likelihood of such suits still further.[7] A health care organization that practices direct and honest communication in the process of supplying references may help to promote a free, open atmosphere in this critical area of human resource activity.

Compensation

Once employees have been brought on board, the organization's approach to compensation and benefits plays a significant role in the new hire's satisfaction and retention (which serves the organization's good) and can demonstrate its fundamental commitment to fairness to employees. Reasonable compensation and benefit packages contribute to competitiveness in the labor marketplace and serve as a concrete expression of an organization's avowed concern for the well-being of those who work for it.

Executive Compensation

Perhaps the most prominent—and certainly the most publicly debated—compensation issue in many businesses arises in the area of executive compensation.[8] In health care, especially in the not-for-profit sector, claims of abuse in this area are less common, or perhaps less vociferous, because executive salaries and supplemental compensation are typically lower than in other sectors of business or in for-profit health care. In the for-profit sector, questions of just compensation can be and have been raised about executive compensation, both in provider corporations and in insurance companies and HMOs. Especially if health care workers' wages are relatively low, it may be important at least to attempt to define what is a proportionally just relationship between top executive pay and that of line staff, and even of middle managers.

Incentives

In addition to questions of executive compensation, broader compensation issues can arise at all levels of an organization. For example, if the organization uses incentive bonuses as a means to reward collective performance (as a complement to the incentives built into its individual performance appraisal system), questions about appropriate structuring of the incentive program inevitably arise.

If the incentive plan is one in which all or nearly all employees can participate, potential ethical questions may include (1) selecting goals that serve as incentive criteria in a given year; (2) weighting criteria when several of them come into play; (3) the threshold of collective achievement necessary to trigger an incentive payout; and (4) for systems such as PHC, of which St. Somewhere Hospital is a part, the distributive relation of an individual facility's performance to the system's performance in determining the payout level to facility employees. Not all these possible issues can be discussed here, but it is important to keep in mind that all of them are likely to deserve the organization's ethical attention. In general, discussion of such issues is likely to focus on balancing the organization's goals in establishing an incentive program in the first place against issues of fair and just distribution of incentive funds among employees, and perhaps across sites or facilities when the overarching setting is a health care system.

An additional wrinkle in structuring an incentive program for all employees is the fact that many of these programs have been inaugurated only recently and have been created in organizations that already had some form of senior management or executive incentive plan. Senior management plans are likely to involve a significant percentage of the manager or administrator's salary and are sometimes viewed as a covert means of artificially lowering high-level salaries by transmuting a portion into deferred, contingent compensation. By contrast, an all-employee plan typically involves a far smaller percentage of the employee's annual wages or salary; it is likely to be viewed more as a benefit than as anything resembling core compensation. However, in some organizations (or in especially good years) incentive payments may exceed the wage or salary increase an employee is eligible to receive through the performance review process.

Questions then arise: Do incentive payments in fact function as a substitute for core compensation by driving down merit pay increases? Is such a result ethically acceptable? Introducing payments that are contingent on collective performance may position an incentive program as a de facto partial substitute for an established program that bases pay raises on individual performance. Staff who perceive such a connection might with some reason wonder whether the unwritten employment contract has been changed without real notice, and whether such a change is fair, especially to staff with a strong performance record.

Pay for Performance

Another compensation issue is introduction of merit pay, or "pay for performance," in an area previously employing another system to assign compensation.

Recently, St. Somewhere introduced a pay-for-performance system among its nonexempt (hourly-wage) staff. This was a change that many employees had long sought from the organization. The old system did make use of performance reviews, and a combination of good reviews and seniority gradually moved most employees through a series of steps in which each successive one placed the employee into a higher pay grade and hourly rate range. In addition, each year the organization made an adjustment in the pay ranges on the basis of the current rate of inflation. The problem was that many senior employees had largely topped out on the highest step. As a result, the annual pay adjustment attributable to inflation was the main source of increase available to them.

Thus, when the new merit pay system was rolled out (with considerable fanfare), there was general approval among nonexempt employees. This system tied pay raises much more closely to performance ratings because there would be only one (much wider) pay range for each position. Presumably, such an arrangement would benefit good performers and serve as an incentive to even better performance. What many St. Somewhere associates did not understand, however, was that the new system also required rerating each position to establish its new pay range.

At their first performance review under the new system, some of the senior nonexempt employees discovered to their chagrin that because of their progress through all the steps of the old system, they were already being paid at or even above the top end of the newly established range. Not a few found that, despite high performance ratings, they received increases of less than a dime an hour. Some received no increase at all after their first review.

Might such an unwelcome outcome be avoided, or its impact at least minimized? Administratively, perhaps better planning can anticipate the potential for hourly rate problems to emerge. In any event, once the undesired effects of the new compensation structure become apparent, prompt and direct communication about the likely gap between expectation and reality make both administrative and ethical sense.

Surveys have shown that good pay is not usually a major contributing factor in employee satisfaction with work, but compensation issues do hold significant potential to become a source of dissatisfaction and "demotivation."[9] In the instance discussed here, moreover, the issue is not only employee disgruntlement with pay itself but also apparent betrayal of trust. Creating mistrust is a serious ethical and management problem with long-lasting, far-reaching consequences (see Chapter One). Insofar as management hype for the new pay system contributes to employees' high expectations, prompt administrative disclosure of the problems can at least minimize the mistrust that is sure to follow when employees discover the compensation shortfall. Ethically, such an acknowledgment signals that the organization values a trusting relationship with employees and that its leadership regrets any disappointment or hardship that earlier poor planning may help create.

Diversity

Most health care organizations have recognized that an optimal ethical and practical response to the many forms of human diversity must go beyond meeting equal opportunity, affirmative action, and other legal or regulatory requirements. Once these requirements became law, and especially after early instances of enforcement were publicized, health care organizations (like those in other sectors) focused on policy and practice in the areas of recruitment, retention, and promotion as means to meet the requirements and avoid sanctions. This essentially reactive approach effectively became the first line of response by health care organizations to the challenge of building workforce diversity. Such an approach eventually proved too narrow to meet the expanded challenge, for diversity was and is a pervasive reality encompassing all aspects of workplace life and experience.

In addition, the tendency of government programs to focus on specific quantitative measures of diversity led some organizations to settle for playing a numbers game and to ignore the more profound concerns that the federal initiatives meant to address. Perhaps most important, organizational responses to affirmative action and equal opportunity requirements, and even some early "cultural diversity" programs, seemed to treat human diversity in the work setting primarily as a *problem* to be overcome, not a resource to be valued and cultivated or an unrealized opportunity in need of better management.

The ethical perspectives that should inform an approach to diversity on the part of a health care organization or human resource function are essentially the same ones that shape human resource and employee relations activity in other areas. Promoting the good of the organization—that is, treating people in ways that enhance (or at least do not undermine) its health care mission—is the primary value that organizational attention to diversity should serve. At the same time, treating employees as ends in themselves—not only respecting but cultivating diversity because doing so promotes individual flourishing—is also a guiding consideration.

Moreover, the organization should approach workforce diversity in a way that is consistent with the values inherent in the health care enterprise. It has been said that, in the business world, diversity programs can have lasting success only if they are grounded in a conviction that they serve business values, for example, a belief that supporting diversity affords a competitive edge.[10] Diversity efforts in a health care organization probably require a similar but augmented faith if they are to flourish over the long term. Executives and human resource leaders need to see not only the potential business advantages (greater market share, improved patient satisfaction, optimal use of employee gifts and talents) of an excellent diversity program but also the potential benefits for patient care (improved recognition of unique patient and family needs, better communication across languages and cultures, and movement beyond mere tolerance to respect for and appreciation of difference).

Because affirmative action continues to further important societal values, an organization should still attend to recruitment, retention, and promotion practices and outcomes as a matter of justice for underrepresented groups. But it should also act out of an expanded vision of diversity as an actual and potential resource: a source of new ideas, creativity, talent, and richness of experience, and a resource that can contribute to improved patient care as well as enhanced work life quality. It is already true that caring for an increasingly diverse population of patients, residents, clients, and their families virtually requires the presence and experience of a diverse caregiver population. In addition, with so many of those served speaking first languages other than English, the value of cultural and linguistic diversity among caregivers is an indisputable, if largely untapped, resource worthy of cultivation and appreciation.

To fulfill such a vision, diversity programs should seek to integrate diverse employee populations into a cohesive workforce, and to develop a more encompassing work culture—rather than assimilate all difference into a melting pot whose eventual flavor resembles that of the persistent dominant culture. At the same time, recognition and even appreciation of cultural differences should avoid the pitfall of unconsciously assuming that each individual reflects the distinctive stamp of—or bears all the presumed characteristics of—the cultural group to which he or she "belongs." Only then can programs in diversity serve as an optimal means "to make the most of each employee"[11] while "managing disparate talents to achieve common goals.[12]"

Employee Relations

The need to oversee certain interactions between management and employees, and sometimes between employees and other employees, is a continuing source of ethical concern. Miscommunication and failure to communicate, disagreement and even outright conflict, and actual or perceived misuse of power are just some of the dynamics that can create ethical problems. Human resource staff and experienced line managers know all too well that human relations problems are inevitable, and that addressing them promptly, directly, and judiciously is in general both the wise and the ethically advisable course.

Consistency

One of the common problems that human resource departments encounter is managerial inconsistency. It takes many forms, such as inconsistent application of policy and procedure, inconsistent treatment of employees in any realm not covered by specific procedures (for example, scheduling holiday work or vacation periods), and seemingly inconsistent standards for employee performance. As a practical administrative matter, the relevant standard of consistency may be contextual rather than absolute.

> The manager of St. Somewhere's laboratory has forbidden her staff to take two consecutive weeks of vacation during the year-end holiday season. The

radiology department's manager, however, permits his staff to take two weeks if the request is made well in advance and adequate coverage can be arranged.

This interdepartmental discrepancy in managerial practice may not present a significant problem from an HR perspective. The most germane question may not be whether the two managers are consistent with each other or with other managers throughout the organization, particularly if they can articulate a staffing rationale, based on the need in their areas, that justifies their specific practice. Instead, the question may be whether each manager's practice *within* her area is consistent. If in fact some employees in the same lab receive a different answer to their request than other employees making a similar request, an ethical problem may exist and the situation may constitute cause for grievance.

The practical and ethical issue raised by such differential treatment within a department might appear simply to be a form of discrimination in which, whether deliberately or unaware, the manager treats employees with what looks like partiality. The standard corrective answer to perceived partiality is a form of impartiality that does not take personal differences into account. But such impartiality may satisfy neither affected employees nor the requirements of a nuanced ethic. For example, even if a lab employee's request for a period of time away is outside the lines that the manager has previously drawn, the employee's reason for asking may evoke the manager's compassion and at the same time suggest that an exception is called for because of distinctive circumstances.

In such a case, the manager may justly agree to the request, not because it has evoked impartial egalitarian justice that blinds itself to personal differences but because a more encompassing justice moves beyond equating fairness with blind impartiality.[13] Such justice can take individual differences and needs into account; it is not bound solely to a principle of impartial distribution. As a matter of the heart, it merits recognition as a virtue,[14] an expanded sense of fair play that, in this instance, is enriched by the virtue of compassion.

At the same time, the just manager would do well to recognize how such differential treatment may be perceived by those who would like to breach the manager's stated policy for their own reasons, or by those who are simply unaware of the unique circumstances behind the anomalous granting of this request. Moreover, a manager's exercise of compassion resulting in differential treatment of an associate may be complicated by the need to hold in confidence the circumstances giving rise to the exception. From a pragmatic viewpoint, such an exception may seem questionable: What is the effect on the department's morale of differential treatment that to some or all of the staff is unexplained and thus, apparently, unjustified?

Negotiating trust and confidence in exercising managerial authority over personnel in such situations is not simple—practically or ethically. It may require considerable creativity, and indeed as much ingenuity as a manager can muster. In such a situation, especially when thorough explanation might do harm to others, the best aid to trust may not be explanation (especially if it is truncated) but rather a virtuous manager, one who already has a reputation for fair dealing along with compassion, open communication, and loyalty to all her staff.[15]

Managerial Competencies

Fortunately, not all employee relations issues involve such intricacies. Many involve more basic human relations problems. Such problems may result from a manager's questionable relational competency in exercising the authority of his role. A manager may become mired in personality conflict with staff, manage in an authoritarian way (or abdicate authority in the guise of providing democratic leadership), fail to communicate significant information to staff, permit an atmosphere that some staff experience as harassing or discriminatory, or display intractable insensitivity to the cultural and racial diversity of the staff. To compound matters further, should problems arise such a manager may delay in engaging the expertise of the human resource function to serve as a sounding board, gather or offer additional information, or intervene with employees directly. Then the manager may unrealistically expect HR to step in and shoulder the burden of cleaning up the mess.

Such situations may initially seem to be no-brainers because the common presenting problem and its remedy (significant behavioral change by the manager, or removal and replacement) seem obvious enough. A deeper question, however, may be the nature of the organization's commitment to the training—or, perhaps better, formation—and sustenance of its managers.

It remains true in health care that promotion to a managerial position often comes to staff who have no formal training in management or the art and skill of supervising others. Typically the new manager is well aware that she lacks such a background. Thus the investment of human and financial resources in forming and supporting managers and supervisors can meet a need that is strongly felt by those who are new in their roles. A development program can seize a strategic opportunity to form new managers' relational attitudes and approaches while they are most ready to learn—and, some cynics might add, before they have had time to solidify nascent bad habits.

Grievances

Although training programs can enhance managerial skills in employee relations, they alone are unlikely to prevent conflict between managers and employees or eliminate the employee dissatisfaction and suspicion that conflict engenders. Even substantial managerial effort to be fair in decision making may encounter dissatisfaction, at least in part because fairness is a matter of perspective, and differences not only of responsibility but of power inform individuals' perspectives on fairness. Thus fairness is not just about the substance of decisions but also about process: increasingly, employees are likely to view fairness as a *procedural* matter.[16] The opportunity to have voice, "to provide input into decisions that affect them" and thus "communicate their interests upward," heightens the perception of fairness for many employees.[17]

In response to this reality, businesses have increasingly instituted various types of formalized grievance procedures. Health care organizations, which initially lagged behind this corporate trend, have gradually followed the lead of business. In effect, a grievance process is a form of due process, although standards of due process are quite diverse and typically far less stringent than legal standards.[18] Grievance procedures can vary widely in their degree of formality, their visibility within the organization, and the structure of their appeals process.

Ethically, the existence of genuine opportunity to raise one's voice and of sound grievance procedures enhances the *perception* of fairness along with the likelihood that the power differential between management and employees does not unduly bias or overwhelm the process of conflict resolution. Widespread adoption of formal grievance processes in response to changing employee perceptions of fairness, however, does show that standards of justice or fairness in responding to employee grievances are not simply static. Even if basic notions of justice are relatively unchanging, in the workplace changing expectations on the part of employees do have an impact on the notion of fairness-in-practice and must be taken into account.[19]

A seemingly reasonable level of fairness and substantial employee satisfaction with grievance procedures have been reported in organizations using a variety of practices for resolving conflict. The most effective processes, however, make a demonstrable difference in employee trust, confidence, and morale. They appear to have several characteristics in common. First, they are readily accessible and easy to use. Second, they frequently result in findings that support the employee's perspective rather than the original management decision; if, for example, only 5–10 percent of manager decisions are reversed, the process is skewed in favor of management (and hardly likely to achieve employee respect). Third, the process has significant visibility within the organization. Fourth, and of particular importance, employee use of the grievance process does not result in any form of retaliation, either overt or covert.[20]

Unions

Health care organizations seem to have a particular aversion to unionization. Some organizations spend considerable energy detailing its evils to managers and staff. The typical antiunion message runs something like this: the day-to-day reality of a union shop drives an unnecessary, adversarial wedge between those who should be cooperating in a shared commitment to patient care; moreover, the specter of a health care workers' strike places patient care and safety in needless jeopardy. An organization may also school its managers in how to offer legally permissible and pragmatically effective responses to "union talk" among staff or to rumors of impending efforts to organize a department or an entire institution.

Optimally, in approaching the possibility of union organizing, a health care organization strives to offer responses that are both legally permissible and ethically sound. Sometimes an administration asks its human resource area to launch a new employee development program or inaugurate other benefits in an effort to counteract the dissatisfaction perceived to be driving the interest in unionization. Such efforts may be legally acceptable, but their underlying aim—to convince staff that "we're good to you already, so you don't need a union"—may be quite transparent and signal an insincerity that undermines the very trust those efforts seek to inspire.

A more adversarial approach can raise other ethical questions. An organization may, in effect, say to would-be unionizers, "Go ahead, you're free to *try* to organize here; we'll respect your legal right to assemble and speak to our people. But if you do, we'll reveal the real dirt about your track record elsewhere and make it costly for you to win your case." Whatever the legal status of this approach, by playing hardball administrators rely on muscle flexing and a form of coercion to achieve their antiunion aims (which is not to deny that those seeking to unionize may resort to similar tactics and indeed may use them first). On balance, it seems that the ethical organization would prefer a strategy of cooperation and bridge building and choose its tactics accordingly, not simply as a matter of principle (taking the high road and treating employees as ends in themselves) but also because in the long run its relations with employees and its ability to elicit their best performance is better served by cultivating a cooperative environment.[21]

Termination of Employment

When a person's employment is involuntarily terminated for any reason, the loss of the job almost always results in significant distress for the employee; regret, bitterness, and recrimination often follow all who are involved in the termination process. Such high human cost (not to mention the short-term financial costs that termination may entail) argues against terminating employees as anything other than a last resort.

Nevertheless, the reality of employment termination, whether for cause or not, is an inescapable feature of the human resource landscape. In part this reality exists because, legally speaking, discharging employees is relatively easy: forty-nine states[22] recognize "employment at will," which means that in most circumstances an organization has no legal obligation to give either notice or reasons in discharging an employee. In meeting what they consider overriding goals, organizations frequently find the option of discharging one or more employees preferable to other alternatives, especially if the law does not impede such freedom of action. At the same time, the fact that an employee as a fallible human being may not perform a job adequately or may engage in serious misconduct means that discharge for cause is an inevitable fact of life in every organization.

Discipline and Discharge for Cause

Termination for cause is emotionally traumatic for all involved; it also has substantial financial implications. The financial drain may include severance; the cost of resources spent to orient and develop the employee; the continuing accrual of retirement or other benefits; and sometimes the cost of litigation or, alternatively, spending time and money on an internal grievance process that may be protracted by appeal.

Sound disciplinary procedures, usually structured as a formal progressive discipline system, can avoid or mitigate such costs of terminating an employee for cause. Even though employment is still largely subject to the legal doctrine of employment-at-will, both federal regulations and case law have admitted some exceptions to this doctrine in recent years.[23] Establishing disciplinary procedures that are fair and following them consistently is, from a pragmatic perspective, a first line of defense against the excessive costs that termination can entail. An adequate grievance procedure can also help to achieve this goal, but a grievance may be filed only after the drama of discipline and termination has already played out. Moreover, the very effectiveness of a sound due process system can mean increased expenditure if a terminated employee's grievance is found to have merit.

In any event, an organization cannot ethically justify using its disciplinary procedures only as a means to ensure that firing results in minimal legal exposure and expense. The disciplinary process should not be used simply to rationalize a termination decision that has already been made or create "official records to justify dismissal."[24] If the organization retains a focus on the good of the employee as well as its own aggregate good, it will shape its progressive discipline process with the redemptive intent of recovering productive staff rather than ensuring easy dismissal. If terminating a given employee does become unavoidable, the organization—especially one that wishes to reflect the values of health care in its internal environment—seeks to create the most humane atmosphere possible for the termination.[25] It seeks to minimize or at least not to aggravate the distress (financial or psychological) that termination normally causes a departing employee.

Consistency in applying the formal discipline process is crucial. Such consistency is central to procedural justice and to employee perception of fair treatment in a situation of unequal power.[26] If a terminated employee's claim of unfair treatment in the disciplinary process seems plausible to former colleagues, the morale of the remaining employees is undermined. If their reaction is to "resist and create negative inertia . . . in the form of dysfunctional behavior," such "resistance is not always effective, but it is always expensive."[27] Thus an organization that insists on appropriate, consistent, and well-documented managerial use of disciplinary procedures may be prudent even as it demonstrates commitment to reasonable justice through its management of those procedures.

Downsizing and Position Elimination

Sometimes termination is not for cause. It is not precipitated by any form of misconduct or by performance deficiency serious enough to warrant termination. In particular, downsizing or eliminating a number of positions (some of which may give way to new, reconfigured positions, as in a reengineering program[28]) can be a primary means of reducing cost or redesigning a work process to meet new challenges.

As already noted, there are many pragmatic reasons to avoid workforce reduction if at all possible. The proximate financial cost of downsizing, which is often underestimated, ranges from the expense of increased unemployment taxes to the costs of early retirement incentives to the support required for an outplacement program.[29] Moreover, the effects of downsizing on the morale and productivity of remaining employees may be overlooked or underestimated, and addressed ineffectually if at all.[30] As a result, in the business world the yield of corporate downsizing has often fallen far short of expectation. In the words of one corporate consultant, "Lots of bullets were fired, but few hit their targets."[31] Other commentators have referred to "the dismal success rate of downsizing initiatives."[32]

Some health care organizations have also experienced less-than-satisfactory results from downsizing. In addition, even if downsizing achieves short-term results in the form of cost reduction, concern about the effect of workforce reduction on the quality of care and even patient safety may reflect more than mere disgruntlement on the part of nurses or other clinical caregivers with increased workloads. Like other enterprises, a health care organization may have the experience of suddenly finding itself under-staffed to meet unanticipated needs (sometimes, arguably, needs that better planning might have foreseen).

These and other practical concerns count among the relevant considerations in making an ethical assessment of any contemplated downsizing initiative. If, for example, St. Somewhere decides to respond to its impending financial constraints by reducing workforce and wishes to evaluate the plan in light of ethical considerations, it will surely take these concerns into account. At the same time, an ethical perspective considers other issues and values, especially selection of positions to be eliminated and the manner in which the reduction is conducted.

Even in its downsizing initiative, St. Somewhere will keep in view both the good of the organization and the good of the employees being released (as well as the good of employees who remain). Questions of fairness and justice, in other words, treating people in accord with their relevant similarities and differences, and treating them as they deserve, are highly relevant here.[33] From the employees' perspective, those who lose jobs are quite likely to feel unfairly and unjustly treated. That is, they wonder why *they* were singled out for job loss while others were not: Why are *they* less deserving of keeping a job?

Many, if not most, organizations say that they select categories of positions to be eliminated on the basis of organizational needs and goals, and then individuals within those categories on the basis of seniority (in effect, last hired, first fired). If St. Somewhere proceeds on this basis, the question of how categories of positions are selected to undergo reduction arises. Relative to other positions in other departments, is the selection made on the basis of salary and benefit cost, or current or projected productivity or revenue generation, or the ability to fulfill the organization's goals?

As for the individual employees whose positions are eliminated, are the organization's needs best served by selecting the newest (and often youngest) employees in a department for discharge? Seniority may have the advantage of being the least controversial criterion; many employees are less likely to question seniority than other criteria just because it is widely used and accepted. But in what way is seniority a claim to special consideration? Perhaps it is typically an indicator of strong (or at least consistent) work performance over time. Or it can be argued that seniority is an index of loyalty to the organization, and that loyalty deserves recognition through retention.

But is durability necessarily a sign of strong performance, or a sign merely of perseverance? Is organizational loyalty in itself worthy of this kind of reward? Some would argue that those with the best track record of performance, as documented in their performance reviews, are more deserving of retaining their jobs and would better serve the organization in the long run—even if seniority is a less controversial and hence easier criterion. On the other hand, employees who discover during downsizing that their formerly competent performance has suddenly become a rationale for dismissal might feel both penalized and betrayed by the belated introduction of job-retention criteria that are now being used against them.

It is not possible here to analyze fully these questions of fairness and justice (and they are hardly an exhaustive list of the questions that can be raised[34]). These questions do, however, constitute a sampling of the issues and values that the administration and the human resource department at St. Somewhere may want to consider— perhaps with consultation from the ethics mechanism—as they assess their options for cost and workforce reduction.

Fairness and justice do not stand alone as a counterpoint to pragmatic considerations in ethically assessing workforce reduction. In whatever downsizing decisions it makes, St. Somewhere presumably seeks to respect the dignity of all employees who lose their jobs[35] and to treat them with compassion. Dignity and compassion are expressions of the humaneness that any health care organization should seek to show internally, consistent with the care and compassion that it wants its employees to show to the patients and families for whom they care.[36]

Moreover, St. Somewhere should pay attention to the *process* by which eliminations are carried out. Leaders and human resource personnel should address questions of timing; of clear, complete, and (especially) prompt communication; and of emotional and practical support (for example, outplacement) for those who lose jobs, to name only some of the relevant issues.[37] As far as possible, it is advisable to involve in the decision making those who are directly affected; at the least, they should be kept well and promptly informed, especially insofar as the timing of the downsizing and any communication about it may affect their ability to explore other job options.[38] Sometimes there may be plausible reasons for secrecy, or for partial or delayed disclosure of information; but since delay or concealment often works to the detriment of terminated employees' ability to plan their future, it would seem to require strong justification. In this regard, a principle proposed by Drew Hinderer deserves full consideration: "It is always ethically preferable to avoid sacrificing important interests unnecessarily."[39]

In addition, both prudence and compassion should lead St. Somewhere's leadership to consider and address the needs and feelings of the layoff survivors during and after the reduction process itself. The human impact of survivor guilt[40] and the effects of workforce reduction on morale and productivity can be addressed by a variety of means, among them regular, complete, and empathic communication. Experience in other organizations suggests it is possible to lessen the stress and strain on remaining employees, but not without commitment by organizational leadership, line managers, and human resource personnel to devote significant attention, thought, feeling, and effort to this relational process.[41] Neither an unfeeling, financially based statement justifying the reduction nor an unbelievably sunny announcement of personnel departures ("John is enthusiastic about this new opportunity to pursue his personal and professional goals") can allay the guilt, fear, and anger of the staff who remain.

Another issue arises if St. Somewhere imitates many organizations in using planned elimination of positions as an opportunity to eliminate some positions—especially managerial—whose occupants happen "coincidentally" to be suboptimal performers, "have an attitude," or are perceived as members of an old guard. This use of the position elimination process raises ethical questions in several respects. For one thing, is it actually the position, or is it really the person in it, who is targeted for elimination? If the answer is the latter, then to label discharge of the employee simply a position elimination is hardly honest; it is at least a partial cover for what management is actually doing.

If performance is in fact an underlying cause for dismissal, is there clear and documented evidence of performance shortcomings? Or is someone in authority acting on instinct, or perhaps on the basis of a long-held negative perception of the employee? If one of the latter applies, releasing the employee may appear arbitrary at best, and an unjust abuse of power at worst. Perhaps those in authority are circumventing the complexity of the performance appraisal and discipline processes (and the possibility that a meritorious grievance will be filed), or avoiding the unpleasant confrontation that even appropriate use of the discipline process might necessitate. Indeed, it may be that the employee has performed marginally but no supervisor has seriously identified, confronted, and documented the performance issues. The at-will nature of most employment may permit such practices from the perspective of the law, but it does not remove the obligations of justice and honesty that are a moral condition of offering and administering employment.

There are other sides to this issue, however. Documenting that termination is for cause usually means the employee is ineligible for unemployment compensation.[42] It can be argued that portraying termination as a position elimination is a more compassionate approach. But is this argument sufficient justification for such a practice? St. Somewhere's leaders should also consider whether, as a matter of social responsibility, it is legitimate to circumvent the exclusionary rules of the unemployment benefit system by disguising the reasons for dismissal. From a pragmatic standpoint, however, an employee who discovers she is thus denied unemployment compensation may be doubly inclined to file a grievance (and might prevail if adequate notice and documentation of performance questions did not precede her termination) or to sue St. Somewhere if she remains dissatisfied with the grievance findings. These concerns for the organization's good, the employee's good, and the interests of the federal government (and, ultimately, of taxpayers) should be weighed, together with previously noted obligations of justice and honesty, in assessing the possible uses or misuses of the position-elimination process. On balance, it is hard to see sufficient justification for a covert and essentially dishonest use of position elimination as a substitute for established processes of performance appraisal, discipline, and termination for cause (see Exhibit 5.1.).

Careful weighing of the considerations discussed here might lead St. Somewhere's leaders to the reluctant conclusion that downsizing is practically necessary and ethically acceptable. As a last test of their resolve, and of their confidence in the moral reasoning behind the decision, the leaders might mull over the minority view of writers who attack the moral basis of downsizing and personal participation in it. In this view, the undeniable taint of self-interest renders all who participate in downsizing guilty of collusion. Leaders and managers who implement a reduction in force are, in effect, ready to sacrifice the jobs of others—to commit "little murders"—to preserve the organization that pays their own salaries. Other managers and staff are also complicit; the same self-interest controls those who regretfully support the downsizing as the only thing to do, as well as those who silently assent to the reduction by remaining in the organization's employ.[43]

The inescapable element of truth in the charge of self-interest may be emotionally unsettling, even if ultimately it does not prove practically and ethically persuasive. Given the gravity of a decision to reduce the workforce, it is appropriate—and perhaps crucial—that leaders let themselves face such unsettling thoughts about their contemplated plan of action. If they can tolerate this kind of moral disturbance for as long as it takes to reach a decision that considers the widest possible range of variables[44] (see Chapter Two), the organization and the staff—both those who might be released and those who would be retained—are likely to be better served than they would be if leaders avoided such reflection.

Exhibit 5.1. American College of Healthcare Executives' Ethical Policy Statement on Issues Related to Downsizing.

Statement of the Issue

As the result of managed care, declining admissions, shorter lengths of stay, higher productivity, new technology, and other factors, the capacity of many health care organizations exceeds demand. Consequently, a large number of organizations will reduce their work forces. Additionally, mergers and consolidations will result in further reductions and reassignments of staff. Financial pressures will continue to fuel this downsizing trend. However, patient care needs should not be compromised when determining staffing requirements.

The hardship and stress of downsizing can be lessened by careful planning. Formal policies and procedures should be developed well in advance of the need to implement them.

The decision to reduce staff necessitates consideration of the short-term and long-term impact on all employees—those leaving and those remaining. Decision makers should consider the potential ethical conflict between formally stated organizational values and their downsizing actions.

Policy Position

The American College of Healthcare Executives recommends that specific steps be considered by health care executives when initiating a downsizing process to support consistency between stated organizational values and those demonstrated during and after the process. Among these steps are the following:

- Provide timely, accurate, clear, and consistent information to the stakeholders when staff reductions become necessary.
- Review values expressed in mission and value statements, personnel policies, annual reports, employee orientation material, and other documents to test congruence and conformance with downsizing actions.
- Support, through retraining and redeployment, if possible, of [sic] employees whose positions have been eliminated. Also, consider outplacement assistance and appropriate severance policies, if possible.
- Address the needs of remaining staff by demonstrating sensitivity to their potential feelings of loss, anger, and survivor guilt. Also address their anxiety about the possibility of further reductions, uncertainty regarding changes in work load and work redesign, and other similar concerns.

Health care organizations encounter the same set of challenging issues associated with downsizing as do other employers. Downsizing decisions should reflect ethical values.

Approved by the Board of Governors of the American College of Healthcare Executives (Aug. 15, 1995).

Source: Reprinted with permission of the American College of Healthcare Executives, copyright 1995.

The Employment Covenant

The high incidence of downsizing in business generally, and recently in health care, has led to claims that a "new employment contract" or a "new relationship agreement"[45] with employees is now called for. In reevaluating its approach to human resources under ever-greater fiscal constraints, St. Somewhere may wish to reconsider its own approach to employees and employment. If the old employment contract promised, or seemed to promise, career-long employment (and often advancement) to employees who were productive and loyal, keeping this promise has become an increasingly tenuous matter. An organization should not, in this view, perpetuate the unrealistic expectation, and even "codependence," that such an explicit or implied promise has evoked in many employees.[46]

On the contrary, in this analysis a new employment contract should support the right and ability of both employees and organizations to be free, temporary contractors with one another. The organization should as a matter of course recognize good work with rewards other than promotion (or even retention), and employees should recognize that it is not the organization itself but the possibility of doing good work that matters most. The organization should give employees abundant development opportunity, both to enhance their contribution in a current position and as a benefit that can equip them for their next position, *whether or not* they remain in the organization.[47]

Before adopting such an analysis, however, St. Somewhere may be wise to consider whether this framework is itself beyond criticism. For example, this analysis implicitly, and at some points explicitly, assumes that the fault in the old employment contract has rested in the codependent expectation of the individual employee and in the organization fostering that expectation. It does not entertain the possibility that something has gone awry in the massive turn to downsizing that so many organizations have taken. Is there anything of disloyalty, even betrayal, in using this mechanism as the primary means to right so many corporate ships (including health care organizations) that have sailed into rough waters? The answer may prove to be no, but it seems inappropriate for an organization to assume without question that turning to downsizing or a temporary employment contract is essentially a no-fault move required by the irresistible tide of systemic macroeconomic change.[48]

Perhaps a more substantial question about the ad hoc employment contract is its apparent assumption that the good work the autonomous employee finds or creates is somehow independent of the organizational context in which it occurs. There are at least two problems with this assumption. First, it undervalues the importance of the organization itself as a means to achieve the various goods that its employees want to achieve—the good work that they have come there hoping to perform. An organization can do what individuals alone cannot, and individuals may value the organization for that very reason.[49]

Second, if through its articulation of a new employment contract an organization signals that it cannot and does not make a long-term commitment to employees, then employees' commitment to the organization and to their colleagues as well may be weakened as a result. "As organizations weaken their commitments to their people," observe Christina Maslach and Michael Leiter, "staff members have less of a basis for making commitments to one another."[50] At the least, this dynamic "impoverishes the social environment" of the organization; at worst, it may undermine the organization's work because that work is so closely tied to the relationships between the people who must cooperate to accomplish it.

Nevertheless, the idea of developing a covenant between the employing organization and its employees has genuine possibilities. A clearly stated covenant may serve as a helpful tool in clarifying employee and organizational expectations. It may answer at least some employees' questions about the organization's attitude—both toward their work (their "doing") and toward them as persons (their "being")—in times that for many health care organizations and employees continue to be quite uncertain. The covenant can outline the organization's understanding of its obligations to the staff and also describe how it intends to value them even when permanent employment is a fading norm and the rewards given for good performance may not include promotion or even higher pay.

The covenant can also articulate what the organization generally expects of all employees on the job and how it expects them to be in their relationships with patients, colleagues, and the organization. It is possible for statements of employee responsibility to be generated entirely by management, and thus for the organization's leadership to be the actual and sole authors of the covenant or "new relationship agreement with employees."[51] For this part of the covenant to carry real weight among staff, however—for them to own it—the process by which it is developed should involve maximal, meaningful employee participation. Optimally, the ideas this part of the statement expresses and the language it uses should represent a consensus of employees as those who are in some sense bound to the responsibilities articulated in their "side" of the covenantal agreement.

At the same time, perhaps both sides should remind themselves ever and again that in a large businesslike enterprise (health care organization or otherwise) the interests of labor and management are never fully harmonious and may at times sharply diverge. Insofar as human beings are creatures of will and therefore capable of defining and pursuing their purposes while resisting external attempts to restrain or redirect such efforts, there are always differences, and indeed conflicts, between the two sides that no covenant can simply erase.[52] One potential fruit of the covenant-building process, however, is that a truly owned covenant results in internalization of the commitments made, including the limits that any covenant inevitably imposes. Thus, those who are party to the covenant *voluntarily* govern themselves in ways that show their good faith and call forth a similar answering response from their partners in the covenant. At its best, the management-employee covenant can be a vehicle that not only articulates particular commitments and binds the parties to fulfilling them but also motivates them over time to go above and beyond, by striving to exceed the commitments they have made.[53] Viewed in such a light, covenant making with employees may indeed be a worthwhile process for an organization to undertake.

Notes

1. Rosen, S. D., and Juris, H. A. "Ethical Issues in Human Resource Management." In G. R. Ferris, S. D. Rosen, and D. T. Barnum (eds.), *Handbook of Human Resource Management.* (Blackwell Human Resource Management Series.) Cambridge, Mass.: Blackwell, 1995.
2. Feuille, P., and Hildebrand, R. L. "Grievance Procedures and Dispute Resolution." In Ferris, Rosen, and Barnum (1995).

3. Rosen and Juris (1995).

4. Harshman, E., and Chachere, D. R. "Employee References: Between the Legal Devil and the Ethical Deep Blue Sea." Presentation at "From the Universities to the Marketplace," Fifth Annual Conference Promoting Business Ethics, sponsored by Vincentian Universities in the United States, Chicago, Oct. 30, 1998.

5. Rosen and Juris (1995).

6. Harshman and Cachere (1998), p. 10.

7. Harshman and Cachere (1998), p. 10.

8. Rosen and Juris (1995).

9. Herzberg, F. "The Motivation-Hygiene Concept and Problems of Manpower [sic]." *Personnel Administration*, 1964, *27*(1), 3–7; cited in D. M. Noer, *Healing the Wounds: Overcoming the Trauma of Layoffs and Revitalizing Downsized Organizations*. San Francisco: Jossey-Bass, 1993.

10. Thomas, R. R., Jr. "From Affirmative Action to Affirming Diversity." *Harvard Business Review*, 1990, *68*(2), 113.

11. Chen, C. "The Diversity Paradox." *Personnel Journal*, Jan. 1992, p. 32.

12. Thomas (1990), p. 114.

13. Hinderer, D. E. "Hospital Downsizing: Ethics and Employees." *Journal of Nursing Administration*, 1997, *27*(4), 9.

14. Solomon, R. C. *Ethics and Excellence: Cooperation and Integrity in Business*. New York: Oxford University, 1993.

15. Hinderer (1997).

16. Feuille and Hildebrand (1995), p. 341.

17. Feuille and Hildebrand (1995), p. 341.

18. Ewing, D. W. "The Corporation as a Just Society." *Business Ethics*, Mar.–Apr. 1990, p. 21.

19. Ewing (1990).

20. Ewing (1990).

21. Herman, S. W. *Durable Goods: A Covenantal Ethic for Management and Employees*. Notre Dame, Ind.: University of Notre Dame, 1997.

22. Furore, K. "Employment AT WILL [sic] Makes It Surprisingly Easy to Fire Workers." *Chicago Tribune*, Apr. 5, 1998, Sect. 6, p. 1.

23. LeRoy, M. H., and Schultz, J. M. "The Legal Context of Human Resource Management: Conflict, Confusion, Cost, and Role-Conversion." In Ferris, Rosen, and Barnum (1995).

24. Coye, R., and Belohlav, J. "Disciplining: A Question of Ethics?" *Employee Responsibilities and Rights Journal*, 1989, *2*(3), 160.

25. Reiser, S. J. "The Ethical Life of Health Care Organizations." *Hastings Center Report*, 1994, *24*(6), 31.

26. Ewing (1990).

27. Pastin, M. *The Hard Problems of Management*. San Francisco: Jossey-Bass, 1986; cited in Coye and Belohlav (1989), p. 160.

28. Hammer, M., and Champey, J. *Reengineering the Corporation: A Manifesto for Business Revolution.* New York: HarperCollins, 1993.
29. Heisler, W. J., Jones, W. D., and Benham, P. O., Jr. *Managing Human Resource Issues: Confronting Challenges and Choosing Options.* San Francisco: Jossey-Bass, 1988.
30. Noer, D. *Healing the Wounds: Overcoming the Trauma of Layoffs and Revitalizing Downsized Organizations.* San Francisco: Jossey-Bass, 1993.
31. Bennett, A. "Downsizing Doesn't Necessarily Bring an Upswing in Corporate Profitability." *Wall Street Journal,* June 6, 1991, p. B1.
32. Whetten, D. A., Kaiser, J. D., and Urban, T. "Implications of Organizational Downsizing for the Human Resource Function." In Ferris, Rosen, and Barnum (1995), p. 283.
33. Hinderer (1997).
34. Hinderer (1997).
35. Rosen and Juris (1995).
36. Reiser (1994).
37. Noer (1993).
38. Noer (1993).
39. Hinderer (1997), p. 11.
40. Noer (1993).
41. Noer (1993).
42. Heisler, Jones, and Benham (1998).
43. Harvey, J. *The Abilene Paradox and Other Meditations on Management.* San Francisco: Jossey-Bass, 1996.
44. Messick, D. M., and Bazerman, M. H. "Ethical Leadership and the Psychology of Decision Making." *Sloan Management Review,* 1996, *37*(2), 10.
45. Giganti, E., and "Think Tank" Participants. "A New Social Contract: Catholic Healthcare Leaders Rethink Their Relationship with Employees." *Health Progress,* 1995, *76*(5), Special Section, 1–5.
46. Noer (1993).
47. Noer (1993).
48. Noer (1993).
49. Maslach, C., and Leiter, M. P. *The Truth About Burnout: How Organizations Cause Personal Stress and What to Do About It.* San Francisco: Jossey-Bass, 1997.
50. Maslach and Leiter (1997), p. 49.
51. Giganti and others (1995).
52. Herman (1997).
53. Herman (1997).

| **Conflicts of Interest**

In the preceding chapter, we examined institutional ethical concerns through a careful review of the operations of one department: human resources. This and subsequent chapters analyze certain thematic concepts linked to ethical concerns. In this chapter, we define the concept of conflict of interest, illustrate it by examining the general principles underlying the concept, and explore how those principles manifest themselves in behavior throughout the organization, first at the executive or governance level and then at the general administrative and clinical levels. This process demonstrates the pervasive presence of this moral concern throughout an organization and also highlights the depth and utility of the concept itself.

The concept of conflict of interest is grounded in the nature of institutional action. Each organization acts through its agents and employees. To fulfill the mission, it depends on the associated individuals to adhere to the mission and to the promulgated policies. In carrying out their jobs, associates have varying degrees of discretion about how they perform their assigned tasks. They have to judge which actions to adopt or reject. The more discretion an associate has in the exercise of his or her judgment, the more important it is that the goals and mission of the organization guide that judgment (see Chapter Seven). There are times, however, when the appropriate decision or course of action is not clear.

Associates do not operate in a vacuum or as automatons of the organization. They have their own interests, such as career advancement, the desire for honor and prestige, family obligations, and independent financial interests. In most cases, they attempt to honestly perform their jobs and find a way to harmonize independent interests with their obligation to the organization. A conflict of interest arises when these outside interests begin to intrude (or appear to intrude) on the associate's judgment about how to perform the job and how to conform to the mission of the institution. This is one of the most pervasive and important issues in organizational ethics.

Defining Conflict of Interest

The classic definition of a conflict of interest focuses on the existence of a personal interest, held by an employee possessing administrative authority for an organization, that runs counter to the interests of the organization. As defined by the 1993 Code of Ethics of the American College of Healthcare Executives,

> A conflict of interest may be only a matter of degree, but exists when the health care executive:
> A. Is in a position to benefit directly or indirectly by using authority or inside information, or allows a friend, relative, or associate to benefit from such authority or information [and]
> B. Uses authority or information to make a decision to intentionally affect the organization in an adverse manner.[1]

According to this definition, a conflict of interest exists only if the health care executive with a competing interest intentionally uses his or her position for personal benefit at the expense of the organization. The definition represents the historical understanding of conflict of interest based on the potential for the agent to use delegated authority in order to profit at the expense of his or her principal. Although it can help to identify many—though not all—instances in which an outside interest of an employee agent adversely affects an organization, there are three difficulties with this definition.

First, there is the problem of intentionality. In defining a conflict of interest as involving a decision to "intentionally" affect the organization adversely, this definition may presume both too much and too little. It presumes too much in positing that an employee willfully violates his or her duty of loyalty and honesty. It presumes too little in saying that the harm caused by a conflict of interest occurs only as a result of an intentional act. In practice, however, failing to act to avoid a conflict of interest can be equally harmful.

Second, the definition invites us to understand harm too narrowly. This definition speaks of acting in ways that affect the organization "in an adverse manner." This would clearly apply to an action that causes an organization to lose money, but there are other harms with which a health care organization is concerned. For example, if a doctor orders an unnecessary test in a hospital-owned facility, the patient is harmed in violation of the hospital's mission—even though the hospital may benefit financially.

Moreover, the mere appearance of a conflict of interest can be harmful. A health care organization depends on the good will of the public and of its employees and agents. It is entrusted with one of a patient's most valued goods—his or her health—and patients must be able to trust that the organization will properly care for them. To learn that employees of the institution have acted (or may have acted) to further their own personal interests rather than those of the organization and the patients it serves can undermine this trust. Similarly, the culture of an institution is powerfully shaped by how employees perceive the actions of fellow staff and administrators. If they come to believe (justifiably or not) that an administrator is putting his or her own interest above that of the organization, this belief can corrupt the culture, breeding suspicion and possibly encouraging others to put aside the organization's interests in favor of their own personal interests.

Third, this definition rests on identifying personal "benefit" to the employee or the employee's close associate(s). What is beneficial to an individual may be difficult to discern, however; individuals may understand *benefit* quite idiosyncratically. Unless supervisors and others are prepared to explore the context of an action and probe the individual's own understanding of what he or she considers beneficial in these circumstances, they take into account only those personal interests that fit within conventional understanding of what is beneficial to an individual. Financial gain is an obvious benefit—and what is usually thought of as creating a conflict of interest—but an individual's desire for power or influence, fear of failure, or even self-destructive impulse can dramatically affect his or her decision making and lead to decisions that cause the organization to act against or outside of its mission.

Thus a more accurate definition of conflict of interest recognizes that a potential conflict exists whenever (1) an employee or an employee's close friend(s), relative(s), or associate(s) has a strong personal life interest, (2) the employee is involved in decision making on behalf of the organization (whether as decision maker or as someone who may influence other authorized decision makers), and (3) the employee's interest may cause (or may be perceived as causing) the employee to exercise his or her organizational decision-making power to further personal interest rather than the organization's mission, (4) to the detriment of the organization.

Because conflict of interest is of such major concern in health care, it is frequently the subject of legal regulation. Rather than discuss those laws in detail, however, we focus here primarily on the moral issues involved in conflict of interest. Four features are of particular concern in analyzing conflict of interest: the interest of the employee/agent; the role of the employee/agent within the organization; the interests of the client; and how the conflict can be addressed. Given the unique nature of health care, particularly important is the issue of what is in an organization's interests, as those interests are defined by the mission.

In considering this issue, we explore three domains or strata of the organization: corporate governance, illustrated by the board of directors; external relationships with doctors; and clinical management.

Corporate Governance: The Board of Directors and Corporate Officers

The overall danger to the organization that is posed by a conflict of interest is proportional to the degree of administrative authority and the level of discretion over job performance held by a staff person. The greater the authority and discretion, the greater the potential harm caused when this authority and discretion are exercised to benefit the interests of the individual as opposed to those of the organization (see Chapter Seven). Members of the board of directors and executive officers typically possess the greatest authority and discretion within an institution. They are the ones charged with defining the mission and guiding operations; it is to them that others within and outside the organization look for guidance and leadership. It is therefore reasonable to demand that they uphold the most rigorous separation between their personal interests and those of the institution.

> A twenty-member board of directors manages PHC. Among its leading members are Stan Kenis, president of the large surgical supply house SS Ltd.; Dr. Susan Philips, chair of a large surgical practice group, with admitting privileges to St. Somewhere, that specializes in plastic surgery; Donna Carlos, RN, head of the nurses' union at Suburban Hospital; Esther Levin, president of PHC and a member of the board of directors of SS Ltd.; and Charles Argent, a stockholder of SS Ltd.

> As a result of reduction in Medicaid reimbursement and its impact on the financial prospects of St. Somewhere, a plan has been submitted to the board to convert a wing of St. Somewhere to serve as a specialized plastic surgery center. It was brought to the board's attention for two reasons. First, it represents a major shift in the services offered by St. Somewhere, which serves a local community that is not a large user of plastic surgery services. Second, because this requires a large investment in new surgical equipment, it involves a substantial shift in resources away from other hospitals within the PHC system, including reduction in services at Suburban Hospital.

As this case demonstrates, the personal interests of board members are as individual as the members themselves, and the importance of those interests can vary according to the situation in which the board finds itself. To minimize abuse arising out of a conflict of interest on the part of executives and board members, organizations adopt five tactics: identification of potential conflict; disclosure; systemic protection and balanced committee decision making; recusal; and exclusion or divestiture.

Identification of Potential Conflict

The potential for conflict arises in a variety of ways and may result not only from the actions or interests of the individual but also by virtue of his or her important relationships (for example, with a family member, a personal friend, or a business associate). The issue most commonly of concern is the existence of a competing financial interest, where conflict usually arises in one of three ways:

1. *Conducting business with the organization.* A director, officer, or close associate or family member contracts with the organization to buy or sell goods or services or to derive some personal benefit.
2. *Usurping an organizational opportunity.* A director or officer obtains for his or her own benefit an opportunity that should belong to the organization.
3. *Competing with the organization.* A director or officer engages in a similar yet independent business.[2]

A fourth form of conflict, particularly germane to nonprofit organizations, can be identified: *using the organization to advance a related activity,* as when a director or officer has personal or professional interests that can benefit from activities of the organization.

In the case of the PHC board, Kenis, the president of SS Ltd., and Argent, an investor in SS Ltd., run afoul of the conducting-business conflict. Both have a strong interest in the profitability of SS Ltd., which can be dramatically affected by the decision to develop a surgical center at St. Somewhere. As a large supplier, SS Ltd. could presumably benefit substantially through the equipment purchases made by St. Somewhere. Moreover, because of the ongoing relationship between SS Ltd. and PHC, almost any action by PHC potentially affects SS Ltd.

Levin, a board member of SS Ltd., also runs afoul of the conducting-business concern, although it is not clear whether she profits individually from her association with SS Ltd. Although she has some interest in managing SS Ltd. well, as a board member there she generally is not compensated on the basis of profitability. Nonetheless, her capacity to influence the behavior of PHC to favor SS Ltd. and her capacity to pass on confidential information about PHC that could benefit SS Ltd. are of very serious concern.

Dr. Philips's interest as chair of a surgical practice group can also be categorized under conducting business. Her surgical group would benefit by having St. Somewhere become a surgical center, though her group would not profit directly from PHC. Like most attending physicians, she stands in the position of a business supplier to St. Somewhere through her capacity to direct patients to that hospital. Indeed, she was probably brought onto the PHC board on the basis of her understanding of how doctors think about hospital admission and treatment as well as her general medical expertise. The board wants and needs this perspective in developing its operating plans. The concern here is that she may seek to use PHC to advance her surgical group's interests, and this may or may not conform to the overall mission of PHC.

Carlos has a somewhat similar conflict. Some of the policy decisions she has to address as a board member may conflict with the interests of the nurses she represents as a union leader at Suburban Hospital. The shift in resources from Suburban to St. Somewhere is one such example. Her membership on the board may reasonably be debated as being improper,[3] but she too was brought onto the board precisely to reflect the interests of nurses within the PHC system. A potential for conflict exists, but she offers important insights for the board to consider.

Disclosure

Disclosure of potential conflict of interest is almost always recommended as the first step in any organization's effort to ameliorate such conflict, though the rationale for this policy is rarely explained. In part, the strategy rests on the corporate officer's or board member's fiduciary duty to act solely in the interest of the organization and thus to disclose to the organization any interests he or she holds that may conflict with those of the organization. There is a tacit understanding that so long as an agent (officer or board member) discloses the potential conflict, the principal (the organization) is free either to reject the agent and seek another who has no such conflict or to accept the agent with the understanding that despite the conflict the agent will serve the principal fairly. Because the organization is aware of the potential conflict, it is in a position to monitor the behavior of the agent with respect to that potential conflict.

Disclosure at the outset avoids the perception of dishonesty that arises if the conflict is discovered later in the relationship, and suspicions that it may have been hidden for a reason. This rationale has some force with respect to executives and board members, where trust is so vitally important.

To be effective, a disclosure policy needs to (1) clearly identify the types of relationship or interest that may constitute a conflict of interest; (2) require ongoing disclosure (generally in the form of an annual statement, and specific disclosure when circumstances change and create a particular conflict); and (3) make the disclosure public to involved decision makers.

PHC has adopted a requirement that all corporate officers (including board members) disclose any affiliation or interest in another company operating in the health care field or providing services to PHC. This includes both their own interests as employees or investors in a company actually or potentially rendering services to PHC and any interest held by a member of their immediate families. This policy forestalls any perception of a conflict created by a special relationship that would be exacerbated if it were hidden; the policy also allows further analysis of the potential conflict. Because one's life interests are not static, PHC's policy requires both that disclosure be made annually in writing and that employees and board members disclose any conflict arising during the course of the year (Exhibit 6.1).

Limits to Authority and Action

As noted in the proposed definition, for a conflict of interest to exist the employee must have some level of authority or control over an action by the organization—including the possibility of the employee influencing the decision(s) of another—that directly affect the employee's personal interest. Thus one way to limit the potential for harm caused by a conflict is to limit the discretion and authority of a particular employee. For example, purchase of goods and services is often of great concern. The most obvious examples of a conflict of interest are purchasing decisions that advance one's private financial interest in an outside business, or a situation in which salespeople offer gifts, bribes, or kickbacks to encourage selection of their products. Employees who do not have direct or indirect purchasing authority are not susceptible to this conflict.

A board of directors, which is charged with the overall administration of an organization, has enormous authority and discretion. Therefore concern over the potential for conflict of interest

Exhibit 6.1. PHC Conflict of Interest Certification.

Conflicts of Interest

I have read the Partnership Health Care conflict of interest policy and agree to abide by it.

Please complete the Conflict of Interest certification below. For all of the provisions, list any instances of actual or potential noncompliance. If there are no such instances, mark "none."

Investments

Neither I nor members of my immediate family* have investments which could result in or constitute a material financial interest in a supplier, provider, competitor, or customer of Partnership Health Care, except:

( ) None

Outside Interest

Neither I nor members of my immediate family* have or hold any interest outside of Partnership Health Care which would result in or constitute a conflict of interest, except:

( ) None

Outside Activities

Neither I nor members of my immediate family* participate in outside activities such as the rendering of directive, managerial, or consultative services to any concern that does business with, or competes with, the services of Partnership Health Care. Neither I nor members of my immediate family* render other services in competition with Partnership Health Care, except:

( ) None

Inside Information

Neither I nor members of my immediate family* have disclosed or used information relating to the Partnership Health Care business for personal profit or advantage, except:

( ) None

Gifts, Favors, Services, Entertainment

Neither I nor members of my immediate family* have accepted gifts, favors, services, or entertainment that might influence my judgment or action concerning the business of Partnership Health Care, except:

( ) None

Exhibit 6.1. PHC Conflict-of-Interest Certification, Cont'd.

Software Development

Neither I nor members of my immediate family* have sold or
distributed system software developed while working for Partnership
Health Care to any other facility, company, or person; inserted code
into or modified any software used by Partnership Health Care for
personal advantage or to the detriment of Partnership Health Care;
used position or knowledge gained at Partnership Health Care to
develop software for sale or to compete against Partnership Health
Care in the marketplace, except:

( ) None

Family Employment

No member of my immediate family* is employed by or has a contract
with Partnership Health Care, except:

( ) None

I have not made or authorized any political contribution or other
prohibited or illegal payments or the like with funds of Partnership
Health Care, nor have I performed or authorized any act which to my
knowledge is prohibited or illegal or which constitutes an irregularity,
except:

( ) None

I do not have direct knowledge of any Partnership Health Care
governing body member, officer, employee, volunteer, or medical staff
member who has or might have authorized or committed any act or
held any position which could or might be prohibited or illegal, and
which has not been reported or disclosed so as to become commonly
held knowledge, except:

( ) None

* Immediate family includes a spouse, child, parent, grandparent,
brother, sister, cousin, uncle, aunt, niece, nephew, grandchild, or in-law.

Signature _____

Print name _____

Title _____

Date _____

is intense. However, even here, the potential for conflict is systemically limited by the nature of the issues submitted to the board. The board is generally called on to exercise judgment over general policies and practices of the organization. It examines budgets and general business plans and is rarely involved in considering specific contracts with suppliers or purchasers unless those contracts have a major impact on the operations of the organization. To the extent that the board members have an interest in another company, they are only rarely called to address a specific transaction involving that outside interest.

The risk of harm to the organization from a conflict of interest can also be minimized through systemic restriction of an individual's discretionary authority. For example, requiring that major purchasing decisions be made subject to an open bidding process where the terms of competing bids are clearly spelled out and accessible to appropriate audit limits the potential for an employee to act on a conflict in relation to that purchase.

The balanced committee decision-making process of the board acts as one such check on conflict of interest that board members hold. For the most part, board decisions are made in a group forum by a majority vote. Individual board members must persuade other members that their position on an issue up for a vote is good for the organization. Insofar as it is clearly disclosed that they have an outside interest that might conflict in any way with their impartiality, it is that much harder to persuade others of the merit of their position.

To make this systemic check effective, care must be taken to be sure that the overall board membership reflects diverse perspectives and is not dominated by a particular interest group. Thus in PHC board decisions that might touch on the interests of doctors and nurses, the board should seek to balance the contributions offered by nurse Carlos and Dr. Philips by having representatives of other, counterbalancing interests. These can include other doctors or nurses, or other business professionals who are aware of the possibility that Philips's and Carlos's judgments may be swayed by their particular outside affiliations. Further, the committee form of decision making reduces the capacity of Philips or Carlos to act solely on outside interest; their judgments must be made acceptable to other directors not sharing that outside interest.

It is this shared decision-making process that allows board membership for a large stockholder like Argent, whose financial interests are problematic. Because decision making occurs in an open committee process, Argent's ownership of stock in SS Ltd. is not considered a severe impediment to membership on the PHC board. A similar stockholding by an operating executive of PHC would be far more objectionable because the decision making of a corporate executive is less open and less subject to check by a committee process.

Recusal

At times, conflict is not ongoing but rather arises in connection with a particular decision to be made by an organization. For example, a family member, a close friend, or a staff person may attempt to persuade an officer of the organization to support or challenge a particular action by the organization. Depending on the delicacy of the decision to be made, on the nature of the lobbying effort, and on the person's relationship to the officer or director, the officer may feel that his or her judgment has been subtly influenced. Or the officer may fear that, although the attempt does not actually influence him or her, many looking on from the outside will be suspicious that it might, thus tainting the decision. The officer cannot participate in the decision without consequence. Therefore, many organizations accept that it is appropriate for the officer to recuse himself or herself by withdrawing from participating in that particular decision.

This is often particularly appropriate for a board member. There are times when the board has to make a decision that does affect a specific action of the organization in which a board member may be perceived as having an outside interest. This situation arises most commonly with respect to executive compensation. However, there is a concern that personal relationships between board members and executives such as the president of the organization may affect the compensation decision to favor the executive at the expense of the organization. Organizations handle this issue by limiting the decision in these cases to those board members who do not have an obvious conflict.

The decision being confronted by PHC is slightly unusual in that it clearly can affect the interests of SS Ltd. More difficult still, it involves the board in seeking to balance two incommensurate interests: a financially motivated change in operations and a nonfinancial interest of the organization relating to its obligation to deliver health care services to the community served by St. Somewhere. Because this service obligation, which is part of its mission, is not strictly valuable according to general business criteria, PHC is uniquely dependent on the judgment of its board. This heightens the significance of any possible financial conflict of interest, in that it involves the board in balancing the financial interests of PHC against the intangible interest of community service.

In this case, it is probably advisable that Argent and possibly also Philips and Carlos, having strong interests in the specific outcome of this decision, recuse themselves and that the board make this decision without their participation. To avoid even the appearance of a conflict of interest, this can include provision that the recused board members not be included in the total needed for an official quorum, along with a request that they leave the room while discussion of the issues takes place.[4]

Exclusion or Divestment

Recusal only works to the extent that the actual (or clearly possible) conflict of interest is a temporary or infrequent problem. Where the outside interest is an ongoing issue of concern, repeated reliance on recusal is not effective. Either the staff person cannot properly perform his or her job or the organization has to tolerate a situation that many would perceive as problematic because the organization cannot maintain a strong barrier between the staff person and the outside interest. In such a situation, the organization must find a way to end the conflict, either by changing the nature of the person's employment (perhaps moving the employee to another department so that the person has no authority in relation to the outside conflict), by having the employee divest himself or herself of the conflict (by selling his stock or resigning her outside position), or by removing the person from the organization.

With respect to the board, the ongoing nature of the relationships between PHC, its various hospitals, and SS Ltd. presents a *very* serious potential for conflict affecting Kenis, the president of SS Ltd., and Levin, a member of the company's board. Yet this type of situation is common. For a long time, many have complained that boards of directors are routinely staffed by a small coterie of old boys, with a single small group of men holding multiple directorships and many chief executives sitting on one another's boards. Critics advocate expanding board membership to include public representatives and "independent" board members. Nonetheless, the prevalent situation is that the board of a profit-making institution includes representatives drawn from the executive ranks of other corporations, often from those operating in related fields.

In part, this reflects the nature of board membership. With the exception of the chairman, board membership is rarely a full-time position. Although it may entail what many would consider to be significant compensation, it does not pay an amount sufficient to compete with what a talented executive can earn as an operating officer of a company or as a consultant. Moreover, an executive in an industry related to the activities of PHC has far more to offer in terms of skill and experience than one drawn from outside the health care field. For these reasons, as a pragmatic matter board reform efforts have never sought to eliminate overlapping board membership completely.

If PHC were a for-profit institution, it might be argued that the potential for conflict is not serious enough to demand the removal of Kenis and Levin. The private interests of the stockholders can, in theory, be protected by their power to elect board members: if stockholders object to a potential conflict, they can remove a director from the board. Yet the reality is that shareholders have limited ability to affect board management.[5] Failure to demand greater freedom from conflict may harm PHC by bringing it under the shadow of suspicion directed toward for-profit health care systems in general.

Regulation of nonprofit boards is generally much more exacting. The board or trustees of a nonprofit organization are charged with managing a public trust for the benefit of the community at large. They are subject to laws governing their management that are generally far less tolerant of potential conflict of interest than is the case with a for-profit corporation. As such, there is less tolerance for even the perception that the institution is being manipulated for private gain. On this basis, many would argue that Kenis and Levin should resign from the boards of PHC and SS Ltd., respectively.

Developing an Adequate Conflict-of-Interest Policy Relating to Governance

As the foregoing discussion illustrates, issues of conflict of interest are often complex, subtle, and pervasive. An organization should seek not only to remedy conflict once it is discovered but also to develop preventive policies and procedures that limit the risk presented by conflict. This includes a number of steps.

First, the organization must clearly identify and educate all affected staff about what constitutes a conflict of interest and the risks posed by the perception of conflict of interest.

Second, the organization should anticipate certain types of conflict and develop safeguards to limit employee discretion in these areas, such as purchasing.

Third, the organization should develop an ongoing disclosure requirement. This commonly takes the form of a disclosure statement, signed annually, along with an obligation for the staff person to give the organization special notice if a conflict arises during the course of job performance.

Fourth, the policy should identify how particular types of conflict are to be handled (recusal, divestiture, exclusion) and the specific means of enforcing these mechanisms.

Conflict of Interest in Patient Care

People often conceive of conflict of interest as a violation of the fiduciary duties employees owe to an organization that result in harm to the organization. There are, however, situations in which a violation of duty affects individuals outside the organization—in health care, specifically the patients. In some cases, harm that results from a violation of duty is not borne by the organization but by its patients. This most frequently involves questions about patient care in relation to financial considerations.

> To remain competitive in the health care market, PHC has focused on creating a totally integrated health care system, including operation of hospitals, home care services, and nursing homes. To induce doctors to refer patients to them, PHC has acquired physician practice groups and entered into joint ventures with a large number of doctors to operate medical labs and medical imaging

facilities (X rays, sonograms, CT scans, etc.). Moreover, because of a shortage of certain obstetricians/gynecologists and pediatricians in the St. Somewhere service area, PHC has begun a recruitment program offering financial incentives (bonuses, office rental subsidies, and malpractice insurance) to encourage these specialists to relocate in the St. Somewhere community. PHC can now meet virtually all of its patients' needs.

In most businesses, PHC's efforts at integration would be unremarkable; they certainly would not give rise to discussion of conflict of interest. But a health care institution has a special relationship to patients, and it creates a special duty.

First, delivery of health care is held to be radically different from consumer transactions. Health is a higher good, and any organization that commits itself to delivering health care is commonly expected to operate according to a higher moral standard. PHC's asserted commitment to deliver high-quality care justifies the claim of a special duty to deal fairly and honestly with its patients in regard to their health care.

Second, all health care organizations act in concert with physicians and other health care providers. Indeed, in modern American medicine the two cannot operate independently. A health care organization can, therefore, be recognized as a participant in the professional-patient relationship.[6] A basic premise of the doctor-patient relationship is that the health care provider undertakes a special obligation to place the interests of the patient above all personal and competing interests.[7] PHC therefore has a twofold special obligation to its patients, with which its institutional interests may come into conflict.

The primary tool in addressing conflict between the interests of the organization and its professional staff and the patients they serve is, again, disclosure. There are additional tools that apply, depending on the nature of the conflict in question.

Conflict Based on the Patient's Payment Obligation

The requirement that a professional, such as the doctor, be compensated for his or her services is not commonly held to present a conflicting personal interest, nor is mere ownership of a facility and receipt of compensation for services rendered. In a free-market economy, all professional relationships are characterized by this exchange. Yet clearly it is in the interest of the patient (or a payer other than the patient) to receive treatment for the lowest possible cost, and in the interest of the provider to maximize income. This divergence of interest is obvious to all. Indeed, because there is no duty to the patient (absent the patient's entering into a professional paying relationship with the caregiver), the relationship itself may be thought of as a predicate to any conflict.

Nonetheless, ethics and often the law recognize that there is a divergence between the interests of patient and caregiver regarding the caregiver's compensation, and this requires that certain disclosures be made by the caregiver to make sure that the terms and conditions of the compensation are clearly set out and are understood by the patient. Because the patient, being ill or debilitated, is in a disadvantaged position in relation to the doctor or health care provider, the latter should not put himself or herself in a position to profit unfairly from that disadvantage. This obligation is implicit in a doctor's duty to deal "honestly" with his or her patients.[8] Under JCAHO accreditation standards, a hospital is obligated to develop ethical practices regarding billing, and commentary suggests that this include clear and precise identification of all the costs of and charges for the services to be rendered.[9] Moreover, because of the power imbalance in the relationship between a large institution and an individual, the health care organization is also required to develop mechanisms to facilitate resolving disputes over billing.[10] Again, this represents an effort to relieve the disadvantage of the patient.

Conflict Relating to Treatment Decision Making

Treating a patient fairly in negotiating the terms of compensation is important. Of far greater importance, however, is the obligation of doctors and other health care providers to offer honest guidance in recommending treatment. Such guidance is the cornerstone of health care. Patients come to doctors because they need expert advice and treatment. The patient is compelled to trust that the doctors and providers are dealing with her honestly and are seeking to provide the best possible health care for her. Any personal interest that might interfere with a doctor's or health care organization's commitment to the patient is, therefore, of great concern.

Potential conflict arises out of two contexts: the institutional system of ownership, and the relationships between the institution and its affiliated physicians.

Conflict of Multi-Institutional Ownership

PHC's efforts toward integration complicate the situation for the patient because the health care industry itself is not integrated. The segments of health care are regulated according to varying rules and often compensated by different sources. Patient needs and approaches to treatment vary by segment as well. Acute care in the hospital, for instance, is quite unlike home care. Likewise, there are a variety of options available in nonacute-care settings, both among competing vendors of that care and in respect to the types of care offered. In long-term care, for example, there are treatment choices to be made among home care, an assisted living facility, and nursing home care. Finally, patients do not initiate the transition from one care setting to another. It comes at the recommendation of doctors or other health care professionals, who may or may not be employees of the health care organization.

Because there is a choice to be made among treatment options and providers, it becomes important to identify the ownership of these alternate facilities. This disclosure allows the patient to consider the possible influence that ownership of the transfer facility may have on a transfer decision. Simple disclosure is, however, only the minimum response ethically.[11] To support the autonomy of patients who are disadvantaged by illness or lack of knowledge, health care providers should also make it clear that the patient has the right to select other facilities and forms of care. This is not required only of a doctor involved in a transfer decision;[12] any morally responsible institution should have a policy to support disclosure of alternatives as well.[13]

Finally, in any transfer decision the doctor is required to make his or her recommendation based on the appropriateness of the type of treatment offered and the quality of that treatment. An organization like PHC, which partner with many caregivers and facilities, can minimize the potential for conflict by making sure that overall its affiliates offer a full range of high-quality services and by developing objective criteria for determining a plan of treatment. It may not be possible economically for PHC to compete with providers of certain types of service; if the patient's needs are better met by a nonaffiliated provider, PHC is morally obligated to recommend that provider rather than an affiliate.

Since all health care providers have a general obligation to provide the best possible services, it becomes crucial for PHC and its affiliates to develop and adhere to uniform, systemwide standards of care and quality. This is already a common practice, but to avoid the appearance of conflict of interest, information about PHC's performance according to these standards should be made publicly available. Similarly, developing clear, clinically sound criteria for treatment that apply across PHC's affiliates, and requiring referring physicians to explain how patients meet those criteria, is at least a desirable goal. Such criteria must, of course, accommodate the play of judgment that is an important part of developing a treatment plan for an individual patient.

Physicians and Their Economic Relationships with PHC

PHC's relationship to doctors is more problematic. It is well documented that doctors have economic relationships with other providers of health care that frequently affect significantly the treatment decisions the doctors make.[14] Patients whose doctors have financial interests in other health care services—for example, imaging services—have been exposed to painful, expensive, and sometimes dangerous procedures more often than patients of practitioners who are not financially involved. Historically, the medical profession has been extremely lax in addressing this issue and resistant to government regulation of practices identifiable as posing conflict of interest (Exhibit 6.2).[15]

In this case and with this reality in mind, PHC has entered into a variety of economic arrangements with doctors. A health care institution stands in a unique position in regard to patients, who are in theory consumers of its services. But the majority of patients do not select a particular institution themselves. Rather, the doctor to whom they have entrusted their medical care refers them to it. Thus a health care institution is uniquely dependent on the doctor as the source of patients. This dependence has given doctors extraordinary power and has considerably shaped the institutional development of health care facilities.[16] Given the economic realities of

Exhibit 6.2. The Federal Anti-Kickback Statute and the Anti-Referral Statute (Stark).

To avoid unwarranted claims under the Medicare and Medicaid programs, Congress has enacted two laws directed against financial incentives linked to medical referrals. The federal Anti-Kickback Statute (1989) makes it a crime to pay or receive compensation that is intended to induce a medical referral for services covered by a federal health care program. As a criminal law, this requires proof of intent and willful action. The sanctions imposed by the law include treble damages (three times the illegal remuneration) plus $50,000 per violation. It can also result in exclusion from participation in federal health care programs.

The second law, the 1993 Anti-Referral Statute (commonly referred to as "Stark," amended in 2000) prohibits all referrals for the provision of designated health services and all claims for federal reimbursement for such services furnished pursuant to a referral, if a physician has a financial relationship with the provider that results in compensation to the physician based on that service through either ownership or other compensation. This covers referrals to clinical laboratories, physical therapy, occupational therapy, radiology, radiation therapy, durable medical equipment and supplies, home health services, outpatient prescription drugs, and all inpatient and outpatient hospital services. (In addition, a number of states have enacted their own antireferral statutes.) The law does not apply to situations in which the services are rendered by the physician or, for the most part, rendered by an employee within the physician's office and under the physician's supervision.

Stark is a civil prohibition, with civil penalties of up to $15,000 per service and exclusion from participation in federal health care programs. Because this is a civil statute, the government does not have to prove intent to commit crime. (To appreciate the difference in these two standards of proof, one need only think of the two O. J. Simpson trials—one criminal, the second civil.)

There are a significant number of statutory "safe harbors" (situations defined by law or regulation that are deemed not to violate these laws) that make the prohibitions in these statutes less sweeping than they might at first appear. For example, under the "sixty-forty rule," physician referrals to an entity in which they hold an ownership is deemed not to violate these laws if:

1. The referring person owns no more than 40 percent of the investment interests

**Exhibit 6.2. The Federal Anti-Kickback Statute
and the Anti-Referral Statute (Stark), Cont'd.**

2. The terms of investment must be the same as those offered to passive investors

3. The terms of investment are not related to the volume of referrals

4. The terms of investment are not tied to any requirement to make referrals

5. The entity and all investors do not market or furnish the entity's items or services to passive investors differently than to noninvestors

6. No more than 40 percent of the gross revenue of the entity comes from referrals from investors

7. The entity does not loan funds to, or guarantee a loan for, a referring investor

8. Payments to investors are directly proportional to the amount of capital investment

To be valid, all eight characteristics must be met.

Given the complexity of the exceptions to this referral prohibition and the extreme severity of the penalties, all compensation and ownership schemes with physicians and other health care providers must be reviewed with great care.

health care, PHC is surely compelled to enter into this type of relationship with doctors to remain competitive. If it does not, it loses patient referrals to competitors who do. The challenge is how to craft ethically sound relationships among PHC's affiliated physicians and facilities.

Two concerns about patient care should inform this effort. First, patients rely on the doctor to evaluate the quality of the institution chosen to render health care. They expect their doctor to refer them to the hospital, nursing home, or lab that best meets their needs. Financial considerations on the part of doctors and health care facilities can conflict with that obligation generally. Second, there are concerns that financial arrangements among particular health care service providers can affect the treatment ordered specially for individual patients.

The first response to both of these concerns is disclosure. Though not mandated, this is supported both by JCAHO[17] and the

American Medical Association's Code of Medical Ethics.[18] How effective disclosure is as a response varies. It may be reasonably effective regarding concern about the quality of a referral to a subsidiary or jointly owned facility because the referral becomes linked to the organization's self-interest in its reputation. A health care institution's reputation in a community is significantly influenced by the physicians it employs or works with, while at the same time, to the extent that the institution has a reputation in the community separate from a particular physician, affiliation can benefit that physician. The two entities (physician and health care institution) can become linked in a common venture, and a prospective patient may be assumed to enter into a relationship with the physician on this basis. Thus, for example, in the purchase of a physician practice group (if allowed by law), disclosure can be very effective. Proclaiming a physician group to be an affiliate of PHC identifies the physicians with PHC, and PHC with the physicians.

Creating a joint venture with physicians may be more problematic. Although PHC and its partner doctors can disclose their affiliation with a venture, the disclosure addresses only part of the concern. Insofar as the doctors remain independent of PHC, there is no joining of reputation that constrains both the physicians and the practice.

To address concern about how business relationships among providers affects patient care, the disclosure obligation may need to extend to the financial terms of the relationship. In what way does the relationship embody financial incentive or disincentive for treatment?[19] Knowing whether a recommended treatment relates to a doctor's financial incentive may alert a patient to the possibility of a conflict.

These disclosure requirements are predicated on the idea of the patient being a knowledgeable and autonomous consumer. The value implicit in disclosure is that the patient is accorded the option of selecting another health care provider; the foundational assumption is that the patient is competent to make that decision. However, this is generally not the case. Patients rely on the recommendation of their doctors.[20] They are unlikely to read documents disclosing the nature of the complex financial relationships between their doctors and PHC. Nor are they likely to be familiar with the studies showing that a physician who owns an interest in a lab or testing facility is more likely to order additional and perhaps unnecessary tests and expensive procedures than is a doctor who does not hold an ownership position.[21]

JCAHO and the AMA Code of Ethics both assert that physicians and providers should not allow financial interest to stand in the way of delivering quality medical care to their patients. But no matter how carefully drafted, and no matter whether the arrangement creates incentives to treat (as in fee-for-service) or to limit treatment (as in capitation), any financial arrangement is subject to abuse. Therefore, PHC has an obligation to develop appropriate treatment guidelines and a system of independent utilization review and quality assurance to guard against conscious or inadvertent abuse. One can hope for good-faith efforts from the physician, but systems must be put in place to correct any lapse.

Physician recruitment practices, such as St. Somewhere's efforts to bring obstetricians and gynecologists into its service area, present a unique problem. The practices do not create an ownership relationship between the parties, or even a contractual requirement that the physician refer patients to the hospital. But a hospital depends nonetheless on a doctor referring patients, whether because the doctor's practice is located in that specific community or from a sense of personal honor. There is, therefore, no ongoing formal relationship to disclose to the patient. Nonetheless, disclosure that the doctor was recruited by and received compensation from St. Somewhere may serve to support a reputation for honesty and fairness on the part of both the doctor and St. Somewhere.

The very possibility of a not-for-profit organization recruiting a physician is of recent origin. Nonprofits were historically precluded from such practices. However, in 1997 the IRS modified its regulations to allow nonprofits to recruit doctors, subject to two requirements: (1) that in the community served by the hospital there is a demonstrable shortage of either general practice physicians or physicians practicing in a particular specialty, and (2) that the recruitment compensation is reasonable and given for a limited duration.[22] Although doctor recruitment may be problematic in that it creates a nondisclosed conflict of interest, it benefits the community in that it secures needed health care services. The compensation offered helps to make up for the reduction in the doctor's earnings caused by his or her move to an underserved area.

In all of these situations, the relationship between the physicians and PHC are difficult and complex, and there are practical limits on PHC's ability to control its affiliate physicians. Nonetheless, since the doctor-patient relationship is central to the whole health care system, structuring the relationship among providers and institutions deserves great attention and care so that it reflects the concern and commitment of PHC. The nature of the relationship between a physician and PHC should, as much as possible, be open for all to see, and extraordinary efforts ought to be made to assure that financial considerations do not adversely affect patient care.

Policy Considerations Relating to Patient Care Conflict

Policies to address conflict in patient care at the multi-institutional level are not usually referred to as conflict of interest. But they should share certain features with policies regarding conflict of interest. First, the policy should identify the patient as standing in a special relationship to the health care organization and its associated health care providers and physicians. Second, it should recognize that the organization and its staff owe patients a unique duty of fair dealing and honesty. Third, the policy should identify areas in which disclosure is necessary, to further its commitment to telling patients the truth (for example, disclosure of common ownership of facilities), and the type of interest that may conflict with this duty, and it should provide guidance about how to deal with those situations (disclosure, explicit adherence to an empirically justified standard of care, referral to a staff person who does not have such a conflict, and so on).

Conflict of Interest in Clinical Management

Conflict of interest arising out of a formal institutional arrangement, such as ownership of a facility or a contract with a facility or provider, impinges on patient care decisions largely through the various financial incentives built into such an arrangement. But serious conflict is not limited to economic issues. At the bedside, the issue of conflict of interest becomes far messier and more confusing, involving concern among caregivers about a colleague's clinical judgment and professional behavior.

Sometimes this conflict is an honest professional disagreement about the best plan of care for a particular patient. An organization has an ethical obligation to develop mechanisms through which to address such dilemmas—for example, an ethics committee or ethics consultation service—but professional disagreements of this type do not concern us here. Rather, our focus is on conflict that arises if the caregiver's personal life adversely affects clinical management of patients' relationships with colleagues and with the health care organization.

> At about 3:00 on a Saturday morning, Dr. Lennox, an emergency surgeon on call for St. Somewhere, receives a telephone call at his home informing him that a car accident victim has been brought into the emergency room and needs immediate surgery. When he arrives at the hospital half an hour later, Nurse Oman notes with concern that he is unshaven, appears very tired, and smells of alcohol, though he gives no indication of being drunk. It is well known that he is in the middle of an acrimonious divorce, which he constantly complains is bankrupting him.
>
> Upon arrival, Lennox consults with Dr. Patel, head of the emergency department for that shift, and Dr. Kim, the senior resident caring for the patient. Both Patel and Kim inform him that subsequent to calling him in, they performed a number of tests that indicate that the injuries are so severe and the prognosis so poor that surgery is no longer indicated.
>
> Lennox reviews the X-rays and performs a cursory exam of the patient. At the bedside, he asks the victim's wife what she wants to do, and she indicates that she wants everything possible to be done. Lennox declares that he will operate. Away from the presence of the wife, Patel reminds him of the results of the tests indicating that surgery is not appropriate. Lennox says he doesn't care and orders the patient taken into surgery. Oman hears him muttering "nigger" under his breath as he walks away.
>
> Oman, who is assisting, notes that Lennox is very slow and tentative in performing the surgery. The patient dies on the table after an unusually long operation. Subsequently, Oman approaches the head of nursing to advise her of her observations and is informed that the legal department is involved and the situation will be taken care of, but they don't want anything in writing.

Two areas of conflict in this case are of concern. First, there is the issue of Dr. Lennox's personal life and the role of the organization in guarding against harm arising from a doctor's (or other employee's) personal problems. Second, there is the question of how an organization can and should address the professional ethical duties of its professional employees and agents.

The Personal Lives of Staff Members

One might characterize Lennox's personal problems as a simple issue of competence and performance of employment obligations. However, understanding them as conflict of interest yields additional insight into the nature of the problems and also offers some guidance as to how an organization may appropriately respond. For example, it is not simply the case that Lennox is an incompetent surgeon, but rather that certain circumstances in his life may be affecting his competence adversely. To address this adverse influence, an organization needs to be sensitive to the situational nature of the circumstances.

Lennox's family problems satisfy all the criteria of the definition of a conflict of interest. First, though technically not an employee, as an affiliated provider Lennox has a relationship with St. Somewhere that creates responsibilities, both for the doctor and for St. Somewhere, in which conflict can arise. By giving Lennox a venue in which to practice medicine and the authority to direct treatment, St. Somewhere has effectively appointed him as its agent in rendering clinical services. Second, Lennox has a number of personal problems or concerns that may be affecting his professional judgment regarding those clinical services. He is going through a difficult divorce; he perceives himself to be suffering financial problems; there are indications of possible alcohol abuse; and he demonstrates racial prejudice.

Third, Lennox's judgment affects a number of interests held by St. Somewhere, including its obligations to patients, its obligations to properly use resources, and its interest in maintaining a work environment free from racial prejudice. (Lennox's actions, however, appear to be motivated not by the interests of St. Somewhere but by his own personal problems and prejudices.) Fourth, these actions actually harm St. Somewhere—and in this instance, presumably a patient.

As with any conflict of interest, to deal with these problems an organization needs to develop mechanisms to seek out and identify them, and it needs to develop safeguards against abuse. These safeguards can in turn be understood as both regulatory and, under a separable duty of organizational care for its employees and agents, remedial in assisting the employee or agent in dealing with personal problems.

Identifying Personal Problems

The role of an organization in addressing personal concerns, such as family issues, is controversial. It is commonplace to distinguish between issues that are public and those that are purely private, with family matters being central to the domain of privacy that is to be zealously protected. Many have begun to question this distinction.[23] Family is a value important to society and to the organizational interests of St. Somewhere; concern for family as a potential source of competing interests cannot and should not be excluded from the workplace. Many aspects of family life can have a significant impact on job performance, which in turn may conflict with other organizational interests. These aspects include not only the extremely problematic elements of Lennox's situation, but also such commonplace concerns as the time and performance pressure on a single parent or a person in a dual career couple.

Based on concern about how family issues affect job performance and about its independent obligation to respect and treat employees and agents with care (see Chapter Five), St. Somewhere needs the means to identify areas in which family concerns may impinge on job performance, so as to develop and implement programs to address those concerns. Discerning possible family problems can occur in a variety of ways. At a fundamental level, a manager can be encouraged to get to know the people who work for her and be open to hearing about their family concerns. A manager or supervisor may also discover problems through conversation with other employees. Also, in quality assurance programs, such as departmental case review and institutional case review, a reviewer should be alert to the possibility that personal problems have affected patient care.

In seeking to identify personal problems, care must be taken against becoming overly intrusive and acting as some type of Big Brother. Such behavior fails to respect employees as responsible individuals. Rather, a policy of openness to hearing about family concerns—one that does not engender fear that those concerns will adversely affect one's career prospects—frequently draws out concerns and allows a manager to work with an employee to address him respectfully and supportively. Some concerns require programmatic support: drug treatment, psychological counseling, day care programs, and so on. Other concerns may be negotiated individually, such as designing a flexible work schedule.

Systemic Safeguards

Efforts to address personal problems through an employee assistance program or through intervention by a supervisor first arose in the context of traditional employment situations. These safeguarding efforts apply best to a situation where the employee operates within a fixed hierarchy, under relatively close supervision by a manager. They may be less effective in a nontraditional, nonemployment situation.

Most physicians are not employees of a health care institution; they are independent contractors. Nonetheless, because they have practice privileges at a hospital like this one, St. Somewhere needs a supervisory mechanism empowered to evaluate personal problems affecting performance. It can be a mechanism of informal cultural controls or a formal system.

Individual behavior within an institution is commonly, and often successfully, regulated by the culture of the institution. Perhaps we discover the inadequacy of existing written policies only when the informal system of control fails. For example, in most hospitals, patients are identified as having a primary care physician, either a private physician or the one assigned to their care on admission—in this case, either Dr. Kim or Dr. Patel. As a matter of professional courtesy,[24] if not of written policy, a specialist like Dr.

Lennox (often referred to as a consultant) develops a treatment plan in consultation with the primary care physician; he does not seek to overrule the primary care physician by independently consulting the family. Possibly under the influence of his difficult personal circumstances, Lennox made a questionable decision about patient care and violated a norm of professional culture. The system of control at St. Somewhere was not prepared to deal with this lapse.

One of the problems with relying on a cultural norm is that if it is violated, there is rarely a mechanism in place to address the specific violation. In the long run, cultural norms are enforced by such mechanisms as ostracism and social censure. But these social tools do not work in relation to a specific patient. Here, Kim and Patel failed to overrule Lennox, which they arguably could have done both on medical grounds and from concern about Lennox's personal problems (if they were aware of them). A policy that clearly identifies who is to be responsible for making decisions about care and a specified method for resolving a dispute between doctors over patient care might help avoid conflict of authority among caregivers.

Policies and mechanisms that facilitate a fellow professional employee raising concerns about a colleague, and that protect anyone who does, can assist in gathering relevant information about personal issues before a problem develops; they also aid an organization's quality assessment procedures after the fact. Oman was concerned about Lennox's behavior and ultimately was willing to come forward. That she did not report her concerns prior to the operation, and the way she was treated when she later brought them to institutional attention, suggests that St. Somewhere's policies in this regard may be inadequate. Her failure to come forward before the operation may have been because St. Somewhere lacks an appropriate method for hearing such complaints, or, possibly because among staff it has a reputation for being unwilling to listen to such concerns. Moreover, the instruction that she not write down her complaint suggests that St. Somewhere's quality review program is not properly oriented toward considering these issues. St. Somewhere should have a policy not only of being willing to hear these complaints but also of actively seeking out and addressing this type of information.

Professional Ethical Obligations

In delivering patient care, St. Somewhere works through the efforts of its professional medical staff. Nurses and doctors operate according to the ethical requirements of their profession and those of the institution. In both codes, a primary concern is the proper care and safety of the patient.[25] A second concern is maintenance of standards within the profession.[26] At the same time, from loyalty nurses and doctors owe it to the institution not to waste assets, for example, by not exposing the organization to unnecessary litigation or exacerbating legal liabilities.

It is in the interest of any health care organization for professional employees to perform to the highest ethical standards of their profession. To ensure that obligations to the profession and to the organization do not come into conflict, St. Somewhere needs to develop clear policies and procedures to facilitate staff in discharging their professional obligations. This would include a mechanism whereby Oman can raise her concerns (ideally prior to the surgery) or at least have them taken seriously after the fact.

There may be short-term legal reasons for which legal counsel recommends limiting postevent reporting. However, this reasoning is often shortsighted, particularly if it is instituted as a common practice, because it can be taken as evidence that the organization is not sincerely committed to patient care and the patient's interest. In turn, a reputation for disregarding patient interests can invite punitive damages being added to a compensatory award for any harm suffered by a patient in a situation of conflict. More troubling, such an approach reflects a distortion of moral values. The nurse has an ethical duty not only to report wrongdoing but also to seek assurance that her complaint is acted on fairly and in a timely manner. To the extent that St. Somewhere fails to support this duty, the message is communicated that it is more concerned with legal liability than with these ethical values.

Summary

As we have seen, conflict of interest or problems relating to competing interest arise in a variety of ways. An organization needs to develop means to identify and address these conflicts:

1. Including within its policy statements clear definition of what constitutes a conflict of interest or a competing interest relative to the tasks engaged in by a particular class of employees or agents.

2. Establishing means of identifying conflict when it arises. In large part, this requires the cooperation of the employees involved, which means that the organization must educate employees about what constitutes conflict and give employees a method of reporting it. At a minimum, employees with administrative authority should be required to file an annual disclosure statement. Other methods, such as having employees help identify conflict, should be implemented as well.

3. Developing means of addressing conflict or potential conflict so as to reduce the potential harm. Disclosure to patients of any conflict based on ownership or financial incentive is one response, if patients have a reasonable way of assessing and acting on the information. In deference to the needs of the patient, the organization should itself seek to limit the potential harm caused by conflict both in terms of quality assurance and utilization review where appropriate.

4. Instituting a policy that a board member, officer, or employee must be recused or removed from the operating functions of the institution when a conflict exists that cannot be addressed by disclosure or mitigated by institutional safety features.

Finally, it should be noted that the appearance of a conflict of interest can be as damaging as the existence of an actual conflict. From the perspective of the institution's public reputation, the distinction between the two is not as significant as might be hoped. The institution's reputation is a valuable resource, a crucial element of its ethical environment that must be zealously protected.

Notes

1. American College of Healthcare Executives. *Code of Ethics*, Section III. 1995. Reprinted as Appendix Three of this book.
2. Webster, G. D. "Board Conflicts of Interest." *Association Management,* Jan. 1993, *45*(1), 151, 155.
3. See, for example, McCormick, L., and Umbdenstock, R. "In Debate: Should Medical Staff Presidents Be Voting Members of the Hospital Board?" *Healthcare Executive,* Sept./Oct. 1993, pp. 12–13.

4. Greene, J. "Appearance of Conflicts of Interest Can Damage, Too." *Modern Healthcare,* Jan. 20, 1992, p. 32.
5. Monks, R.A.G. "Shareholders and Director Selection." *Directors and Boards,* 1995, *9*(3), 9–11.
6. Toulmin, S. "Medical Institutions and Their Moral Constraints." In R. E. Bulger and S. J. Reiser (eds.), *Integrity in Healthcare Institutions.* Des Moines: University of Iowa, 1990.
7. See, for example, AMA Code of Medical Ethics, Principles I, II, III, IV, and V; JCAHO Rule RI.4 et. seq.
8. AMA Code of Medical Ethics, Principle II.
9. JCAHO, p. RI.2.4.
10. JCAHO, p. RI.2.4.
11. JCAHO, p. RI.2.4.
12. See, for example, AMA Code 1.00, 2.00, 8.032, and 8.035.
13. JCAHO, p. RI.4.1.
14. See the articles cited in Chapter Three of Rodwin, M. *Medicine, Money, and Morals: Physicians' Conflicts of Interest.* New York: Oxford, 1993.
15. Rodwin (1993).
16. Starr, P. *The Social Transformation of Medicine.* New York: Basic Books, 1982, especially Chapter Four; Stevens, R. *In Sickness and In Wealth.* New York: Basic Books, 1989.
17. See, for example, JCAHO, p. RI.4.
18. See AMA Code 8.032.
19. JCAHO, p. RI.4.4.
20. Rodwin (1993).
21. Rodwin (1993); Florida Health Care Cost Containment Board. *Joint Ventures Among Health Care Providers in Florida,* 1991.
22. For a simplified discussion of this regulation, see Cejka, S. "Tax-exempt Hospitals Sweeten the Doctor's Pot." *Medical Economics,* July 13, 1998, pp. 28–35.
23. See Elshtain, J. B. *Public Man, Private Woman.* Princeton, N.J.: Princeton University, 1981.
24. AMA Code of Medical Ethics, Principle IV.
25. AMA Code 1.00; American Nurses Association. *Code for Nurses with Interpretive Statements.* Washington, D.C.: American Nurses Association, 1985, 3.1.
26. AMA Code 2.00; ANA Code 3.

Chapter Seven

Discretion and Control

Every day, every employee of a health care organization makes decisions regarding his or her work. Employees decide how to allocate their time and choose ways to accomplish their tasks; they make innumerable decisions about what it takes to get the job done. Many of these decisions are routine and involve no surprises. There are times, however, when an employee must make a decision in the face of uncertainty, confronting a dilemma in which she sees conflicting but justifiable courses of action and does not have the confidence or resources to help sort through the issues.

Employees may also face decisions in which they know the ethical thing to do, but they feel thwarted by particular features of their organization. At such a time, they must exercise *discretion,* making a decision based on their own judgment when they are uncertain of the right course of action. Poor judgment by an employee in this circumstance can produce adverse results for the organization (and perhaps for the employee). Because the organization entrusts the employee with discretionary power, there is the potential for abuse of discretion by that person, as in making a self-serving decision.

These dilemmas do not have to be dramatic, risking the organization's reputation; they often occur among coworkers or within a department. Attention to the challenge that an employee faces in exercising discretion highlights another feature of organizational ethics in health care.

Discretion is an essential component of the health care workplace. But because of the uncertain nature of decision making and the possibility of abuse, organizations set limits. Discretion must be managed. This occurs in three ways. First, management personnel direct, regulate, and coordinate the employee's work. They exercise formal *control*, guiding or managing worker decisions and activities. Managers have to check, test, or verify an employee's work; this exercise of control is an integral part of the world of working.

Second, an organization has formal standards—defined by its mission and values statement, employee job descriptions, and policies and procedures—to define the limits of discretion and guide employee decision making. Third, in addition to the organization's formal control mechanisms, its culture—the informal beliefs, values, and structures—controls employee behavior by shaping perceptions, evaluations, and decisions. The intent of these control mechanisms is to further the organization's goals.

In some situations, management control or aspects of the organization's standards and culture may affect an employee's judgment adversely. First, too much or too little managerial oversight affects an employee's confidence in exercising judgment. Second, employees might be ignorant of, misunderstand, or disregard policies. Third, although a job description outlines the parameters of one's work responsibility and accountability, not all possibilities can be anticipated. Finally, the organization's culture can tacitly permit behavior that is incongruent with its formal values. In these circumstances, how controls operate within the organization may compromise the employee's judgment and job performance, producing outcomes that threaten the organization's mission and values.

This chapter analyzes the benefits and abuses of discretion and control and how their dynamics play out in the culture of a health care organization. It illustrates how the dynamics of discretion and control can create a morally distressing quandary within a health care organization (Exhibit 7.1).

We also suggests ways for an ethics mechanism to address these situations. The suggestions, however, do not eliminate the need for discretion and control within a health care organization. Organizational relationships and structures always include elements of uncertainty, dependence, and power. As a result, every member of an organization faces situations in which the moral course of action is not clear, but he is called upon to exercise his own judgment regardless. By understanding the dynamics of discretion and control, the members of an ethics mechanism can work to minimize adverse effects and bolster an employee's confidence in addressing a morally uncertain situation.

Exhibit 7.1. Ethical Quandaries of Discretion and Control.

1. Cover-up and misrepresentation in reporting and control procedures
2. Misleading product or service claims
3. Overconfidence in one's own judgment to the risk of the corporate entity
4. Lockstep obedience to authority, however unethical or unfair it might be
5. Price fixing
6. Sacrificing the innocent and helpless to get things done
7. Suppression of basic rights: freedom of speech, choice, and personal relationships
8. Failing to speak up when an unethical practice occurs
9. Making a product decision that perpetuates a questionable safety issue
10. Knowingly exaggerating the advantages of a plan to get needed support
11. Failing to cooperate with other areas of the organization
12. Lying by omission to employees for the sake of the organization
13. Abusing or just going along with corporate perks that waste time and money
14. Missing an important deadline to do a "quality job"
15. Blowing the whistle

Source: Adapted by permission of Harvard Business School Press. From *Good Intentions Aside: A Manager's Guide to Resolving Ethical Problems* by L. Nash. Boston, MA. 1990, pp. 8–10. Copyright 1990 by the President and Fellows of Harvard College; all rights reserved.

Discretion

Discretion is a word with various connotations. Descriptively, it suggests that an individual has the authority to act according to his or her own judgment, to exercise the power of free decision that accompanies, for example, a particular job. The person's discretion builds on the parameters established by the job description, and within those limits the employee feels authorized to act as she sees fit. Recognizing that employee discretion is necessary, an organization trusts its employees to make decisions in its best interests, as an incident in our ongoing case study shows.[1]

The CEO of Partnership Health Care is scheduled to visit St. Somewhere Hospital. Wanting to impress the system's chief executive, St. Somewhere's public affairs director orders her staff to produce a book for presentation to the CEO, replete with photographs and illustrations and describing the hospital and its operations. The cost—about $2,000 for the single copy, covering labor, materials, and production costs—will be covered from funds budgeted for promotional materials. Some staffers believe that the money would be better spent on materials promoting the hospital's outpatient programs; they call the hospital's ethics hotline with their complaint that the money is being misappropriated. The institution's ethics officer investigates.

On one level, the public affairs officer's decision seems unremarkable. St. Somewhere Hospital's executives entrust the public affairs director with funds for promotional purposes. She, in turn, has the authority to determine the purpose and the amount to spend. With this authority for decision making come responsibility and accountability within the organization's reporting relationships; the director is fiscally, legally, and morally accountable for her decisions, according to the hospital's stated values (and sometimes the hidden ones).

In another sense, exercising discretion rests on the presumption that a decision involves evaluating various options and values, appreciating that choices have consequences, and being free to act responsibly. PHC assumes that its employees, from the CEO to the public affairs director and the rank-and-file employee, can be trusted to exercise judgment in a prudent and competent fashion, and it permits them to do so. In this case, the director has the authority to allocate money from her budget; the organization assumes that she does not act whimsically, but makes prudent (and justifiable) decisions. When making a decision about how to allocate funds, a manager often faces a choice, reflecting competing and even conflicting values, of one option over another.

Because of the latitude of discretionary authority, it can be difficult to measure its appropriate exercise. In one sense, a "good" decision resolves an immediate issue. The more routine the matter at hand, the more mundane the discretionary challenge and the less likely subsequent problems are. The decision to order one brand of coffee for the public affairs department's coffee pot may turn on taste and price. A "bad" decision about the coffee may result from not having all the facts, or from not processing them adequately, but in this instance probably no one is hurt and the organization's business is not affected.

Other decisions, however, carry weightier values or consequences with more serious or far-reaching implications. A decision to produce a $2,000 book for the system CEO might mean spending less money to promote outpatient services that would benefit the people in St. Somewhere's neighborhood. In this case, some staff believe that the funds are being misused. Is St. Somewhere's public affairs director abusing her discretionary authority? Is she exercising poor judgment in producing the book?

This is an unexceptionable example of discretionary judgment; the public affairs director makes a decision about allocating funds after weighing two options that entail competing values. The director sees the book as an opportunity to impress the visiting system CEO; people on staff think the money should be spent to promote direct services to the public. The members of her staff who have concerns feel strongly enough about her decision that they raise the issue with the hospital's ethics mechanism (in this instance, an ethics officer reporting to the systemwide ethics committee). The officer must explore the competing values that have polarized the public affairs department. In doing so, he should consider the influence of the organizational culture on how employees understand and give meaning to their work. This influence plays a role in exercising judgment.

Discretion and Organizational Culture

An organization's culture plays an important part in determining the meaning of discretion and how people exercise their judgment. A discretionary decision always occurs in the broader context of the needs and values of the organization (see Chapter Ten), which are expressed both formally and informally. An organization's mission, values, and philosophy constitute the overall framework for decisions. Its policies and procedures, covering the many aspects of operations, offer guidance for the individual employee's immediate decision and action.

There also develops within an organization a culture—a shared sense of what is important, of the way things are done around here—that evolves over time and is absorbed into the mind-set of employees (see Chapter Two). The particular moral environment or institutional culture—with its relationships, system of reward and inducement, leadership style and behavior, and opportunity for mischief—has a great deal to do with how people exercise discretion and evaluate its results.

This organizational mind-set, of which an individual may be unaware, shapes the way in which he or she understands, evaluates, and reacts to a situation. The culture permits certain actions and discourages others; it reflects the organization's norms and values as surely as do its policies. The culture and policies of an organization, however, may not be totally congruent. The organization might, for example, espouse the value of "excellence" in its mission and values statement, encouraging employees to act independently to resolve dilemmas. At the same time, its culture might encourage or reward employee deference to the boss.

In this case, St. Somewhere's public affairs director comes from a hospital culture in which one does everything to please the system CEO. Her several critics feel that excellence is better served by spending the money to benefit people in the hospital's inner-city neighborhood. How individuals interpret a situation varies. On the one hand, the public affairs director may be unnecessarily currying favor with the CEO. On the other hand, by bringing favorable system-level attention to the hospital and its programs, the director may benefit her organization and its focus on delivering outpatient care.

After talking with the individuals involved, the ethics officer might suggest that the moral uncertainty in this case can be relieved by better communication between the public affairs director and her staff. Although there is a conflict over the values to be served by the director's decision, she is not overstepping the bounds of her discretionary authority in producing the book. If the effort brings the good work of St. Somewhere to the CEO's attention, the expenditure of funds may pay off across a broader front, to the ultimate benefit of the neighborhood.

Benefits of Discretion

As a feature of work, discretion offers advantages for the health care institution, promoting creativity and maximizing initiative within the parameters of the role or job description. Micromanagement of employees is inefficient, and it is difficult for those in authority to know all the particulars of subordinates' actions or decisions. By including and upholding discretion in the workplace, therefore, a health care organization allows its employees a measure of independence to solve problems and develop projects. Discretion also fosters their personal investment in the success of the organization's work and the implementation of its mission. "We trust your judgment" is a powerful, supportive message for an employee. At the same time, trust implies a situation involving risk, in which the outcome is uncertain. Therefore, an organization also incorporates responsibility and accountability into its expectations of the employee.

As with responsibility and accountability, discretion is a basic feature of decision making that exists at all levels of the health care organization. Latitude for decision making at lower levels, however, is usually constrained by clearly defined job descriptions, managerial oversight, or performance standards (for example, see Case Three). By contrast, at higher levels these organizational features are generally less well defined, and the gray or uncertain areas about which an employee must exercise his or her judgment demand a finer sense of discretion (see Case Five). As a rule, however, at any level the more inconsistency between expressed values and actual behavior, or tolerance for ethical misconduct within the institutional culture, the more discretion might be abused.

Abuse of Discretion

Let's look at an example that reflects clear abuse of discretion.[2]

> A food vendor has recently offered the purchasing agent at Partnership Health Care's Suburban Hospital four tickets to the hometown pro football team's game with a traditional rival. As the vendor's primary contact, the agent wonders if the tickets are something he should refuse, use himself, or give to his organization. After deliberation, the agent decides this gift is the vendor's thank-you for doing business and accepts the tickets.

This case reflects a conflict of interest and a clear example of poor judgment (see Chapter Six). The purchasing agent has discretion in choosing and negotiating with vendors. Ideally, he pursues those negotiations within the organization's established purchasing guidelines, which reflect the organization's goals and values when it comes to, say, the proper standard regarding gifts.

The purchasing agent at Suburban Hospital accepts the tickets as an expression of the vendor's gratitude. Such a gift creates a conflict of interest when decisions or actions regarding patients or the institution are influenced by personal (or professional) interest (see Chapter Six). A gift that shows gratitude, however, should be corporate, not personal. A gift intended for the personal benefit of an employee conveys the impression that the vendor is seeking to buy favor, create a preference, or undermine the employee's judgment.[3] The purchasing agent should ask himself what other coworkers and vendors would think if they knew about the tickets. If there is any chance they might think that his objective business judgment on behalf of Suburban was being impaired, he should turn down the gift. In all cases, he should report anything greater than $100 to his supervisor and PHC's corporate compliance officer (see Chapter Four and Case Six). In this case, the agent has chosen a course of action that abuses the trust that he acts in accordance with the organization's goals and values.

If someone reports the purchasing agent's action to the hospital's organizational ethics mechanism, responsibility for disciplinary action will rest with human resources. If brought into the matter, the ethics officer or committee might consider reviewing the institution's system of checks and balances for conflict of interest, as well as conducting an educational program (with attention to values, including corporate compliance) for employees who find themselves facing a similar situation. Given the hospital's clear policy regarding gifts and conflict of interest, the purchasing agent's moral culpability is clear.

In other situations, where the limits of discretion are less defined, abuse is harder to identify. Also, an individual may have problems implementing organizational norms and values if the guidelines and latitude within which she exercises discretion are not clear or are hidden in the woodwork. Typically, a problematic situation develops if the employee is troubled by the choices she faces, if outcomes are not clear, or if the values of the affected parties cannot all be accommodated in a way that is satisfactory to each of them.

> The new chief financial officer of PHC's Long Term Care (LTC) division invites the division's only full-time chaplain to lunch. During the meal, the CFO reveals that, in spite of every effort to trim costs, a number of positions will be

eliminated. The LTC divisional CEO, a hard-driving executive brought in to "straighten things out," has assigned to the CFO the responsibility to formulate a downsizing plan; she has told him to keep the project secret until "we're ready to move."

The CFO tells the chaplain that their conversation is confidential. The information about the downsizing upsets the chaplain because he knows that morale is suffering as rumors of staff reductions spread, and he feels that the site executive should tell employees of the upcoming layoffs. Since the chaplain reports to her, he considers seeing the CEO to express his concerns. However, this conversation is confidential. Being a member of the new ethics committee in the LTC division, the chaplain decides to bring the matter up in that forum.

Staff reductions are occasionally necessary for a health care organization, usually owing to financial pressure. (See Chapter Five for a discussion of ethical issues involved in downsizing.) In itself, such a decision is not the province of the ethics committee. Since decisions are made about whom to keep and whom to lay off, however, downsizing always involves an apparent sacrifice of some interests in favor of others. All of ethics is in essence a concern for managing interactions and relationships in which not all of the affected parties' values can be accommodated in ways that are satisfactory to each of them.[4] A manager's discretionary judgment requires carefully weighing a variety of factors to enhance, to the extent possible, the quality of those interactions and relationships. As the ethics committee begins to analyze the situation in terms of the values and behaviors involved, the members find several examples of employee abuse of discretion.

First, an employee abuses discretion when he exceeds the bounds of professional knowledge and role authority. In relationships such as the one between the CEO and the CFO, and between the CFO and the chaplain, problems arise for the organization when a subordinate assumes that his knowledge or professional expertise qualifies him to act contrary to his superiors' expectations. The chaplain questions the CEO's judgment and motivation to keep the downsizing secret and brings the matter to the ethics committee; but in doing so, has he overstepped the bounds of his role and professional expertise?

As an expert in his field of pastoral care, the chaplain interprets the actions of the chief executive from his own frame of reference. He has an expectation of his boss based on his perception of the obligations and responsibilities she should owe to the organization, its employees, and the people it serves. Yet for many people, the moral standards of a religious representative, or even ordinary moral standards, do not apply to business decisions and practices. Instead, common business practice (satisfying the legal statutes governing business activity) sets the standard of ethical conduct. In this view, a manager acts ethically as long as she conforms to the general practice and acts within the letter of the law.[5] Given the extent to which administrative concerns in a health care organization are increasingly affected by financial considerations, a CEO's focus on business practices is understandable. To the chaplain, however, the CEO appears to be a person steeped in the culture and ethos of business organizations in which managerial professionalism (to be distinguished from pastoral professionalism, perhaps) trumps moral concerns.

The dichotomy between the two types of professional, however, may be too easily drawn. One mistake commonly made by those who warn that a strict focus on the bottom line converts health care professionals, including managers, into "mere" business people is the unwarranted assumption that business people have no commitment to values such as excellence, honesty, or compassion. The chaplain's assumption is that management cares about the quality of LTC services only insofar as such quality contributes to maximizing the organization's profit. However, one of the basic ethical tasks of a conscientious manager operating in a competitive environment is to provide the best product or service for the client or customer while at the same time achieving an acceptable bottom line. Given the information that the chaplain presents to the ethics committee, there is no evidence that these values are not important in the CEO's decision regarding downsizing.

An important factor affecting the chaplain's judgment is his desire to respect the CFO's confidence. A pledge of secrecy alters a person's freedom of action. He or she "promise[s] to perform some action that will guard the secret—to keep silent at least, and perhaps to do more,"[6] as Sissela Bok writes in *Secrets*. Generally, a person feels that it is wrong to divulge a confidence to which others possess no legitimate claim. When one promises to keep a secret, he or she is obliged to do so unless there is an overriding reason not to keep quiet.

The question of confidentiality, however, raises an interesting issue involving both the chaplain's and the chief financial officer's roles, and their understanding of discretion (also see Case One). The CFO receives the information about the downsizing by virtue of his position, and the CEO tells him to keep quiet about the upcoming layoffs. Has he abused the CEO's trust by telling a colleague? On the one hand, the CFO is insubordinate; he reveals privileged information and violates his superior's instruction. Yet he is troubled that the layoffs will adversely affect the LTC division's quality of services.

The CFO, in turn, asks the chaplain to keep their conversation in confidence. If others learn that the CFO has violated his superior's directive, his position could be jeopardized. The CFO's comments also might undermine others' trust in him and their trust in the CEO. His conversation with the chaplain, therefore, might indicate a lack of prudence on the CFO's part. His ethical quandary would have to be sufficient to overturn the control placed upon him by his superior. Similarly, if the chaplain breaks the CFO's confidence, why should his colleague, or others, trust him again? (Clearly, the commitment to confidentiality on the part of the ethics committee is crucial if people are to trust its members with their problems.) The question of whether to break a confidence depends on when reasons count enough to make a difference.

There is no doubt that the LTC employees would want to know of impending layoffs; they may want to plan for contingencies by looking for other jobs. Again, if the chief financial officer and the chaplain violate their respective confidences by revealing their information to others, even to the ethics committee, have they overstepped the bounds of their authority, or acted appropriately? The ethics committee suggests that the chaplain (and the CFO) consider the structures in place to help guide or control how employees tackle dilemmas. In organizational ethics, the nature of the control structures is important for people exercising discretion.

Control

Because a health care organization entrusts its members with discretionary power, the latitude of which is not always clear, a system of controls or guidelines directs exercise of discretion. The manager is responsible for monitoring, regulating, and accounting for a subordinate's activities. Standards, policies, and procedures function as a benchmark for the manager and the employee in exercising discretion.

The Meaning of Control

As with discretion, there are various ways in which control can be understood within a working relationship (as this case study for purposes of our PHC discussion illustrates).

> Responding to a memo from corporate headquarters, the LTC division CEO asks an information services consultant to review the division's e-mail system to determine to what extent employees use the system for personal reasons. The IS consultant reports back that a number of e-mail messages are of a personal nature—and some are derogatory toward her and other executives at the system and local levels. The CEO directs the consultant to develop a policy on electronic surveillance, which basically reserves the employer's right to monitor electronic mail and Internet use, promulgates guidelines for using electronic resources, and states the penalties for inappropriate use. She also tells the consultant to install monitoring software.

The LTC division policy on using company-owned networks, software, equipment, and electronic surveillance is an example of one type of formal control of employee behavior that can be adopted by an organization. Once counsel has reviewed the proposed policy, the appropriate body has approved it, and the CEO has posted the guidelines, then employees are accountable for strict adherence to the rules. Also, the law generally is a powerful measure of control over employee decisions and actions. In the case of electronic surveillance, the law to date supports workplace monitoring.[7] To craft as fair a policy as possible, the divisional CEO should consider involving representatives from the ethics mechanism and employees in discussion of the design of the policy. This process helps ensure that various values are reviewed and reflected in the policy, which then better functions as a form of organizational control over employee action and is better received by the employees themselves. Close attention should be given to employee education about the new policy.

Benefits of Control

Normatively, control functions as a positive check or restraint on an agent's decisions and activities and is a necessary foundation for job performance. For example, the JCAHO did not design its standards both for patients' rights and organizational ethics to be punitive but rather to establish benchmarks for satisfactory performance. In the example of electronic surveillance of employees, the division's standards of conduct inform and guide the decision making and conduct of its employees regarding use of company hardware and software. To protect the interests of the organization and its employees, the standards must be understood and consistently enforced. They exist to reduce employee uncertainty and anxiety in a difficult situation. Some employees dislike the electronic surveillance policy, feeling it is an invasion of their privacy. But at least it gives them a clear idea of the organization's expectations for e-mail or Internet use.

In this sense, oversight, monitoring, or reporting relationships serve a positive function: they set the context by which the organization or personnel can measure themselves. In this way, controls establish the context for autonomy and encourage agents to factor the good of others and the organization into their decision making. The virtues associated with positive understanding of control are accountability, trust, and empowerment. Employees and managers are less afraid of making a mistake when the rules are clear and they feel they can exercise their discretion with the organization's support.

Control and Organizational Culture

A health care organization expresses control in numerous ways, depending on informal processes, structures, and relationships that shape the nature and identity of its culture. The PHC case illustrates several ways in which organizational culture elicits concern about the use of control, as another incident in our ongoing case study shows.[8]

> Having been assigned responsibility by the LTC division CEO to develop a downsizing plan, the CFO recommends that the division make its layoff deci-

sions based on employees' scores on their last three annual performance reviews. While reviewing the evaluations, the CFO notes two departments in which the directors have marked "n/a" for several employees where evaluation scores should be. Because these few employees have not been evaluated according to the divisional performance criteria instituted systemwide three years earlier, the CFO feels that he must treat them as special circumstances in the downsizing plan. Since he wants to be fair to all employees, the CFO meets with the department directors to discuss the "facts of the matter."

When asked about the scores, the department directors tell him that these are long-time employees. When the organization instituted the new performance review system, they agreed to the employees' request that they keep receiving informal evaluations as they always had.

Up to this point, it is unlikely that the issue would reach the LTC ethics committee. The CFO, in fact, follows the steps recommended in Chapter One for a case analysis; he poses the moral question of fairness and seeks the facts to better understand the situation. After talking with the directors and the employees in question, the CFO feels that within the organizational culture of the LTC division unclear lines of authority encourage managers to set their own rules. In spite of a new performance review policy and procedure, therefore, when faced with employee concerns the department managers acted within the decision-making limits established by the informal culture ("the way things are done"). They also acted this way because within the LTC division, when faced with troubling choices, managers said that they have no one "safe" with whom they can share their uncertainty or misgivings. They sought to control the situation by agreeing with the employees' request in order to make the problem go away. Now the CFO confronts two tasks: first, what to do about the immediate situation; and second, how to revise the culture so those managers who face choices feel secure and encouraged in asking for guidance or feedback. He decides to talk over his concerns with the CEO.

Abuse of Control

Continuing with the CFO's dilemma, we see a variety of examples that reflect the various ways in which members of an organization can abuse control.

The CFO raises with the CEO the inconsistent application of performance reviews as a problem for his downsizing plan. She responds that, given their good retirement benefits plus the severance package that the CFO has developed, laying off these employees saves jobs for younger people. She tells the CFO to handle the situation and reminds him to keep the layoffs secret.

When the directors agreed to their subordinates' request for informal evaluations, they did not abuse their discretion. Instead, their agreement signals shortsightedness on their part and lack of consistency in applying the new performance review system to all employees. It also cheats the employees themselves of accurate information about their own performance. The department directors apparently did not consider how this special arrangement might affect the feelings of others, especially if layoffs threaten. The CFO needs to address their failure to fully implement the performance review plan.

Taking the opportunity presented by downsizing to eliminate several people may illustrate an abuse of managerial control. Apparently, the divisional CEO perceives these employees to be expendable. As part of the fact finding of an ethics analysis, it is important to clarify these possibilities. It may be that the employees in question are excellent workers, quite productive, and highly regarded by their coworkers. If, alternately, the CEO feels that they are just "too old," or that their elimination allows younger people to be hired at lower salaries, then there are legal and moral questions to resolve. If encouraging and supporting integrity and truth telling are concerns of organizational ethics, as an ethical officer the CFO should consider two values that are threatened in this situation.

The first is respect, specifically, respect for others with whom one has entered an ongoing relationship. The two department directors agreed to the informal reviews. Although in hindsight their agreement may have been unwise, out of respect for the employees and the agreement under which they have been working they should not be penalized now. In any voluntary relationship, people are expected not only to honor their agreements but also to hold others accountable to do so as well.

Put simply, accountability is a form of control whereby individuals check to see whether others have complied with explicit and implicit terms governing their agreements and then reward or punish them accordingly. People are morally culpable to the degree that they fail to communicate clearly to another person their judgment about how the other honors, exceeds, or fails to honor these expectations. Holding others accountable involves more than calling attention to flagrant violation of organizational rules and values. It involves letting people know where they stand and how well they are doing. To do otherwise is unfair.

The second threatened value is fairness. If performance standards are the basis for a decision regarding workforce reduction at PHC-LTC, is it fair to evaluate the longtime employees according to these standards? From the case description, they may have been comfortable with the informal evaluations because the old system did not hold them to any particular standards. It may be that they simply did not like the new performance review criteria and persuaded their managers to continue the old process. Under the present arrangement, however, they clearly are not accountable to the same standards as other employees under the new system. They are receiving preferential treatment—although that treatment may in the end be to their detriment.

To permit these few to carry on under a different performance appraisal is unfair to other employees in the LTC division. The ethical values of justice and fairness require that people be treated as they deserve and that similar cases be treated similarly. If performance review is to be the basis for a downsizing decision, out of respect and fairness the CFO should inform these several employees that they are being held to a different standard.

After reviewing the case from the perspectives of all those who have an interest in it, and after considering different resolutions, there is still one aspect of the case to which the CFO should attend. A manager can exercise control by misleading or deceiving other employees through controlling information. The earlier conversation between the CFO and the chaplain illustrates another value that an abuse of control undermines: honesty.

The chaplain is concerned about rumors and the effect that they have on organizational morale, on working relationships among employees, and on resident care. A number of rumors have circulated among the staff about possible layoffs. Employees have asked the chaplain if he knows anything about downsizing. If asked about a new downsizing, what should he do? Following the dictates of the Golden Rule, the chaplain has always felt it wrong to lie. Operating with the moral rule of universalizability, if he is willing to lie then he is willing to allow all others in similar circumstances to lie. In a time of rumors (when trust is somewhat suspect, anyway), is it all right for the chaplain to remain silent or prevaricate if asked about layoffs?

There are occasions when being silent is not only an acceptable but also a morally preferred course of action. At other times, however, not disclosing what one knows amounts to the same thing as lying. When one holds in silence information that others would consider vital if they knew about it, not disclosing can be as intentionally misleading as uttering a direct lie.

When a development such as downsizing arises that affects the organization as a whole, controlling information is risky. If news of the layoffs leaks, employee reaction might include feelings of anger and betrayal; it could even have an effect on residents of the long-term care facilities, who are sensitive to the organizational climate. A downward spiral of mistrust between management and employees can ensue, with workers retreating into sullen passivity, fatalism, and poor morale. There may be instances of costly negligence. Such retribution erodes management's trust of workers, precipitating more mistrust on both sides.

As in many situations regarding organizational ethics, in this example the chaplain feels pulled in several directions as he considers what to do. He takes the downsizing matter before the ethics committee, which serves primarily in an educational and advisory capacity. At the same time, the chaplain hesitates to approach the chief executive with his concerns because of his promise to the CFO. The chaplain also perceives that the CEO's orientation is to the bottom line. If he approaches the CEO, he risks acting without full knowledge of the situation, and if she asks him how he learned of the downsizing, he might violate the CFO's request for confidentiality. If he does not speak with her, the chaplain is perhaps perpetuating a style of management-employee relations characterized by distrust and distance. With the ethics committee, he explores options running the gamut from violation of confidence to perpetuation of the current situation.

The Dynamic Tension of Discretion and Control

Because of the discretion that accompanies their jobs and the control strictures within which they operate, the people in these cases face a variety of ethical issues. Among these issues are cost containment, allocation of resources, partiality toward certain employees, respect for people, privacy, integrity, downsizing, honesty, truth telling, confidentiality, employee morale, and quality of patient care. These issues can provoke a variety of reactions. Several people must deal with a tough situation of moral uncertainty that confuses them about values or the right thing to do. Others confront a moral dilemma in which they see conflicting but justifiable courses of action and do not have the confidence or resources to help them sort through the issues. Finally, individuals experience moral distress in situations in which discretion and control are unbalanced.

This distress is the painful feeling caused by a situation in which one knows the ethically appropriate action to take but feels that one cannot carry out that action because of institutionalized obstacles: lack of time, supervisory lack of interest, lack of authority, institutional policy, or legal limits.[9] Employees and managers find themselves exercising discretion or asserting control (making choices that they may subsequently rationalize as the lesser of two evils). They may violate some moral standards while pursuing actions they feel obliged to perform. Advancing the company's interest is not an indifferent matter; they have promised to do this as part of their job, and it is wrong to break promises. Yet at times advancing the organization's interests may mean not honoring commitments formed in individual relationships. Their decisions exhibit discretion or control that may put people out of work or endanger the good name of the organization.

Some measure of moral distress is inherent in the relational character of human life and action, and therefore a fundamental feature of the moral ecology of a health care organization. It is a positive sign that these judgments matter to employees. Such distress can be debilitating, however, if people feel their superiors or their institution constrains them from rendering decisions or taking a course of action. People are upset by not knowing how to draw a line between what they judge to be legitimate practices and questionable ones.

Moral judgment hinges on multiple factors: openness to the input of concerned stakeholders, the "facts" as they appear at the time, full consideration of consequences, and the organization's values and rules. Clarity about discretion and support for its exercise (within well-thought-through limits) enhance employee confidence about moral decision making. This is why discretion is a good thing—so long as it takes place within an organizational culture characterized by openness, fairness, and trust.

Integrity-Preserving Compromises

These stories illustrate problems that develop for individuals within a health care institution where people find discretion and control pitted against each other. As the members of an ethics mechanism wrestle with ethical concerns, there are virtues that can guide their deliberation: integrity, respect for people, honesty, and fairness.

Integrity is defined as the personal commitment to be honest and trustworthy in demonstrating and evaluating how one balances discretion and control in relationships with others. When parties in a working relationship find themselves facing a tough choice, teasing apart the elements to understand the locus of disagreement can be beneficial. In each of the various PHC cases, the ethics committee or officer should ask if there is a course of action to redress the balance of discretion and control, to preserve one's integrity and protect the values important to others in the dispute.

In the case of electronic monitoring, management's concern about use of PHC computer and telecommunication resources for personal telephone calls, e-mail, or Internet access is a legitimate business interest. Despite organizational concerns about productivity, the legality of employee monitoring does not foreclose discussion of appropriate limits of control over employee behavior. From an ethical point of view, an employee does not give up all of his or her privacy on entering the workplace.[10] The message that such monitoring sends to employees and the kind of workplace culture that it suggests should concern employers who closely monitor employee behavior.

To the degree that managers and employees maintain open communication, in an atmosphere of trust a monitoring procedure can serve as a means of keeping in touch, rather than a way of trying to uncover misbehavior (or employee criticism of an executive). Ironically, under these circumstances, trust erodes and the organization moves to explicit control over employee behavior. Then employees perceive management's control as an attempt to limit noncompliant behavior.[11] Involving employees in creating a monitoring policy is a good way to find common ground. By bringing employee and manager together to develop principles and guidelines for electronic mail, and by effectively communicating a policy on electronic surveillance to the staff, the CEO of the LTC division fosters better balance between discretion and control.

In a second example of an integrity-preserving compromise, the ethical values of *respect for people, honesty,* and *fairness* argue that the CFO and the chaplain should find a way to clarify and resolve their ethical concerns with their CEO fairly and openly. If the CEO terminates the several longtime employees based on her perception that it's time for them to go, then she allows a small subset of values or interests to determine a decision without regard for others' important interests. Her statement suggests disregard for due process and distributes the burden of downsizing unfairly. The ethics committee wonders if special circumstances might allow the executive team a way to resolve the dilemma of the longtime employees. The CFO could enlist HR to inform the associates of where they stand and then allow them to choose for themselves whether they will retire or, over the next year, invest their time and effort to move up in the performance rankings.

The values of respect for people, honesty, and fairness also suggest to the ethics committee that the chaplain should voice his concerns to the CEO. Finding that voice requires courage. The easy temptation is to remain quiet and complain or murmur in the background. To speak up involves risk: of going on record, of facing the consequences, of losing standing, of humiliation. To remain silent and resentful, however, does not foster the values that the organization espouses for its employees. The chaplain's position and standing within the organization's culture (built on its history and mission) give him a power base from which to present his views on the justice and fairness of the evolving downsizing plan. If the chaplain chooses to maintain confidentiality (an important value in a relationship, the ethics committee acknowledges) and not reveal the source of his knowledge, he can encourage the CFO to incorporate his concerns into the downsizing plan. It is within the CFO's discretion to include the chaplain on the planning team.

For Partnership Health Care's LTC division to fulfill its mission while controlling costs, the chief executive might treat the employees with respect by acknowledging the tough times and enlisting their aid in finding ways to keep down costs. With a sound and sensitive plan in place, and kept informed of developments and reasonably notified of upcoming cuts, employees might well feel that necessary layoffs are as fair as possible. A fair severance package and a solid outplacement program demonstrate organizational concern. Morale might well take a positive turn, if employees are informed of the necessity of the cost-cutting measures and feel respected as members of the organization having some power to affect the course of events. Combined with reassurance for residents and their families, these steps may produce the best outcome possible, while promoting the integrity, honesty, and trust on which good working relationships depend.

The point of balance between discretion and control varies from position to position and person to person—one size does not fit all. If discretion and control are at odds, distrust and suspicion characterize working relationships. Trust flourishes when discretion and control are appropriately balanced (Exhibit 7.2). Organizational ethics begins with the question of how trust is established—how participants in a corporate structure can come to trust the intention and action of other individuals carrying out their roles.

Recommendations for Balancing Discretion and Control and Building Trust

To build a strong organizational ethics mechanism, we recommend addressing the dynamics of discretion and control and building trust across the organization.

It is important to acknowledge the vital yet precarious nature of discretion and control in the work of employees. In a health care institution, routines, procedures, managerial oversight, and

Exhibit 7.2. Trust as the Basis for a Balance of Discretion and Control.

Attention to trust is an essential component of organizational ethics and the basis for a flexible balance of discretion and control. A business enterprise, like any other human activity, presupposes some established patterns of reliance and commitment. Trust is confidence in or assured reliance on the honesty, dependability, or character of someone or something that does not rest solely on investigation or evidence. An element of risk always accompanies it. In spite of the risk, or more accurately because of it, the trusted person or thing becomes a locus of belief, expectation, and hope. Trust rests on honesty, openness, consistency, and respect, but it also involves commitment in spite of uncertainty. It then becomes the strongest—and the weakest—foundation on which to exercise discretion and control within organizations.

Trust results from a climate that includes four elements:

1. Honesty: integrity, no lies or exaggeration

2. Openness: willingness to share, and receptivity to information, perceptions, ideas

3. Consistency: reliable, predictable behavior and responses

4. Respect: treating people with dignity and fairness

As the bond that allows any kind of significant relationship to exist between people, trust is perhaps the most pervasive element in social interaction. Once broken, it is not easily recovered.

established ways of doing things help guide one's judgment. But since the dynamics of discretion and control always involve contingency, people ordinarily trusted to act within the organization's guidelines might violate them. Equally, people and the events to which they respond do not always lend themselves to being controlled. The first recommendation, therefore, is to develop standards of authority and accountability about the amount of discretion attached to a position (for example, what an employee can and cannot decide).

The second recommendation is to *educate all participants* about their appropriate role and professional responsibility. New employee orientation should include attention to the role of discretion and control within the organization; it should also involve periodic review. Those responsible for the health care organization's ethics mechanism should give special attention to training that helps managers appreciate the pitfalls of discretion and control. Examples and cases can clarify policy and standards having to do with discretionary decision making. Management and employees should regularly discuss such policy. Every employee should know the discretionary standards for the organization and how they affect his or her job.

Third, establish a strong system of *checks and balances* to routinely evaluate use of discretion and control. Grounded in the health care organization's mission and values, policies and standards of conduct inform and guide employee decision making and conduct. To protect the interests of the health care organization and its employees, the organization should consistently enforce its policy and standards. Finally, designing performance reviews to include attention to the organization's mission and values serves as a strong endorsement of the organization's commitment to ethically appropriate exercise of discretion and control.

Fourth, we recommend developing *systems for communication* throughout the organization (Exhibit 7.3). When a situation arises that the organization's formal standards of control do not clearly address, there should be a safe means to raise concerns publicly or to seek advice from a manager or designated ethics resource person. These systems should have significant visibility and include a grievance process for the resolution of conflicts involving the exercise of discretion and control.

The fifth recommendation is to establish and hold additional *forums as a safe place* to clarify expectations, to evaluate the balance between local and central control, and to assess possible conflict of interest. The ethics committee can be a forum for sharing concerns. The important point is to protect and respond to the person within the organization who brings up ethical problems and questions. Ignoring, hushing up, or punishing those who raise concerns spreads an obvious lesson through the organization, as Emily Friedman warns: "We claim to have ethics, but we do not use them."[12]

The sixth recommendation is to *encourage ethical achievement*, not just avoidance of ethical failure. We raise two points here. First, there is a pervasive attitude of organizational self-assessment within

Exhibit 7.3. How to Cultivate Good Conversation.

Generally

- Encourage people to speak up because it matters and makes a difference.
- Make moral discussions and decision making part of the everyday culture.
- Allow and encourage dissent.
- Help people develop their ability to hear and be attentive.
- Allow conversations to develop, and avoid premature closure.

Organizationally

- Define speaking up as a part of every manager's job description, not just as a troubleshooter but as a manager of quality.
- Transform the auditing function from one-way policing to two-way interactive activity.
- Institute regular discussion of ethics in each unit.
- Establish multiple media for employees to voice concerns, questions, ideas, and so on.
- Establish training programs in conflict resolution.

Source: Adapted from Bird, F. *The Muted Conscience: Moral Silence and the Practice of Ethics in Business.* Westport, Conn.: Quorum, 1997, p. 239.

corporations, including health care organizations, that not being caught is sufficient for ethical success. However, as sociologist Robert Coles has observed, "character consists of how you behave when no one else is around."[13] There needs to be a system to support people who contribute to the organization's goals and objectives regarding ethics. Second, contrary to the typical practice of pushing responsibility for a decision as far down the organizational line as possible, the model for ethical use of discretion begins with the leaders.

Summary

Integrating ethics into a corporate culture is not easy. To develop values through which to pass the facts that become one's judgments and to stick to those values in the face of opposition can be risky. Entrusting people with discretion involves the possibility of abuse; they inevitably face decisions requiring them to judge between competing interests, under uncertain and ambiguous circumstances. Recognizing and acting on ethical concerns, trying to do the right thing, may produce moral distress—indeed, such action may even entail losing one's job.

However, there also are risks associated with *not* doing the right thing. Perhaps the greatest risk is poisoning the culture in which one works. An ethical organization cannot stand on cowardice.[14] The courage to act comes more easily if systems are in place to facilitate ethical behavior. It is hard to be ethically courageous when one feels alone in an organization that does not encourage and support fair and appropriate exercise of discretion.

As with mission and the bottom line, the question is not merely a choice between discretion and control. A manager who controls information and manipulates people signals distrust. He may tell himself that he is acting in the best interests of others, but his actions are paternalistic. Employees react to this form of control with alienation and suspicion. Cultivating trust and appreciating interdependence become increasingly problematic to the extent that the intricate patterns of dependence and power encourage the individual in a corporate setting to use discretionary authority to carve out a zone of self-seeking control.

Strict emphasis on checks and balances can easily become a controlling mechanism and exacerbate the pull toward distrust. Structures need to be in place as a guide to balancing discretion and control, but the manager's attitude is important. Other people's ethical standards cannot be controlled, legislated, or managed; they can only be encouraged and modeled. The organization cannot ignore unethical behavior, and there may be situations that require direct prevention or intervention. To produce a positive expression of discretion, one can only create an atmosphere that is conducive to and that rewards such behavior. The good manager commits to open and honest communication, willingness to manifest the values that the organization espouses, and trust as the basis of relationships with others.

Notes

1. This case was adapted from Jackal, R. "Moral Mazes: Bureaucracy and Managerial Work." In T. Donaldson and P. H. Werhane (eds.),

Ethical Issues in Business. Upper Saddle River, N.J.: Prentice Hall, 1996, p. 64.

2. This case was adapted from Edwards, G. "Addressing Ethics Accusations." *Healthcare Executive,* 1997, *12*(4), 49.

3. Edwards (1997).

4. Hinderer, D. "Hospital Downsizing: Ethics and Employees." *Journal of Nursing Administration,* 1997, *27*(9), 9–11.

5. Gillespie, N. C. "The Business of Ethics." In W. Robison, M. Pritchard, and J. Ellin (eds.), *Profits and Professions: Essays in Business and Professional Ethics.* Clifton, N.J.: Humana Press, 1983.

6. Bok, S. *Secrets.* New York: Pantheon, 1982.

7. Schulman, M. "Little Brother Is Watching You." *Issues in Ethics,* Spring/Summer 1998, *9,* 11–15. It must be noted that employer monitoring of employees is controversial; it is upsetting to many employees who protest on the grounds of a right to privacy. Courts have upheld the employer's right to monitor its employees, but legal challenges undoubtedly will continue to occur.

8. This case was adapted from Shanks, T. "The Case of the Performance Appraisal." *Issues in Ethics,* Summer 1997, *8,* 22.

9. Shanks (1997).

10. Schulman (1998).

11. Bird, F. *The Muted Conscience: Moral Silence and the Practice of Ethics in Business.* Westport, Conn.: Quorum, 1997.

12. Friedman, E. *Choices and Conflict: Explorations in Health Care Ethics.* Chicago: AHA, 1992, p. 111.

13. Friedman (1992), p. 111.

14. Friedman (1992), p. 113.

Chapter Eight

Evaluating the Moral Life of an Organization

The Case of Resource Allocation Policies

Understanding the moral choices of an organization seems daunting, if not impossible, in comparison to observing the moral actions of any individual who works within it. To get an accurate account of an organization's moral choices, do you look to the actions of the trustees and shareholders, the executive leaders and management, or the workforce? Examination of any or all of these actors who affect an organization's moral life might reveal the complexity of that life, but it remains unclear whether these individual choices can accurately be described as reflecting the moral choices of the organization as such. One good proxy to estimate the moral choices of an organization is to probe formal policies and procedures that direct the choices of every member of the organization.

Policies affect everyone in an organization. Management proposes policy; trustees approve management's recommendations; and workers are guided by management's plans. Whether every member of the organization follows policy or not does not detract from the fact that the organization has written that it intends to act in this manner. Thus, policy is a mirror in which to see the organization's moral nature. This chapter offers a method for analysis for organizational moral choices: exploring policies.

Some of the most influential organizational policies are those that direct resources. In almost every choice made within a health care organization, some mix of human and technological resources are marshaled to pursue the goals of healing and comfort. Choice about resources becomes a focus in examining the organization's moral norms.

The resource choices can be made formally or informally. The organization makes obviously formal choices through policies on purchasing, admission and retention on units, futility, appropriate care, and drug formularies. Less obvious but no less formal allocation decisions are made through contracts, decisions made by technology assessment and clinical effectiveness committees, and hiring and staffing patterns. The organization displays an informal pattern of allocation with choices made not according to policy but dictated by influences such as organizational culture (not following stated policy); professional ideology (physicians given large discretion for ordering tests and procedures); and employee bias (for instance, being more or less generous depending on the personalities of the patient and his or her family).

Adequate moral analysis of an organization's allocation choice includes understanding formal and informal choices. Moral analysis of informal organizational choice is difficult because the task requires time-consuming observation. A less complicated method for understanding organizational choice is to focus on formal policy, as this chapter does.

In the current financially competitive climate, a health care organization needs to be especially concerned with policies that contain health costs. These policies help meet the primary mission of patient care that cannot be accomplished without prudent use of resources. Since access to and the costs of health care are a public concern, the organization is being held to a high level of social accountability. Allocation policy is a natural place to examine organizational accountability. This chapter examines a means to evaluate existing resource allocation policy, and it offers considerations necessary for developing new policy.

The chapter also asks questions that make explicit the moral nature of institutional decisions to direct resources. We proceed on the assumption that the new challenges to manage resources, as onerous as they first appear, can, if properly managed, produce an equitable and socially responsible health care system by examining whether the organization's policies are ethically defensible.

A Case and Method

The situation at PHC offers a case straddling clinical ethics and organizational ethics and suggesting a method for analyzing policy.

PHC needs to reduce patient length of stay in hospital if the system is to remain competitive and maintain a high bond rating. PHC's cost per adjusted discharge is the highest in the region, making it noncompetitive. Compared to the other hospitals, the intensive care unit (ICU) at St. Somewhere has an unusually long length of stay with poor patient outcomes. To address the organizational ethics problem, the chief executive creates a systemwide task force to examine resource management policies to see whether they can generate savings and simultaneously reflect PHC's mission.

The first step for the task force is to examine cases and determine whether the policies that direct them are appropriate. The task force finds the record of a man who stayed six weeks and eventually died in the ICU. The medical record notes: "Long-stay patient died in intensive care unit with multiple organ systems failure. Patient utilized exorbitant resources—staff time and numerous tests, drugs, and interventions. (Staff believed early on that most of the patient's treatments were useless.)"

The note is part of a chart of an otherwise healthy seventy-eight-year-old who came to the emergency department with a pain in his throat and difficulty swallowing. He was found to have a turkey bone lodged in his throat. When the emergency room physician attempted to remove the bone, the patient's esophagus ruptured. A surgeon attempted several repairs, starting with a thoracotomy. The patient developed an acute infection and was treated with numerous antibiotics but became septic. He experienced acute liver and kidney failure and respiratory failure and required mechanical ventilation and hemodialysis. The patient was restless, grimacing, and neurologically unresponsive. The staff believed he should be transferred out of the ICU because he was moribund.

The issue of appropriate ICU resource management has been raised because staff were aware that for rupture of the esophagus the literature reflects nearly a 100 percent mortality rate. The patient's surgeon has had good—but unpublished—results with patients of this sort; he regularly defends his position with other consultants who maintain the patient is likely to expire early on during the course of treatment.

The hospital ICU transfer policy provides many criteria for moving a patient from the ICU, among them: "Any patient may be discharged from the critical care unit who is determined to be moribund in the assessment of the attending physician and for whom no extraordinary medical measures will be used to prolong life or prevent death." Some staff judge that because this patient was moribund no more treatment other than palliation should have been given, and that the patient should have been transferred from the ICU.

This case may seem atypical, perhaps extreme. Nonetheless, in this and other cases, clinicians and managers fret about whether there is inappropriate utilization of health care resources. Employees throughout any organization make choices about resources; however, the issue is more conflictual in a health care organization with allocation decisions that directly affect patients. A situation of providing care to an individual patient captures our attention and, unfortunately, blinds us to the fact that with very few exceptions all resource choices affect patients—some obviously, others less so. Clinical ethics committees have long considered cases of this kind, which show great overlap with organizational ethics. The differences between the two modes of analysis are significant: how the moral questions are framed, how facts are gathered, the values that need to be balanced, the justification for a decision, and identification of alternatives.

Clinical moral analysis is usually confined to the relationship among the patient, family, and providers. Rarely is consideration given to ethical issues that reflect organizational decisions. In such a case, how should an ethics mechanism proceed? What difference in approach, if any, is observed in comparison to the work of a clinical ethics committee? The method used in clinical ethics, with its emphasis on certain elements, is a useful place to start. This includes focusing the moral questions, obtaining the facts, clarifying elusive concepts, identifying and analyzing the moral values in dispute, evaluating the moral arguments, and looking for integrity-preserving compromises.

Identifying Questions

In ethical analysis of a case, the reader is often quick to identify what the moral problem appears to be. It is important to be cautious in framing the question, because if only one question is asked—for example, Who should make the decision?—the moral analysis might revert to a traditional bioethics analysis, which can short-circuit organizational ethics. From an organization's perspective, several questions present themselves. Is it defensible to limit treatment to this patient? What criteria are used to trigger allocation of resources? Are the criteria clear, agreed upon, and applied fairly? Who should make a decision to limit treatment? Who has participated in developing the policy?

Before moving to fact gathering, an ethics mechanism would find it useful to see whether there is any natural priority in answering the questions. Some questions and facts need to be answered before moving to others. For example, before it can be determined whether it was defensible to limit treatment for the seventy-eight-year-old man, a prior question needs exploration, namely, Are the criteria that determine allocation fair? Also, whether or not it is legitimate to limit treatment in this case depends on beliefs about limiting ever being defensible. The moral questions determine what facts are needed for the analysis.

Observing the Facts

Fact gathering about resource allocation requires work different from what is typical for a clinical ethics committee. As described in Chapter Two, gathering the facts entails interviewing those whose job it is to carry out the policy. Questions need to be asked about resource allocation: Is there a clear policy? Is the policy always followed? Are there exceptions to the policy? Do staff have practices or routines that violate the policy? Who follows the policy?

The answers to these questions partially describe how resources are allocated. Observation is also necessary to confirm the answers or to clearly understand how resources are actually allocated. It is important to know whether in the day-to-day life of the organization there are instances when the policy should be followed but is not. In these cases, why is the policy not followed? Is it irrelevant, or inconvenient to follow, or simply ignored? Does a policy have binding force, or is it left to the discretion of the physician? Is a process available for speedy appeal in an exceptional case?

As the facts are gathered, it is important to identify concepts in the policy that determine decisions about allocation. In allocation policy, such concepts are expressed by "dispensed p.r.n." (as needed) and "the intervention is medically necessary." An observer would want to understand the range of possible interpretation of the concepts. Is there an unequivocal understanding that is shared by all in the organization, or can various individuals interpret the concept differently? For example, in p.r.n., how is need assessed? The greater the clarity of the concept(s) and the more there is shared understanding of meaning within the organization, the better the chance that the allocation mechanism is applied consistently. One test of a policy's fairness is its consistent application.

In the PHC case, staff disagreed about whether the patient was moribund. Notwithstanding the grim mortality rate in the literature, for which reason some staff believed the intervention to be futile from the beginning, the surgeon's experience with at least some success in repairing this problem left him feeling obligated to try to heal the patient. This difference in opinion about the patient's prognosis led to a difference in views of what was appropriate treatment. In other words, the concept that determines resource allocation (moribund condition) can be interpreted differently by each clinician. This situation creates a moral risk: varying interpretation leaves open the possibility that similarly situated patients can be treated differently. Clearly there are ethical implications for policy development. Concepts that determine resource allocation should not inadvertently create the possibility for unequal treatment.

Other facts are needed if the moral question is framed as, Who should make the decision about resource allocation? This question applies equally to initially formulating the policy and implementing it. As is most often the case, there is very little legislative history about how the policy applied in this case has come to be and who has participated in its formation. This is not a benign moral issue. It has been argued that some choices are so tragic that they need to be made quietly, away from public scrutiny, in the least damaging way for the good of the institution or society. Others argue convincingly that policies should be in clear view of those most affected by it (patients). Although this latter view may prove to be difficult or taxing for an institution conducting initial policy formation, this consideration demands at a minimum that patients be informed of mechanisms that materially and importantly affect their course of care.

Unfortunately, the policy used in the PHC case makes no mention of whether or how the patient and family are to be party to the decision to transfer the patient. The case example is silent about how the patient or family is to be informed of relevant medical information (the man is moribund) and how their wishes are to be integrated into a decision to transfer and limit care. For example, they were not informed either that the literature reflects nearly a 100 percent mortality rate or that the surgeon has had unpublished positive results. Although the case report does not describe whether the family knew of the dispute over transfer or whether the physician felt an obligation to inform them of it, it is safe to suggest that the policy should have required more active family participation. The lack of explicit requirements indicates a moral weakness in the policy as written.

Clarification of Concepts

Concept clarification can run the gamut from a single term (moribund) to clarification of the scope of the resource management policy. When examining a policy, the organizational ethics mechanism must clarify what kind of policy it is examining. For example, is the policy about human resources, investments, institutional partnerships, or resource allocation? Each kind entails its own moral questions. For example, an investment policy raises the question of how far an institution should pursue socially responsible investments (see Case Nine). Even though the PHC task force has a single case and policy concern, its overall mandate is analysis of resource utilization policies generally. Therefore, the task force needs clarification of several issues: What does it mean to manage resources? Which resources count as health resources? Which health resources should be managed?

As the task force begins its work, it questions the concept defining its mission: managing resources. To some task force members the term *management of resources*, which is used interchangeably with resource allocation, is doublespeak for rationing—that is, denial of care. In its least inflammatory and nonmoral definition, *resource management* or *allocation* means more than simply taking a retrospective review of resource utilization. The term means prospective control and direction of health resources. Prospective management involves setting priorities among patients' conditions. Services must be provided consistently with organizational commitments and, under some circumstances, limited or denied if inconsistent with those commitments. In this concept clarification, the task force recognizes that a definition of *resource management* or *allocation* is an issue separate from judging whether the limitation of resources is morally justified. With this clarification, the task force sees the aim of later tasks more clearly, namely, to identify and distinguish morally justifiable limitation of resources from the unjustifiable.

Since the task force's commission is to examine resource management polices, it needs to clarify the meaning of a "health care resource." What counts as a health care resource is a contentious issue. At a minimum, the most precious health resource is time—that of the provider. Extra time spent with one patient and family is time not spent with another patient and family. Rarely, however, do formal structures address allocation of time. Informally, the choices made by staff to spend more time with one patient as opposed to another merit consideration, especially the choice of the basis on which staff allocate time.

A health resource is commonly thought of as a machine, a bed, a drug, a diagnostic test, or some therapeutic intervention. Here, the moral analysis changes considerably if one is looking at policy to manage a simple intervention, such as a physical diagnosis, as opposed to policy to manage a long, drawn-out episode of care. The latter entails many services, as seen in the case of a long-stay patient in the ICU.

The task force, seeing the wide array of health care resources, needs to further clarify whether all or only some resources must be managed. Little agreement exists among the task force members about which unit of resources ought to be managed, but it concludes that it is a mistake if only certain oxen are gored. If some services are selected simply because of high cost and others are not examined, the aggregate cost of the unexamined services might be as morally relevant as those that are scrutinized. If there must be limitation or denial of services, every resource in the hospital should be considered. Otherwise the burden of the process falls disproportionately and unfairly on those patients currently in need of expensive treatments. The task force concludes that the mark of morally responsible policy making is to be consistent. If some health care resources are managed and others are left unmanaged, then there is some room to criticize the organization's policy and moral choices.

Alternatives and Consequences

In evaluating the policy, the task force must imagine policy alternatives and the consequences for constituents and cherished values. At this point, alternatives present themselves. One is the status quo, which simply leaves the policy as is and concludes it is, on balance, morally acceptable. Another policy alternative is alteration of the decision-making process, when it is developed and when it is implemented.

If the policy is left as is, some of the organization's cherished values are protected, and others are tested. One protected value is stewardship. No doubt PHC is interested not only in financial solvency but also in remaining competitive. An equitable resource management mechanism is concerned with promoting equity of care—to ensure that the right of each person to basic health care is respected—and the good health of all in the community. To these ends, the mechanism must at the least ensure that no resources are wasted. The Golden Rule requires all persons to be good stewards over available resources; there is a general expectation that a person conserves resources because she or he, in fairness, expects others to do so as well. Practically, this means that a resource management mechanism must ensure that waste has been eliminated. In this case, the general intent of the policy is to ensure good stewardship and avoid waste. This argues against staying with the status quo.

If the policy remains as is, there may be concern about whether the policy recognizes and protects the value of the common good. The common good is realized when economic, political, and social conditions ensure protection for the fundamental rights of all individuals and enable them to fulfill their common purpose and reach their common goals. A resource management policy that operates on equity might distribute resources on the basis of meeting the basic needs of the whole population but inadvertently treat patients with special needs as if their interests do not count. Attention to the common good balances the needs of the community and the individual, never neglecting the individual and especially being attentive to individuals who are frequently, or for no good reason, denied access to care.

Therefore, any resource management mechanism should consider facilitating service to and advocacy for those people whose social condition puts them at the margin of society and leaves them particularly vulnerable to discrimination: the poor, the uninsured and underinsured; children, single parents, and the elderly; those with incurable disease and those with chemical dependency; and racial minorities, immigrants, and refugees. In particular, someone with a mental or physical disability, regardless of the cause or severity, must be treated as a unique person of incomparable worth, with the same right to adequate health care as all other persons. The case of the seventy-eight-year-old man is ambiguous when considered in light of the common good, but some room exists to infer that there is little advocacy on his behalf. The policy mentioned in the case is silent on the matter; however, moral analysis of the policy, with protection of the common good in mind, might call for revising it.

If the policy remains as is, the value of due process is put at risk. A principle of due process sets guideposts for resource management. Due process requires powerful bodies to act according to established rules and to give notice, an opportunity to be heard, and access to a reasonable appeals process. For example, due process generally requires that like cases be treated alike. It calls for consistency in treating patients in a resource management mechanism. If resources are tightly managed in one unit but not another, questions may be raised about possible unfairness. It is important to ask whether one group of patients might be bearing a disproportionate share of the limitation or denial of services. It is not clear from this policy or case whether all other services are under similar resource allocation mechanisms. If further investigation reveals that other services are not treated similarly, then there may be reason to consider the current policy alternative unfair.

Finally, if the policy remains as is, the value of respect for people is placed at risk. In health care, respect for people is a highly prized value, sometimes translated as acting for the good of the patient. At a minimum, this principle promotes some behaviors and excludes others. Respect for people has been used traditionally as a means to direct treatment and can be traced back to the Hippocratic maxim of *primum non nocere* ("first do no harm"). This maxim restricts the physician from giving or withholding resources if the result is likely to harm the patient. Of course, a central question this principle raises is, What counts as harm? Respect for people in resource management requires that all persons, and not just some, be respected. For example, any resource management mechanism that, arbitrarily or without justification, denies or limits treatment to some persons is morally indefensible. In this case, it is not clear whether this seventy-eight-year-old man was being treated arbitrarily; however, to the extent the concept of *moribund* is used malleably, this alternative is open to allegations of unfairness.

Alternatives to the current policy entail some alteration of decision making. For example, one alternative is to consider where resource decisions should be made—at the bedside between the physician and patient (in other words, with no policy) or at an institutional level (in the boardroom). The disadvantage of institutional policy making is that patients' choices are limited and physicians' prudential judgments are constrained. Especially in a situation where the budget is limited or aggressively managed, the choice to offer one patient a service might have the consequence of denying services to other patients. It is essential that clinicians advocate for services they believe benefit patients, but it is also true that in the face of limits there must be a public discussion and decision about what to limit and on what basis. The case for policy-based resource management is strong; it lessens an individual clinician's bias and offers access to institutional information about resources—such as cost, efficiency, and effectiveness—that an individual clinician would find it hard to be constantly apprised of.

Another alternative to the current policy and process in this case is to enhance informed decision making for the patient or an appropriate surrogate decision maker. The policy and the case display little attention to decision making by the patient or surrogate. Certainly health care professionals do not consciously hide either the development of resource management mechanisms or individual decisions generated by them. Yet in their good intentions (or discomfort about discussing the limitation of service), clinicians might keep patients and families in the dark about the formulation and implementation of a resource management mechanism. Is there any reason to think that this practice or policy is defensible? As noted earlier, any mechanism should be in clear view of those people most affected by it, so that patients can make other arrangements, such as transfer to another health care institution, if they disagree. Any well-ordered society, including a health care organization, must be animated by a notion of "fair terms of cooperation and mutual advantage."[1] Fair cooperation is possible only if all the parties to the cooperative agreement know where they stand; this is possible only if the relevant considerations are known by all involved. In this policy and case, only one party to the agreement (the medical team) has all the relevant information.

There is another argument for patient participation in resource management: that our society is to some extent held together by openness and honesty. To exclude from decision making those who have the most at stake dissolves the glue that binds us as a community. Additionally, it can be argued that a resource allocation decision is anything but a mere medical decision, where all the data are clear and complete (the patient is moribund) and need only be entered into an agreed-upon equation by skilled minds. Rather, a resource management decision rests firmly on people's values—about disease and disability, about treatment and palliation, about costs—and these are the issues about which individuals will reasonably disagree. It is assumed that medical experts can identify what effect an intervention ill produces, but clinicians cannot be presumed to have more insight than patients about which effects to value. Hence, patients must be informed of resource limitations so that they might make alternative arrangements.

Justification

At this point in the policy analysis, one pervasive question remains: Is resource management necessary or defensible? The allocation mechanism has long been part of the territory: a hospital formulary committee is only one obvious mechanism that has long existed with the mission being, in part, to limit distribution of highly expensive drugs. Less obvious but more pervasive are the mechanisms involved when staff face a shortage—traditionally, a bed shortage—and must select which patients shall receive the scarce resource. The rapidly changing health care market is pressing health care organizations to ensure quality services—providing effective care at a reasonable cost and avoiding ineffective care. In the competitive health care environment, organizations have been forced to adopt policies to manage health care resources. But are these actions justified?

Perhaps the least satisfying justification for managing resources is that it is inevitable. Some argue that public resource management plans such as Oregon's rationing experiment are too politically unacceptable, especially for publicly elected government officials. Public officials shy away from choice about limiting or denying services. But these choices are not disappearing; they fall instead to health care providers. Those who pay for health care, such as employers and the government, ask providers to render access to care at lower prices. Decisions to limit and perhaps deny services are likely to be pushed out of public view, to hospitals and managed care organizations—places where the difficult choices have to be made in the context of resource limitations imposed externally by competitive forces.

Others justify resource allocation mechanisms on the grounds that they reduce irrationality. The inevitability of the current cost containment trend is troubling; the health care organization has inherited the traditional moral commitment of patient advocacy that once belonged to the medical practitioner. Yet in the nature of the allocation cases, managing resources can, and often must, pit the interests of patients against each other and those of cost-conscious organizations. These are indeed severe threats; a decision to limit access to health care resources can seem capricious and indefensible. Anxiety about this can be reduced. Moral analysis such as that modeled here, when put to work in organizational policy, can effectively address the threat to competing interests. Limitation and denial of services will not be eradicated, but sound policy can ensure that capricious and indefensible decisions can be.

Another justification for managing resources is that it creates system support and checks and balances while promoting good medicine. This particular case demonstrates how a lack of checks and balances and accountability can promote bad medicine. As is often true, patients are cared for by a team, each member having expertise in care for a physiological aspect of the patient (heart, kidneys, lungs). Each member focuses on a particular physiological system of the patient, and the need to fix it can come at the expense of a comprehensive view of the patient's well-being. For example, the chain reaction of a patient undergoing multiorgan system failure may precipitate involvement of many subspecialties: a cardiologist may be able to maintain adequate cardiac output, a pulmonologist may deal with lung functioning, and a nephrologist may be able to dialyze a dying patient. Any one of these interventions could work, yet an individual clinician might lack the broader view that the patient is in multiorgan system failure and is going to die.

The lines of accountability and authority are clearly fragmented. After the patient's death, it is sometimes asked whether there was appropriate resource utilization and whether there is a need to rethink existing strategies for directing resources. Clinicians often lament that unnecessary or harmful intervention can be avoided if there exists a concept to determine more judicious use of a health care resource. Good resource management means good medicine. Comprehensive processes with checks and balances can help craft a care plan that serves the whole patient.

A further bolstering justification is that being explicit about managing resources eradicates the perception that an organization is unfair or lacking in social responsibility. A majority of the present mechanisms are out of view of the patients and—too often for comfort—simply informal. Whether explicit or hidden from view, these mechanisms deeply affect the physician-patient relationship, staff relations, and community relations. If patients and families have the notion that the rules for resource utilization are applied inconsistently among patients, or if staff think formal processes are being gamed or overruled by informal mechanisms, or if the community imagines that there is little accountability for the existing process, this consternation and resultant adverse publicity is likely to force the institution to reconsider the present way of doing business.

Cost Is Not a Justification

Even if there are circumstances under which it is legitimate to allocate care, there are always arguments about whether cost should justify allocation policy. It is therefore imperative to analyze a policy to understand how costs function in the background, even though they might not be explicitly mentioned in the policy. First, it is well known that clinicians are generally reimbursed for a specific procedure, not an entire episode of care. It is important to be realistic in policy development and take into account any incentives that run counter to the purposes of rational resource management.

Second, the moral adequacy of knowing which costs to include as part of a mechanism is nicely understood in the case of dialysis and kidney transplantation. At first blush, it seems extravagant to some that a significant amount of money is spent on kidney transplants; however, their true cost can only be evaluated in relation to alternative procedures and cost, such as the annual cost of keeping a person on dialysis. In moral evaluation of a policy, it is important to examine the costs of alternative treatments and nontreatment.

Third, under prevailing health care finance systems, the amount of an organization's health care resources do not expand indefinitely. Most reimbursement schemes are not open-ended; costs in one area reduce expenditures in another. As a result, it has become imperative to morally evaluate a policy by means of the question, What costs are diverted from other socially desirable goals of the institution?

Fourth, since costs are relevant to resource management policy, the patient must be informed if more expensive alternatives are not offered, and given the reason why they are not (for example, the more expensive service has only a marginal effect).

Directions for Integrity-Preserving Compromises

The task of evaluating resource policy is daunting because organizations have so many formal and informal, obvious and not-so-obvious, mechanisms being used by a variety of professionals. Developing an evaluation process that accounts for every allocation circumstance is impossible, but sufficient tools exist to begin a general process of policy evaluation.

As a preliminary step, a health care organization should be guided by an ethics mechanism that comprises interdisciplinary participants. It should be evident from the range of topics raised in this chapter that professionals with a range of analytical talents— sociology, anthropology, organizational development, ethics, policy making, and economics—are necessary.

Second, as is evident from this particular policy, one source of tension stems from the question of who should decide about resource management. As has been noted, this question occurs both in initially developing a policy and in implementing it day to day. In both situations, several issues are not publicly contested. First, the policy and how it works must be made public to all parties who have an interest in the resource management decisions. Second, because there are values that are imbedded in resource management policy, decisions about these values should not be left solely to health care professionals. Rather, the values of patients (and families) must be taken into consideration. Third, there must be a means for all interested parties to appeal the resource decision. Any policy that does not meet these minimal conditions is morally inadequate.

Third, as is evident from this discussion, allocation polices are often criticized for limiting the patient's choice. Although a condition of resource management is to direct and narrow patient and provider choice, policy should offer alternative treatments where feasible, adequate flexibility for professional clinical judgment, and in all cases opportunity for appeal. For example, if out of necessity a health care organization decides to limit services, patients should be informed, and where necessary assisted, in making alternative arrangements.

Fourth, since allocation policies should respect patients' values, provision must be made for reasonable accommodation of patients' wishes. For example, in some situations, such as supplying ICU care to a brain-dead person, many would agree to halt treatment. However, there is an exception to this general rule. The law acknowledges that religious requests for resources must be accommodated within reason. A case in point is provision of care for brain-dead Orthodox Jews whose families do not acknowledge legal criteria of whole brain death.

Fifth, there is ample social science evidence to suggest that a clinician's bias on class, ethnicity, religion, and gender importantly influences management of resources.[2] Policy should include ways to lessen the amount of bias that is integrated into the final decision to allocate health care resources. A resource policy might want to prompt the clinician to ask herself whether an individual resource decision can be applied to all patients. If not, this inability to universalize the decision should trigger a question in the clinician's mind about whether she is being fair in this case.

Sixth, for a resource management policy to work, it must be used. Sociological evidence suggests that clinicians are less likely to use concepts (for example, moribund) where the rationale for their use is not clear. Is the mechanism presented in such a way that the clinician thinks the health measurements used are valid and reliable? Does the clinician find this policy useful because it addresses real problems in allocating resources? Are the recommended outcomes from employing the policy credible—that is, do they have an impact on good clinical outcomes?

Debate concerning the ethics of health care resource management policy is in its infancy. Because of the heterogeneity of the mechanisms used to manage resources, most early attempts at moral analysis employ a variety of measures against which to judge policy. A process of trial and error will persist for the near future. Nonetheless, everyone concerned about organizational ethics must begin to identify certain necessary features of ethical analysis.

Notes
1. Rawls, J. *A Theory of Justice.* Cambridge, Mass.: Harvard University, 1972.
2. Zussman, R. *Intensive Care: Medical Ethics and the Medical Profession.* Chicago: University of Chicago, 1992.

Chapter Nine

Resource Allocation and Utilization
Structural Issues

Questions about resource allocation are among the most important in organizational ethics. Not only do they reflect the quality and availability of particular services; at a deeper level they offer a concrete expression of the organization's values. They are the most powerful tools a manager possesses to set the moral tone of the organization. The old cliché "Put your money where your mouth is" expresses the simple truth that the willingness to commit one's economic resources to a task is compelling testimony to profound commitment to the task.

The preceding chapter focused on the traditional understanding of resource allocation as specifically applied to clinical decision making. The concern of this chapter is how allocating resources within an organization can shape the moral culture of the institution, and how the moral culture and political environment can affect decisions about allocation. Once one moves beyond focusing on the formal practices and policies of an organization (rational systems theory) to include consideration of how cultural, informal systems and the external environment can affect the organization's behavior (natural systems and open systems theories), how resources move through an organization becomes vitally important. Careful analysis also reveals how allocation affects the informal culture of the organization. Tracing resources can show how the informal culture alters the movement of resources toward ends not necessarily intended or understood by the formal allocation plan.

In a fixed economic system, where income cannot be infinitely expanded, an organization must allocate available resources among its many mission goals. The key in making these judgments is how an allocation decision conforms to the organization's mission, including treating fairly all of the claimants to the institution's resources (patients, the public, associates, and the institution itself).

This chapter focuses on systemic interaction regarding resource allocation decisions. The first case examines how resource allocation affects institutional identity. The second case considers the effect of informal systems and cultures on judgment in clinical resource allocation. Finally, the third case highlights the expressive function of resource allocation (what an allocation decision communicates to employees and others about the values of the organization) and its effect on the moral ecology of the organization.

Organizational Identity and the Social Environment

One of the most potent tools senior management has in defining and shaping the identity of an organization is its power over the purse. Broad decisions on resource allocation convey a powerful message about the overall character of the organization; an organization that allocates the bulk of its resources toward marketing and financial activities, for example, is radically different from one that funnels most of its resources to providing services. Because the broad parameters of resource allocation are reasonably stable over time—overall budgets do not generally change radically from year to year—how subtle shifts are made in response to changing circumstances is incredibly important. Such decisions reveal the current intention and thinking of an organization.

PHC owns a number of hospitals operating in a variety of economically and socially diverse communities in the metropolitan area. The decision by Medicaid officials to reduce reimbursement rates for a specific class of procedures by 25 percent, though applicable to all hospitals owned by PHC, in fact has a significant effect on the potential income of only St. Somewhere Hospital. The board could make income adjustments among all of the hospitals and other services to meet this Medicaid shortfall. Instead, it determines that despite the change in circumstances, St. Somewhere is still obligated to maintain its projected return on assets (in other words, its profitability).

The decision to require St. Somewhere's managers to maintain their projected return on assets despite a significant change in income projections has a substantial impact on the hospital's ability to deliver services in its community and on its relations with employees, patients, and other members of the community. The board is ethically responsible for the consequences of its decision.

In reflecting on this decision, we find two levels of analysis. First is the question of whether it is appropriate for the board to demand the projected return on investment. Second is the question of how any necessary adjustments are to be made within the system. Specifically, how does this decision affect the moral culture and identity of the organization? How do these allocation decisions fit within the broader social context in which they are made?

Institutional Identity and Moral Culture

At the outset, the board needs to reflect on the nature of the organization itself in relation to the individual hospitals within it. Who within the organization is best situated to decide how the moral demands of service and responsible fiscal management are to be balanced? How does delegating authority to make this decision affect institutional identity? A complex health care organization like PHC might be structured in one of three ways: radically decentralized decision making among its constituent operating units; a single entity with centralized decision making; and some—but not all—decision-making authority delegated to subsidiary operating units.

Radical Decentralization
Let's assume Partnership Health Care follows the decentralized model, so that all substantive decisions are made at the level of the operating unit, with the PHC board having little or no moral responsibility for, or authority over, the acts of those units. For example, PHC might have been created as a holding company whose purposes are limited to providing consolidated administrative services. In such a situation, the board's demand that St. Somewhere meet its return on assets target is analogous to any business or service provider demanding payment for goods delivered or services rendered. How the payment is to be generated is within the dis-

cretion of the payer, in this case St. Somewhere. The demand is morally neutral.

If operating units are truly autonomous, however, it makes little sense to say that PHC exists as a coherent moral organization. As a loose association of independent entities, not only does PHC have no moral responsibility for the acts of its constituents but it has no more authority over them than might any other external organization.

Such a scenario is extremely rare. It is much more likely that St. Somewhere is an operational unit *within* PHC. Although there may be greater or lesser degrees of identification between St. Somewhere and PHC, there is some sense in which PHC is thought of as a single, integrated organization with one locus of decision making on how systemic resources are allocated.

Identity

In contrast to a radically decentralized model, let's assume that PHC is structured as a single entity guided by the authority of the board and senior management. Although the entity's activities span a variety of settings and formats (for example, it operates hospitals, nursing homes, labs, and so on), the board conceptualizes PHC as unitary. The board thus takes all the employees of PHC's various operating units to be working for the single organization.

This again is an extreme position and fairly rare in practice, except in the smallest of organizations. To act consistently under this model, the board cannot delegate authority to St. Somewhere to determine how it meets its financial goals. That direction has to come from the board or senior management.

Subsidiary Delegation

A model of delegation seeks a constructive balance between the foregoing extremes. It grants individual operating units substantial authority in their operations and how they make allocation decisions. But this autonomy is exercised as part of an overall strategy set by the senior leadership of the organization. Instead of central management trying to impose detailed business plans on individual operating units, it offers general guidelines and grants operating units a certain degree of freedom in fulfilling those plans. This action allows innovation and gives the local manager flexibility to operate in accordance with the particular conditions of the local market. It results in a sort of institutional diversity in which the localized unit creates its own identity to serve the individual market.

This model of management is analogous to what is referred to as "subsidiarity" in Roman Catholic social thought.[1] Briefly, this principle asserts that in any large social organization, decision making should devolve to the social group most affected by that decision. It is a way for the larger social organization to honor and empower identifiable communities.

In health care, the virtue of this approach is that the administrators of individual facilities, such as St. Somewhere, are arguably in the best position to assess the needs of their community and to seek to deploy institutional resources in ways that best meet those needs. Moreover, by allowing the operating unit to make these decisions, this approach facilitates developing a certain character that is reflective of the local community. In its best sense, such a character can shape and inform the services that the constituent institution offers to its community. For example, St. Somewhere may elect to direct its resources toward providing low-technology community health care as opposed to high-technology health care that may not be suitable for the needs of its community.

To be consistent in this approach, in the present case the board has to delegate authority over how to address the change in Medicaid reimbursement and also has to allow St. Somewhere to participate in determining how those changes affect its return-on-investment target. As in any allocation decision, subsidiarity does not mean that St. Somewhere decides alone. Just as it has obligations to the community it serves, so too it has obligations to PHC. Subsidiarity simply requires that St. Somewhere be involved in negotiation with the board or senior management as to how to meet and balance these varying obligations.

Thus the first, fundamental question for the board to answer is what type of organization they are seeking to create or support in their allocation of resources. In this case, the board must balance its interest in the unity and overall identity of PHC against its support for subsidiarity and local control. A policy of radical decentralization may be at odds with the objective of creating a corporate identity for PHC and advancing corporate goals and mission.

Taken in isolation, the mandate for St. Somewhere to meet its target return on assets regardless of the change in circumstances acts against creating or maintaining a shared PHC identity. Employees have a certain affinity for the institution in which they work—they see it in operation day to day, and they know their fellow employees. Their affinity with the larger entity PHC is, in a sense, mediated through St. Somewhere.

How PHC and St. Somewhere interact helps shape the relationship that an individual employee at St. Somewhere has with PHC. It is difficult to imagine a more powerful message that one is *not* an integral part of the whole than that sent by PHC, which in effect says that St. Somewhere is on its own in terms of the consequences of this turn of events. Instead of communicating that all parts of PHC share in both the pain and the reward of joint operation, the message is that St. Somewhere simply stands alone.

If PHC asserts that St. Somewhere is an integral part of the overall organization, then to act ethically the board needs to take cognizance of the ethical implications of its decision. All of St. Somewhere's employees must be made aware of how the institution participates in a larger whole. In line with the ideals of subsidiarity, it may be appropriate to place the primary responsibility for meeting this economic challenge in the hands of St. Somewhere's managers. They are the ones closest to the delivery of health care services and are in the best position to assess which reductions best allow St. Somewhere to continue to deliver quality health care. If the authority to make allocation decisions is delegated to St. Somewhere, PHC must assure itself that such delegation does not harm the identity of the whole or violate its moral values.

A number of tactics can be adopted to accomplish this. First, PHC can educate employees about why it has been decided that despite reduced Medicaid reimbursement St. Somewhere is to be held responsible for meeting fiscal targets; PHC can help them understand how this decision fits within the mission and operation of the whole. Establishing a moral identity and educating associates about it is a way of respecting employees and helping to create and simultaneously serve the desired organizational identity.

Second, the board can adopt strategies to inform itself of the ethical consequences of reductions made at St. Somewhere and, in its deliberations, make a conscious effort to weigh the consequences against those of reductions that can be imposed on other parts of the organization to meet the shortfall. In an integrated system, a board that is seeking to support and sustain a coherent institutional identity and moral culture cannot isolate itself and consider only financial issues. There has to be a "moral accounting system" in place as well (Exhibit 9.1).

The exact nature of such a moral accounting system may vary.[2] Some authors have suggested that the system should be quantified to make it comparable to existing financial accounting systems and therefore easily understood by directors and administrators trained in quantitative financial analysis. But one can question the validity and value of such an effort. How one quantifies a value requires a judgment about that value. If properly presented, there is no reason to think that board members are any less qualified to make those judgments from the raw data of moral accounting (whatever form they take) than those who seek to interpret and quantify the data for them. The important point is to devise a system that gives directors relevant information about moral values and concerns as well as the usual financial and managerial information routinely presented to them.

Considering Social Context

PHC does not operate in isolation. The decisions it must make are grounded in the social context of modern American health care. Every action it takes—for example, how it allocates resources among many competing interests—can have consequences that touch many others. In making these socially consequential choices, PHC faces a basic moral stipulation: that these allocation decisions conform to the demands of distributive justice. Although there are many technical and theoretical formulations of this principle, in the simplest one distributive justice is an effort to determine whether the distribution of certain goods or services is fair.[3] However, the question is not just whether the transaction by which the consumer acquires the good or service is fair (did the consumer freely agree to the price paid?), but also whether such social or systemic factors as the nature of the good or service involved, or how it relates to other goods, alter our understanding of fairness. For

Exhibit 9.1. Values Audit and Accounting.

As the field of business and organizational ethics evolves, a number of thinkers have begun to highlight the need to make ethics visible within a system that traditionally relies upon financial principles as its unifying language. Ethicists have therefore adopted the language of audits and accounting as a means of bringing ethics into the discussion. These efforts come in various forms and involve a number of targets of concern.

Values Audit

A values audit attempts to identify the values held by an organization and its employees and how organizational values are communicated to the employees and to the public at large.[1] This requires, first, that an organization explicitly identify its values (in the mission statement or other forums) and second, that the organization review its policies and public statements to see how they relate to the organizational values and to test whether there is consistency among its various statements. Third, the organization engages employees in a discussion to seek their understanding of its values and their opinion as to how the values are being enacted in operations. (This is a way of understanding the informal culture of the organization.)

Once the initial audit has been completed, the organization can structure its values implementation effort to address existing discontinuity between espoused values and behavior, as well as rectify systemic obstruction to living out its values.

Social Accounting

A social accounting looks at the social values served or affected by an organization, directly or indirectly. This includes not only valuing the specific services offered but also looking at the impact of the organization's operation on the environment, on employment within a community, on affirmative action efforts, and other social goods. In health care, issues of public health, community service, and human relations all fit within this effort.

In carrying out a social accounting, the organization first identifies appropriate stakeholders—employees, funders, customers, media, community members, suppliers, and so on. With their participation, as needed and in various forums, the organization identifies its internal values, external objectives (what social goods it intends to address), and the values expected of it by others. The organization then attempts to measure its effectiveness, or effect on these goods, using financial auditing standards applied to nonfinancial information.[2]

Notes: 1. Trickett, D. "How to Use a Values Audit." *Training and Development,* Mar. 1997, *51,* 34–38.

2. See, for example, Raynard, P. "Coming Together: A Review of Contemporary Approaches to Social Accounting, Auditing, and Reporting in Non-Profit Organizations." *Journal of Business Ethics,* Oct. 1998, 7(13), 1471–1479.

example, poverty and historical patterns of discrimination are commonly recognized as impediments to fairness in distributing many social goods (including health care).

Health care services are subject to these demands of distributive justice. They are commonly defined as "social goods" because they involve socially important values (health) and also because they draw on social resources, including government funding for such things as medical research, medical education, and medical care and insurance. In addition, the medical market is regulated in such a way that medical services are not available simply according to market demand but according to socially determined needs. As such, a hospital has a certain social obligation in connection with delivering services. (See the discussion in Chapter Three.)

In terms of distributive justice, the drop in income from St. Somewhere represents a net loss to PHC. How the corporation meets that loss can affect others. If PHC elects to recoup the loss from other units in its system (perhaps the other hospitals), the recouping comes at the expense of programs, services, or benefits attributable to those other units. This may mean, for example, that Suburban Hospital has to reduce the services provided to its patients to cut costs. In essence, because the income is being diverted away from Suburban to cover the losses at St. Somewhere, Suburban's patrons subsidize the patients at St. Somewhere by losing services they would otherwise receive.

This fact mirrors a traditional form of medical resource allocation that has come under increasing criticism: the one in which hospitals charge paying customers (generally through their insurance company) higher fees for services as a way of underwriting costs of uninsured, nonpaying patients.[4] The criticism is that paying customers are being charged more than the value of the services they receive in order to benefit others, without their consent or participation in the allocation decision. Critics argue that to the extent such "uncompensated" costs are to be underwritten by others, government should subsidize them. The subsidy then becomes a cost to society as a whole, and those paying the costs (the taxpayers) have some say in how the program is formulated.

There is merit to this argument, but the PHC board can nonetheless justify, on two grounds, responding to St. Somewhere's revenue shortfall by redistributing income from elsewhere in the system. First, it may be that the claimed reduction in services paid for by patients at Suburban is illusory—Suburban's patients may be receiving more services than they actually pay for. Allocation among the member hospitals may reflect a historic decision that does not adequately account for the actual benefits received. For example, it may be that profits drawn from St. Somewhere were used to underwrite the acquisition of Suburban or certain development costs attributed to it. Corporations do not necessarily maintain detailed records of such events because they are not external; they simply represent the contribution of parts to the whole. Similarly, the reallocation in this case may be a form of compensation for past investment by St. Somewhere in Suburban.

Second, although it may be desirable for public health costs (such as covering uninsured patients) to be underwritten by the government, the system that is operative is a "mixed" economic system that blends public funds, not-for-profit contributions, and contributions expected from for-profit entities. This blended system depends on some level of corporate contribution that is drawn from this invisible medical surcharge on paying patients. The moral justification for shifting resources between St. Somewhere and Suburban is that all of the patients are part of the same community. It is an artificial distinction to assert that residence in any one community within a metropolitan area breaks the social and economic linkage with others in the same area. Absent governmental reform to rectify this situation, the board is justified in following this pattern.

Political Practice

Moreover, health care does not operate according to a pure market model. The government is an important participant in health care decision making. In dealing with the government, one does not simply "negotiate" with particular individual officials; rather, one participates in a political process that includes directly negotiating with administrative officials, lobbying legislators and executive officials, and forming political alliances or coalitions. PHC's allocation decisions can affect these negotiations.

In this case, the harm caused by the change in Medicaid reimbursement policy can be linked to a particular community. To the extent that the board elects to ameliorate the harm by allocating costs to the system as a whole, the board loses two political tools in its effort to lobby for change. First, because they become lost in the system as a whole, the effects of the policy are hidden from legislators and government officials. Instead of seeing a significant effect on the services offered by one hospital, regulators see a much less significant loss of services systemwide. Second, by ameliorating the harm to that community, the motivation for community action is eased, and the hospital loses a possible political ally.

Admittedly, this approach raises many troubling moral questions. It all too closely resembles an effort to hold a weak, relatively disenfranchised population (the poor) hostage for political purposes. To be justified, such an action requires both very severe provocation and commitment by PHC to undertake concerted action on behalf of those most severely affected by the change in Medicaid reimbursement.

Insofar as the Medicaid reduction is unreasonable and bad public policy, the board has an obligation to attempt to negotiate changes with Medicaid administrators (if it is an administrative change) and to lobby legislators and executive branch officials to alter this decision. It has a moral mandate for action. At the same time, PHC must act responsibly toward its patients within the community, ameliorating the harm caused by the Medicaid dispute whenever possible. To act responsibly, the board must recognize its responsibility to PHC to address this political problem not only in the short run but in the long run as well.

Summary

In evaluating the allocation decision, the board must consider more than the effect of the decision on individual patients and aspects of the organization's mission. The board must also consider how the decision affects the moral environment of the organization as a whole and how the decision relates to the larger social and political context within which it is made. Some basic questions must be asked:

1) What does this allocation of resources communicate about the values held by our organization?
2) What does it communicate about the nature of our organization and our relationships to associates and community (or communities)?

3) How does this resource allocation decision fit into and affect the broader social and political context of American health care?

These questions do not point to easy answers. Insofar as PHC elects to act as an administrative service organization for largely autonomous subunits, each subunit must have the autonomy to create and sustain its own moral environment. All involved employees, patients, and members of the larger community must consider PHC a secondary entity. If, however, PHC is thought of as the institutional leader of the system, it must seek to demonstrate moral leadership. It needs to be cognizant of the moral costs of its decisions and should communicate concern about the moral effect of the decisions to all involved, within and outside of the organization. Whereas in the end St. Somewhere may be forced to bear the brunt of sacrifice caused by this drop in income, the rationale for such a scenario should be clearly articulated within the context of the organization as a whole, lest the message be communicated that PHC is only concerned with the bottom line.

Cultural and Informal Systems Interaction

Strategic planning by a board of directors or senior management is based on a particular assessment of needs and certain assumptions about how those needs can and will be met. This includes assumptions about how employees comply with the directives of the strategic plan. In clinical health care, the fact that the employees or agents of the organization (doctors and nurses) are professionals who operate with a significant degree of autonomy and according to the ethical standards of their profession complicates the assumption of employee compliance. Implementing a strategic plan (a form of resource allocation) effectively requires that the leaders of the organization be cognizant of these alternative sources of authority and that the leaders find a way to engage them within the processes of planning and implementation.

> Dr. Alicia Kay, the medical director of St. Somewhere's intensive care unit, has a problem. The ICU has ten beds; they are all full, and she is beginning to receive calls from the floors requesting new admissions. Among the ten current

patients, three are appropriate candidates to be transferred to Hospice House, the St. Somewhere hospice unit. However, attending house staff disagree with this assessment of one of the patients (Patient A), and the private attending physicians for the other two (Patients B and C) have a well-known policy of refusing to refer their patients to hospice. Kay believes that Patient C, who is intubated and therefore cannot be sent to the floor, should undergo a terminal wean from life support.

According to the office of the general counsel, it is the policy of the hospital that in the absence of a valid advance directive a patient may not be removed from life support without a written order by the attending physician and the written consent of the patient's next of kin. In this case, neither the private attending physician nor the next of kin are willing to sign the consent form.

Finally, there is one patient who Kay does not believe is sick enough to be in the ICU. This is a private patient of Dr. Stanley, the head of the largest physicians' group associated with the hospital, who repeatedly has asked that her patient be allowed to stay "one more day" (her standard request until the day before a patient is released from the hospital).

In some ways, this is a classic case of clinical allocation: there is a limited resource (intensive care beds) and a demand that exceeds that resource. As with most hospitals, St. Somewhere's written policy is that all patients are subject to triage to assess their objective medical need for intensive care, and at the determination of the appropriate medical officer (in this case, Kay) patients can be refused admission or transferred out of the ICU. Nonetheless, there are some systemic impediments to implementing this policy fairly. These include the services mix, inadequate integration of services, a potentially flawed policy toward removal of life support systems, problems in the relationship among medical house staff and private medical personnel, and possible conflict of interest.

Mix of Services

Before examining individual patient allocation decisions, one must ask whether St. Somewhere has made adequate provision for its ICU. Does it have sufficient beds to meet service needs? The problem is that demand is elastic, and the question of estimating need is difficult. Research has shown that the more ICU beds available, the more they are filled.[5] However, ICU beds are extremely expensive, and it is wasteful to create more than are needed. To address the issue of legitimate need, St. Somewhere must implement a policy of ongoing assessment of use to take account of possible changes over time. It should also consider treatment options other than admission to the ICU, such as referral to hospice and creating ventilator-support facilities and intermediate care facilities.

Systems Integration

St. Somewhere was not created *de novo* according to a single, comprehensive plan. As is often the case, many features of the hospital evolved over time and were loosely incorporated into the system. The ICU was created in the early 1960s, though the hospice unit was not developed until 1997. It is unclear whether St. Somewhere's planning committee has ever considered the relationship between these two units.

St. Somewhere's managers could decide that the units should offer coordinated treatment and that those patients for whom hospice is appropriate should be encouraged to transfer into hospice. For example, Kay assumes that a hospice is better equipped to treat the terminally ill patient in terms of meeting that patient's physical, emotional, and spiritual needs than are the ICU and the wards. Moreover, she believes that to delay a patient's transfer to a hospice until the very end (as is often the case) prevents the patient (and the patient's family, who are also considered in the treatment plan) from receiving all the benefits of counseling and treatment extended by the hospice. In relation to her triage decision, complicating this issue for Kay is the fact that Hospice House has expertise in palliative care that is not available on the wards—indeed, Hospice House has expertise exceeding that available in the ICU. Yet in a comparison between the wards and the ICU, the latter offers better palliative care (strictly in terms of pain management) than the wards.

In considering the hospice option, the administrative staff add that there is increasing pressure from Medicare and other funding sources to reduce excess treatment of a terminally ill patient in a critical care setting. Hospice can meet the needs of those who are terminally ill at a far lower cost than that incurred in the ICU.[6]

The stumbling block for Kay is that transfer to Hospice House requires the consent of both the treating physician and the patient's family. Here the physicians involved have refused to authorize such a transfer. Particularly striking is the fact that the two private physicians have a well-known policy of refusing to transfer their patients to hospice. Why is that?

In discussing transfer decisions with people working in a hospice, one hears a number of reasons for this all-too-frequent phenomenon. For some, the culture of medicine trains doctors to think of death as a failure, and the decision to transfer a patient to hospice is to admit that there is nothing more that medicine can do for the patient. Finally, there is some concern that if a doctor transfers a patient to hospice, the physician loses the right to continue caring for the patient (significantly, as is often suggested on the wards, they fear that they will lose the fees involved).

If St. Somewhere thinks that hospice offers more appropriate (and even better) care, it needs to find a way to address this type of potential resistance. It can do this in a number of ways, perhaps by developing educational programs to address the points of resistance. The simplest to address is, of course, the fact that a transfer to hospice does not terminate the primary care physician's relationship with a patient. That relationship can—indeed, should—continue. To overcome physicians' fear of failure and to understand hospice care as an alternative form of treatment (as opposed to nontreatment) requires a strong effort to lead physicians to a new way of thinking about death.

It may also be possible to influence this process through a change in medical record keeping whereby any member of the hospital staff (including nurses, who are frequently identified by hospice personnel as being a good source of referrals) can enter a notation in the medical record that a patient is suited for transfer to a hospice. The attending physician can then be required to answer the notation with a written justification for continuing treatment in the ICU or on the wards. Although a physician who is ideologically opposed to hospice care can still resist transfer, he must be willing to put his concerns in writing, where they are subject to review by the medical records committee.

Many hospitals seek to control ICU use through triage. As medical director, Kay can be empowered to assess the appropriateness of each patient to receive ICU care and to transfer (or refuse to admit) patients not deemed appropriate for ICU. This power can be used coercively to push patients toward hospice. Assuming that hospice is a better alternative than transfer back to the floor, it might force doctors and their patients to accept a transfer to Hospice House.

However, there are a number of significant problems with this approach. First, it does not offer the opportunity to truly educate the doctors involved about the virtues of hospice. Second, it does not facilitate good patient care planning. It may not allow patients adequate time to talk about the possibility of transferring to hospice. Finally, it ignores the possibility that the physicians who disagree with the ICU director's assessment may not be motivated by bias against hospice but instead honestly disagree on what the best clinical care for this patient is. Given that prognosis is not an exact science and hospice care requires a prognosis of less than six months to live, this is a serious concern. But unless the overall bias against hospice is addressed, Kay cannot be sure of the role that bias (as opposed to differing professional judgment) plays in an individual decision.

In short, as St. Somewhere makes its needs assessment and allocation decisions on critical care beds according to an understanding that ICU and hospice are both integral elements in meeting patients' needs, it must implement the systemic changes necessary to assure that these services are integrated in practice.

Termination of Life Support Policy

The resource allocation decision can also be affected by policy that is inadequately thought out with respect to the implications for resource utilization. For Patient C, who is on life support, the policy on withdrawal creates a question about who controls continuing expenditure of ICU resources. If there is a clearly terminal prognosis where death is simply being delayed by life support, who should decide whether to continue to expend ICU resources (including allowing a patient to remain in a needed ICU bed)?

The policy put forward by the general counsel's office, which requires the signed consent of the attending physician and family, is legally very conservative. As a prophylactic measure against a possible lawsuit, it is understandable. But is it morally justified? Such an extreme position is not required by law in most states.[7] Moreover, with respect to the physicians who have refused to issue removal orders, are they refusing out of concern for the accuracy of the diagnosis, out of personal moral concern about removing life support, or out of their own fear of legal liability? Regarding this last concern, the conservative nature of St. Somewhere's policy may in fact contribute, consciously or unconsciously, to the doctors' resistance to discontinuing treatment.

It is often easier to refuse to put a patient on life support for medical reasons than it is to remove the patient from life support once it has been initiated. Yet ethically the two decisions are not that different. The St. Somewhere policy narrowly focuses on the issue of consent to treatment (which includes the concept of refusal of treatment) as a way of defining treatment options. Consent is clearly an important ethical concern, but most experts agree it is also necessary to consider the appropriate goals of treatment and the utilization of resources necessary to achieve those goals.

A comprehensive policy statement differentiates among these values. In terms of consent, the policy identifies the role of individual patient consent, the role of advance directives, and the role of the family. With regard to the family, the policy can determine whether the hospital is seeking the family's consent as representative of the patient's wishes (in other words, asking the family to exercise substituted judgment) or as a way of eliciting and acknowledging the family's own values (their desire to keep their family member alive "no matter what"). A policy should suggest how each interest is to be valued.

At the same time, a truly comprehensive policy identifies the role of medical judgment in the treatment decision, as well as what criteria may be used in a decision that does not necessarily follow the wishes of the family. With respect to this latter concern, there may be considerable variation from one jurisdiction to another, resulting from differences in state law. It is important to clarify the level of medical discretion allowed within the context of the law. With such clarification in hand, St. Somewhere is in a better position to address the practice standards of its physicians, whose decisions may be based more on legal than on medical concerns.[8]

Moreover, by focusing attention on the appropriate goals of treatment, this type of policy may facilitate negotiation with a patient's family regarding any qualms they have about the appropriate course of treatment. Instead of talking about removal of life support, the discussion can focus on the less emotion-laden concept of appropriate treatment and the objectives of that treatment when there is no hope of recovery.

House Staff Versus Private Attending Physicians

A resource allocation decision can also be influenced by the informal culture of the organization. As suggested by the natural systems theory of organizations (discussed in Chapter Two), groups of employees—especially those sharing a particular professional identity—tend to create informal decision-making systems that vary from the official procedures of the hierarchical, rational system. One bit of hallway wisdom in health care holds that if you want to get something done or want information, go to the nurse, not the doctor.

In this case, Dr. Kay's concern is the difference between staff physicians and private physicians. There is no written policy at St. Somewhere privileging private physicians, but Kay cannot avoid being aware that they are commonly accorded a high level of deference. Historically, they have been a primary source of admissions for hospitals.[9] They are therefore courted by hospitals and given a wide degree of autonomy and privilege.

Given this culture of deference, it is not surprising to find that with respect to the three patients appropriate for hospice (A, B, and C), Kay may be more inclined to attempt to persuade the staff physicians who express doubt about the appropriateness of transferring patient A to Hospice House than to approach the private physicians of patients B and C. Yet the staff physicians stand on firmer ground medically in that there is disagreement about prognosis. The difficulty with Stanley, whose patient is suitable for transfer back to a ward but who heads the largest physicians' group, is politically problematic because Stanley is arguably more important economically to St. Somewhere as a source of patient referrals than are the other private physicians.

It is unrealistic for the administrators of St. Somewhere to expect Kay to address this issue on her own; nor can a simple written statement of policy address it. Employees often assume the difference between "real politics" and paper policies. To address this problem, St. Somewhere's administrators need to find a way to genuinely involve the private physicians in policy making and to obtain commitment from them to abide by the decisions that are made.

One policy change that might be effective here is to modify the medical records requirement to include an entry of a medical challenge (a statement from a staff person questioning whether continued treatment in the ICU is appropriate), which requires that the attending physician enter a response justifying his or her request for continued treatment. These justifications are then subject to review by the medical records committee. This approach engages both formal procedures of decision making and informal cultural practices. Formally, it is general practice in health care that a medical policy decision, whether on the basis of individual review or policy, is made by a medical committee. Informally, making a doctor's behavior subject to peer review brings to bear the force of the informal culture of doctors and the power of peer opinion. Doctors do not want to look bad in the eyes of their fellow physicians.

Summary

Questions about resource allocation, such as that of ICU beds, require coordination and integration among a large number of individuals, programs, cultural norms, and institutional policies. These decisions, a form of rationing, must be made systemically or else the decisions made may be distorted by factors such as the informal culture of the institution or incompletely thought-out policies. Patients might then receive substantially different treatment according to who their doctors happen to be, who they are related to, and whether a certain treatment has or has not been initiated.

To ensure that decisions are well coordinated and that all patients are treated fairly, the health care organization can consider adopting these practices:

1. *Systemic services review.* This is an effort to review the total mix of services offered by the organization and the allocation of resources among them, and to determine how they interrelate.
2. *Education.* The organization then needs to educate staff about the relationship between services and methods of allocation.

Simple promulgation of written policies is not enough to change institutional behavior. To effect change requires active educational engagement.

3. *Policy reform.* The organization also generally has to review the effect clinical policies have on allocation decisions and modify those policies that unintentionally restrict resources.

4. *Engage the informal culture.* The organization may need to find a way to draw on the strength of its informal culture to support institutional goals. This can involve the cultural group in decision making, planning, and "public" review of practices.

In all cases, what is required is sensitivity to the fact that the system, its historic evolution, and its cultural components can have a profound (although often unarticulated) effect on allocation decision making.

Communicating Values Within the Culture

An allocation decision about an apparently routine business matter can have significant ethical ramifications for other areas of the organization. The challenge is how to bring ethical concerns to the table at the time the initial decision is made and to continue being open to those ethical concerns as the business plan evolves.

Four years ago, with great fanfare, PHC announced a five-year plan to update its information processing capacity by developing an integrated network, making workstations widely available, integrating financial and patient care files to provide better service to its patients, and making its operations more streamlined and efficient. As the head of information systems for St. Somewhere, Alma Reis has a number of problems. First, despite her complaints at meetings of the information systems working group that expanding availability of workstations and consolidating patient records present a risk to the confidentiality and security of those records, the committee was unable to adequately address those concerns prior to implementing the system.

The seriousness of this problem has been brought home at the last working group meeting, when it was revealed that the records of two patients who were coded DNR did not reflect that fact, although the records of two others not so coded indicated that they were. At another hospital, the financial records of four patients were, intentionally or unintentionally, significantly altered.

Finally, at St. Somewhere, Reis overhears a lunchtime conversation about a professional sports star being diagnosed and treated for AIDS at Suburban Hospital. On investigation, she discovers that the source of this information is variously identified as a part-time nurse or a clerk in the finance department.

Although the implementation schedule is rigorously adhered to, Alma has lost four members of her staff whom she has not been able to replace thanks to a hiring freeze at St. Somewhere. Her staff likes and respects her and works very hard for her, but overall morale is poor. She fears losing additional staff because of complaints of overwork and a feeling that their work is not appreciated. Adding insult to injury, two of the staff who left went to Suburban Hospital, a facility acquired by PHC two years previously that does not have a hiring freeze and whose pay scale for comparable positions is significantly higher than that offered at St. Somewhere.

Most of the ethical problems in this situation can be traced back to inadequate attention to resource allocation over the course of this computerization project. The problems are not linked only to the project, however. They are affected by failure to attend to larger systemic concerns as well, and they raise three sets of issues: expression of values, coordination of resources with values, and fair treatment of employees.

Expression of Values

How an organization chooses to expend its resources is a powerful statement about its values. PHC has identified the modernization and integration of its information processing systems as an important company objective that is intended to advance commitment to high-quality patient care and to enhance its operating efficiency. Both of these are strong corporate moral values, the first in terms of the mission to serve the public and the second in relation to the duty of stewardship or financial responsibility to the organization. Achieving this objective requires systemwide compliance, primarily because of the need to centralize much of the financial data, but PHC administrators have failed to ensure that adequate resources are made available to achieve this result.

They have allowed discrepancies to develop in various units. For example, during development of the system, the necessary resources were cut back. As a result, staff are being overworked, and they also feel unappreciated. PHC is not supporting its ostensible commitment to improved information systems with appropriate financial resources.

This failure has a number of adverse consequences. First, employees may be led to distrust PHC's public declarations. Although it has announced the importance of this computer enhancement program, actions do not live up to the words. Second, PHC's failure to respond to Reis's complaints gives her, and those members of her staff who are aware of her objections, the message that the organization does not value their concerns. That the staff feel overworked further exacerbates the situation. In both instances, the allocation decisions seem to contradict the values the organization professes.

Coordination of Values

To advance the moral mission of the organization, the means of monitoring adherence to certain moral standards must be built into the process of resource allocation. In this case, PHC has failed to make appropriate allocations of material and human resources to address ethical concerns arising out of the computerization program. PHC failed to incorporate a review of ethical concerns in its initial development process, and despite the fact that Reis raised concerns over security and privacy after the initiation of the project, the system then failed to make adjustments to allocation plans when concerns arose during implementation. Here, issues of privacy and security have significant moral implication, including the risks of mistreating patients, causing financial losses, and violating patient confidentiality.

Written records carry inherent limitations on what information is available to whom. In the past, financial professionals dealt with financial records; medical staff dealt with medical records. Integrating records and expanding information resources means more people have access to that information. Therefore, many employees who now have access to information undoubtedly lack the necessary background to appreciate the unique ethical and legal concerns hitherto the province of limited groups of professionals. Employees need training to help guide them in dealing with the additional kinds of information—and ethical concerns—to which they now have access.

These concerns could be addressed in a number of ways. Technical safeguards limit access only to authorized people, but it would probably take additional time and labor to develop them. Perhaps more important, the organization could implement appropriate employee training not only to ensure that staff understand how to operate the equipment and enter data but also to train them to respect patient privacy and the confidentiality of patient records. (This type of educational requirement is, in essence, demanded both by JCAHO and by corporate compliance laws.)

Fair Treatment of Employees

This case also reveals an insight afforded by close attention to resource distribution. Tracing resource allocation across a large system may reveal ethical discrepancies not readily apparent in looking at an isolated unit within the system. For example, if PHC considers itself a single, integrated entity, then it has a direct relationship with each employee. This in turn raises moral concern about treating employees fairly and equitably. Is it fair or equitable that employees holding essentially identical positions receive different treatment or compensation simply because they work in one location within PHC rather than another?

This differential is not intentional; it is at least in part an accident of the organization's history. Like many integrated health care systems, PHC is a composite entity created out of the merger or acquisition of a number of formerly independent (or differently affiliated) entities. It has hospitals and other organizational units that are based in a variety of socioeconomic settings, from inner-city hospitals such as St. Somewhere to hospitals operating in affluent suburban areas, such as Suburban. It is easy to understand how pay scales and working conditions came to vary across PHC's operating units. In its corporate mission statement, however, PHC asserts that its associates are the most important assets and that it is committed to treating them fairly and equitably. There appears to be a contradiction between this statement and the experience of the staff.

The contradiction may be one of appearance only. If PHC operates according to a decentralized self-understanding, then employee affiliation may be more closely linked to a particular unit (say, a hospital) than to the whole. Because one cannot judge in solely financial terms the employee benefits conferred by work, fairness may also entail considering what each unit uniquely offers its employees. For example, it is not uncommon for employees in charitable, inner-city hospitals to accept lower salaries because they are committed to the hospital's mission to serve the poor in the community. The challenge for PHC, therefore, is to determine what its relationship is and should be to each employee and to act consistently in that regard.

Summary

For the most part, specific operational needs ground a resource allocation decision. However, each decision can and often does touch on a number of other considerations. First, a decision about what resources to make available and how they are used can tacitly express values that either sustain or are at odds with the organization's professed mission values. The organization needs to be aware of this expressive function in making decisions. Second, too narrow a focus on operating activity in making an allocation decision can provoke ethical problems. Reflecting on potential ethical concerns and being open to employee concerns raised by an allocation decision are two of the ways this problem may be addressed. Finally, tracing the flow of resources through an organization can produce valuable insight about systemic problems that might not otherwise be apparent.

Conclusion

How an organization chooses to allocate resources (financial, material, and human) has a profound effect on its moral and ethical culture and its standing within the community. Such decisions are a compelling expression of where commitments actually lie; if a resource allocation decision does not sustain a commitment professed in the organization's mission, written documents become illusory.

Organization leaders will want to consider certain features of resource allocation questions and procedures:

1. *Identify with values.* Does the resource allocation decision correspond with the values of our organization? To assess this, the

organization needs to define its values so as to clearly express how they are to be put into action. Among these values are the institution's own identity—self-perception and relationships with employees, subsidiary operating units, and the community as a whole.

2. *Coordinate adherence with values.* How does this allocation decision affect other values or operations within our organization? Processes and procedures may need to be modified or developed to ensure that decisions reflect organizational values throughout implementation, by means of such mechanisms as an ethical accounting and tracking system.

3. *Integrate resources.* How do the various units within our organization relate to each other? Ethical problems arise when there is incomplete integration of services or operations. Tracking resource use can serve to identify these gaps.

4. *Identify cultural influences and impediments.* What are the values held by the employees of our organization, and how are they being expressed? How do those values relate to the articulated values of the organization? Tracking resource use can also identify informal cultural systems that impair or alter organizational goals and objectives. Once identified, methods such as educational programs can be developed to use these cultures in support of organizational goals.

5. *Review and reform policies and procedures.* What effect do general policies have on particular use of resources? Policies and procedures that are ostensibly distinguishable from resource allocation decision making can nonetheless profoundly affect the decisions. These unintended effects cannot be addressed until they have been identified.

Although not exhaustive, this list should bring general direction to addressing concerns about systemic issues relating to resource allocation.

Notes

1. Grisez, G. *Living a Christian Life.* Quincy, Ill.: Franciscan, 1993.
2. See, for example, Zadek, S. "Balancing Performance, Ethics, and Accountability." *Journal of Business Ethics,* Oct. 1998, *17*(13), 1421–1441.
3. See, for example, Rawls, J. *A Theory of Justice.* Cambridge, Mass.: Harvard University, 1971.

4. Mann, J. M., Melnick, G. A., Bamezai, A., and Zwanziger, J. "A Profile of Uncompensated Hospital Care, 1983–1995." *Health Affairs,* 1997, *16*(4), 223–225.

5. Zussman, R. *Intensive Care: Medical Ethics and the Medical Profession.* Chicago: University of Chicago, 1992.

6. Murphy, D. J. "The Economics of Futile Interventions." In M. B. Zucker and H. D. Zucker (eds.), *Medical Futility and the Evaluation of Life-Sustaining Interventions.* New York: Cambridge University, 1997.

7. Prip, W., and Moretti, A. "Medical Futility: A Legal Perspective." In Zucker and Zucker (1997).

8. Carlton, W. *"In Our Professional Opinion . . .": The Primacy of Clinical Judgment over Moral Choice.* Notre Dame, Ind.: University of Notre Dame, 1979.

9. Starr, P. *The Social Transformation of American Medicine.* New York: Basic Books, 1984.

Chapter Ten

Mission and the Bottom Line

The proper relationship between delivery of health care and profitability is the most fundamental question in health care organizational ethics. Every act of an organization has a measurable cost and some effect on financial affairs. Yet many people fear that whenever consideration of the bottom line enters into a discussion within a health care organization, all other values are forced to give way—or that ethics is co-opted and used simply to justify pursuit of profit. The question of profitability in health care becomes so controversial that many health care organizations do not address it forthrightly, as if ethics, practice, and the bottom line could be cleanly separated. Whether because they share the suspicion that questions of profitability are ethically tainted or because they are concerned for the organization's public image in a climate of suspicion, leaders of health care institutions are hesitant to explicitly confront the relationship between their responsibility for the financial health of the organization and its mission to care for the sick and injured.

Nonetheless, the question must be asked and answered. Health care in the United States is delivered in the context of a free-market economy, and any institution that fails to be cognizant of this will not survive long. The leaders of a health care organization must find a proper balance between the bottom line and other values it may hold. To do this, they have to answer some questions:

- What is the purpose (or mission) of our organization?
- How do the organization's actions advance (or impede) that purpose?

- How can multiple missions be integrated?
- How should individuals within our organization serve its mission(s)?

The effort to create an ethical organization, one that moves beyond the suspicion that profit trumps ethical values, requires that everyone know the answers to these questions.

The Question of Mission

Anyone attempting to analyze the place of profitability in the ethical life of a health care organization must begin with the question of purpose or mission.[1] One must understand what the institution believes its mission to be and develop criteria to assess the adequacy of the stated mission in shaping the ethical life of the institution and meeting its social obligations.

Every health care institution articulates its mission in some way, as part of the articles of incorporation, as a statement of philosophy, or in a document specifically identified as a mission statement.[2] Although these sources may identify some aspects of the mission, they are generally couched in vague language and fail to offer sufficient guidance for making day-to-day decisions about how to deliver health care. Or a mission statement may be morally flawed, failing to recognize that the organization has moral obligations beyond simply rendering competent, compensated services. It is vital, therefore, to develop a general understanding of mission by which to evaluate the mission statement.

The nature of an effective health care organization presents a model for assessing the mission statement. Three primary features define a health care mission: provision of quality care, service to the community, and assurance of adequate resources.

Providing Quality Health Care Services

The first element of mission is almost universally agreed upon; obviously, it does no one any good to deliver inferior health care. No institution can promise to deliver perfect care, but it is clearly desirable to deliver the best care possible under the prevailing conditions.[3]

Community Service

Health care is not delivered in a vacuum, nor to a theoretical patient. The institution is situated in a particular community and is licensed to serve that community, much the way a doctor or lawyer is licensed to offer his or her professional services. In exchange, it is reasonable to demand that the privilege be exercised competently and ethically, in furtherance of the identified social good to be served. In health care this includes not only offering competent patient care but also adequately serving the needs of the community in which the institution is located. Although an organization can voluntarily expand its understanding of obligation to the community—for example, by committing especially to render services to the poor—all organizations have some obligation to their community. The parameters of this baseline obligation depend on the community being served and the rigor demanded by (and benefit conferred within) the licensing privilege. For instance, the more rigorously the licensing system limits competition by decreeing the number of beds in a particular market, the stronger the obligation imposed on those granted the privilege of operating any of those beds to serve the needs of the community fairly.

Securing Adequate Resources

Although many people question the appropriateness of profit making in health care,[4] a health care organization must be able to marshal sufficient human and material resources to provide quality care to meet the needs of its community. Delivering health care requires the cooperation of many people and allocation of significant resources.[5] To accomplish it requires certain organizational structures, and in a market economy a system of exchange that can support those structures. The reality is that to provide health care services the contemporary health care organization must bring in enough money to survive. Failure to acknowledge this economic need as a legitimate part of the mission may do little more than repress or "hide" this agenda.[6]

The real moral question for a health care organization is not the issue of making a profit but rather determining what *level* of profit can appropriately be earned by a not-for-profit or for-profit

organization. A prominent argument, popularized by Milton Friedman and other free-market economists, is that the role of the business corporation is solely to maximize its profits—it has no moral
duty other than what it owes shareholders in return for their investment in it.[7] Ignoring this duty harms the institution (by impairing
its ability to raise capital) and its investors (by reducing the value of
their investment and the income they expect to earn from it).

Whereas a for-profit corporation does have a legitimate moral
duty to its shareholders, the idea that this is its only social responsibility has come under attack in recent years.[8] The rationale of this
attack is particularly appropriate in regard to health care: health
care managers do have a moral duty to earn a profit appropriate
to the nature of the institution, but they also have a duty to manage the organization in compliance with the moral obligations em-
bodied in its mission.

Other Obligations

As argued in Chapter One, an organization is a moral being with
moral responsibilities that must be met in carrying out its mission.
Because organizational ethics is concerned with means as well as
ends, creating an organization for delivery of health care services
entails further moral concerns about how it is structured and how
it functions. This generates four obligations an organization owes,
to its employees, the community it serves, and the society of which
it is a part.

First, the institution must treat its staff members with respect.
It operates through the efforts of employees or agents. A utilitar-
ian argument that how an organization treats its staff affects how
the staff in turn treat patients is plausible, but it seems an inadequate understanding of the relationship between a *health care* organization and its staff. In the language of Immanuel Kant, we have
a duty to treat individuals "not merely as means, but also as ends
in themselves." People are not simply to be used as tools to reach
certain goals. They ought to be treated as individuals deserving of
respect in and of themselves. (See Chapter Eight for full discussion
of this relationship.)

Second, the organization must offer the staff constructive work.
Descriptively, of course, a health care organization gives personnel

gainful employment. Morally, concern about providing employment opportunities in the neighborhood and avoiding layoffs are therefore legitimate considerations for the organization. There is, however, a deeper moral dimension to the employment relationship. Humans are social animals for whom *constructive* work is a positive good[9]—not simply as an opportunity to earn a living, but as a chance to engage in a productive task. In health care, this moral concern is reflected in an institution's effort to recognize both the role of every employee in fulfilling the mission and the sacrifices that are sometimes made by employees to advance that mission.

Third, the organization must abide by the basic moral rules of society. An institution has an identity independent of its individual staff members. There is a general expectation that all citizens behave morally. Insofar as they undertake public duty and responsibility, individuals are expected to carry out those tasks in the manner promised. Because the health care institution is recognized as a citizen with legal standing (which, as a corporation, it is), one reasonably expects it to live up to the standards with which the organization identifies itself. By law we recognize the right of an institution to enter into contracts, to perform certain services, and to possess certain rights (such as limited free speech). We therefore expect an organization to behave ethically. It must, for example, act with honesty, integrity, and fairness in dealing with others (including its staff).

Fourth, the organization ought to be a responsible institutional citizen. A health care institution is a powerful presence in society. In licensing a health care institution, the state is granting it a place in the vital social service of delivering health care. By accepting the licensure, the institution is arguably accepting the duties that come with this powerful position. Moreover, the organization functions as a mediating institution within our society. Health care organizations are charged with performing essential social functions, and they are also the means by which a democratic society assesses social needs.[10] This includes an advocacy role to inform other elements of society (such as government entities) about the needs of the community the institution serves and to identify appropriate strategies to meet those needs.

The obligations we impose on a health care institution may be greater than what we might expect of an individual. Although society has an ethical expectation that doctors render some public service, there has been some hesitation about legislatively mandating that they do so individually. Instead, doctors have elected to fulfill this obligation collectively through their medical societies as well as through individuals voluntarily acting on behalf of the community of doctors. One might question the adequacy of this effort, but the idea that doctors have a greater duty as a profession than as individuals can be justified. An individual doctor can have only a limited impact on society; doctors as a group are extremely powerful. This supports the principle that the profession is obligated to society. A health care institution is an organizational expression of this profession. It receives the social benefit accorded to the profession (the right to provide health care services) and is a social organization through which the practice of medicine is carried out. It thus shares in the professional's obligation of citizenship in the community.

To say that an organization has other relevant goals does not, of course, determine the weight these goals should have in institutional decision making. This particular balance depends on what criteria justify the competing goals. Surviving in the health care marketplace is crucial to meeting organizational goals and fulfilling institutional mission. But the profit incentive must be balanced with the obligations undertaken by the institution in pursuing the profit motive.

In the context of weighing the competing values of the organization, creating a moral culture within the organization may be a value in and of itself. Any decision that ignores the moral dimension of the mission or violates generally applicable moral standards can be considered harmful to the organization. It can damage the moral culture of the institution itself by conveying the message that ethical values are not important. In this regard, creating a moral organization is "good for business."[11, 12] Being good for business is not a moral ground in and of itself, but the manager's responsibility to the organization and its stakeholders must include a duty to consider the moral dimensions of every decision. Moreover, it may be argued that, particularly in respect to health care, maintaining a good moral culture is a necessary condition for providing good patient care.

Mission in Action

Let's revisit the scenario described in Chapter Nine.

> St. Somewhere is a general tertiary care hospital serving a diverse population. At the beginning of the first quarter of St. Somewhere's fiscal year, Medicaid announces that it is reducing its reimbursement schedule for a particular class of illness by 25 percent. On reviewing the records, the administrators of St. Somewhere discover that those illnesses have historically accounted for 30 percent of the hospital's revenues. Shortly after this, the board of Partnership Health Care, the integrated health care delivery system of which St. Somewhere is a part, announces that despite this change, the hospital is expected to meet its projected return on assets, the method PHC uses to evaluate profitability.

The administrators of St. Somewhere are caught between the seemingly irreconcilable demands of Medicaid to reduce costs on the one hand, and of the board of directors to maintain the projected level of income on the other. They are being challenged to evaluate the role of profitability in relation to the mission of the organization.

Setting the Stage: The Role of Upper Management

Senior management and the board of directors are the principle leaders in determining the role of the bottom line in the life of an organization. They define the mission and set the projected budgets that determine the general scope and nature of operations. The ethical significance of these determinations is rarely considered in the budgeting process. Although budgets may change, they often do so incrementally such that the effects of the change can be obscured by compensating efforts on the part of operational managers attempting to make do with the budgets they are given. It is only when confronted by dramatic and abrupt change in financial circumstances that many leaders first face the challenge of choosing among competing values within the limits imposed by the organization's financial constraints.

In confronting the dramatic change in circumstances created for St. Somewhere by lower Medicaid reimbursements, senior management must answer the second and third of the questions on organizational ethics that we posed at the beginning of this chapter: How do an organization's actions advance (or impede) its mission? How can the multiple missions of an organization be integrated in the event of conflict?

Two events have precipitated the conflict faced by St. Somewhere and its board: reduction of Medicaid reimbursement for the covered procedure, and the board decision to maintain expectations regarding the hospital's return on assets. There are significant moral problems in any attempt to resolve this dilemma, but at the outset it may be suggested that the real moral problem in this situation is Medicaid's payment decision.

We suggested, under the general description of the components of the mission of a health care organization, that PHC and St. Somewhere are institutional citizens of their community. As such, it is within the moral compass of their mission to evaluate the morality of the government's acts. In this case, because the government has undertaken the obligation of providing recipients of Medicaid with appropriate health care, the government should be expected to live up to that obligation. If its reimbursement policies do not fairly compensate providers for the services they render, then the government is in effect attempting to shift this obligation onto the shoulders of providers. As institutional citizens, PHC and St. Somewhere can be said to have an obligation to seek to alter this decision. It is within their mission to advocate for change, not simply to passively accept it.

Of course, PHC must confront the situation as given. It does not control government programs, and even if it can successfully lobby for change, that change is probably going to take time to effect. Thus what is of initial interest here is the *institutional* decision, the board's insistence that management of St. Somewhere meet its targeted return on assets. If we agree that this mandate by the board is immoral, then all of the decisions that flow from it are tainted.

Making a profit is not morally objectionable; however, profit cannot be the only criterion to be considered. In addition to monitoring the financial performance of St. Somewhere, the board should seek information about the impact its decision has on the institution's responsibility to the public and patient care, and how the decision relates to the overall mission and culture of the organization. In this case, the board has failed to do so. It has reiterated its position on the projected return on investment without explicitly addressing—or even soliciting—additional information about the impact of the decision.

At the same time, the board is concerned with the mission and economic viability of the whole system. This decision may be one of necessity. For example, St. Somewhere could be losing money, and the board might make its decision based on the fact that it cannot afford to underwrite additional losses without harming the other institutions within PHC. Or PHC may need to meet particular performance targets as part of the financing agreement(s) it has with certain banks or else face the prospect of losing access to necessary credit (or seeing its cost of credit increased). This in turn can lead to additional cuts in service throughout the system. These systemwide needs may reasonably lead the board to conclude that it is justified in this position because the needs are directly related to the mission of the organization. By contrast, if this determination rests simply on the desire to meet a basic financial target—linked, for example, to industry averages—one could say that its decision-making process is morally flawed because it fails to attend to the other dimensions of the organizational mission.

Middle Managers as Moral Decision Makers

An approach that views the organization solely through the lens of hierarchical, rational systems theory (in other words, where the organization is understood solely according to formal structure and management) might judge the board's decision making according to standards defined by the role of the board member, while lower management is judged according to its role as lower management. In such an approach, it might be argued that the sole moral responsibility of lower management (St. Somewhere's administrators) is to do their best while adhering to the demands of the board—an admittedly vague proposal.

Natural systems and open systems theories may offer a more holistic understanding of organizational ethics (see Chapter Two). Recognizing the role of culture and informal structures in guiding behavior, or the role of the environment within which the organization operates, suggests that all levels of management have a similar, shared role in creating and maintaining the ethical culture of an organization. Although each manager may perform his or her own tasks, they must share basic understanding of the mission of the organization and commitment to support the mission within their individual roles.

According to this holistic approach, in making decisions necessary to achieve the financial bottom line a manager or the management committee of St. Somewhere must be cognizant of the same ethical criteria that impinge on the board's decision. That is, a manager must be sensitive to how financially motivated decisions affect the health care institution's public obligations, moral culture, and mission. This managerial obligation runs in two directions: back toward the board, and out through the organization.

With respect to the board, just as profits and financial returns are not the sole moral duty of the institution, so too a manager's obligation to the institution is not limited to meeting financial expectations and reporting returns. Although the manager has financial responsibilities that must be adhered to, she or he also has a duty to report morally consequential results to the board. To make an adequate moral judgment, the board must have information about the effect of its financial decisions on the mission and culture of the organization. Every manager, having the greatest access to specific information, should attempt to convey it to her or his own manager or the board.

With respect to the organization, one of the challenges of organizational ethics is to bring to light how managers participate in formulating mission and creating the informal culture of the organization so that they are conscious of their role in this process. The manager's understanding of mission can then serve as a guide in considering the available alternatives—and their consequences.

Alternatives and Consequences

Assuming for the moment that the board's financial expectation is reasonable and ethical, how should the manager or management committee seek to achieve the goal? One might suggest a number of responses, each of which must be evaluated according to its consequences for those who have an interest in how the dilemma is resolved. Here are some possibilities:

1. *Change the patient mix.* St. Somewhere might change the mix of patients being treated by reducing the number of Medicaid patients it admits and seeking other, more profitable patients. But what happens to those Medicaid patients? St. Somewhere may be the only hospital serving this community. If it is not, undoubtedly the other hospitals are also considering changing their patient mix for the same financial reasons. Given that the mission of a health care institution includes a duty to help meet the health care needs of the community, refusing to care for these individuals clearly fails to meet this duty.

Moreover, turning away from the needs of this patient group may risk the moral culture of the hospital itself. Instead of supporting a self-identity that is linked with good moral care, such a decision communicates to the staff and the community a sense that financial goals supersede concern for individual patients.

2. *Reduce waste.* This clearly is morally the least objectionable course. It is a moral duty of all managers to avoid wasting the assets placed under their care; the difficulty is in finding expenses that are wasteful. Expenses are incurred and authorized because they are thought to advance the mission of the institution. Absent fraud or abuse, identifying waste is most frequently a question of allocating resources among competing goods for the institution. Identifying and reducing wasteful expenditures may be especially difficult given the health care environment of the last few years. Extensive efforts have been made to eliminate waste, and though it has never been an overwhelmingly large amount, there is probably less waste to be found today than ever. Surely not enough to meet a 7.5 percent drop in revenue.

3. *Reduce or eliminate nonessential functions.* Again, this is a question of resource allocation. What is an essential function? Is it defined simply by the needs of direct patient care? The understanding of mission that we presented earlier argues that maintaining an effective organization is also a legitimate value. Are accounting and information processing essential functions? The institution would not survive without them. Are marketing and advertising? The institution's long-term viability may depend on public awareness.

4. *Reduce capital expenditures.* St. Somewhere has a variety of budgeted capital expenditures directed toward upgrading medical and support equipment, building repairs, and maintenance. Because these represent large sums of money, the manager or management

committee can elect to defer these expenditures. Such deferrals may be necessary at times, but they do not address the underlying problem. In this case, there is no indication that Medicaid will reverse its decision in the next fiscal year. Moreover, capital expenditure represents necessary investment in the future of the institution. It clearly breaches a manager's moral duty to maintain the organization and provide quality care if he or she allows the physical facilities of St. Somewhere to deteriorate. Management should not sacrifice the future viability of the organization to reach short-term objectives.

5. *Reduce or restructure staff.* There are a variety of ethical problems involved in downsizing, a popular path in recent years, among them the organization's duty to its employees, the problem of staff overload and burnout, and the adverse impact of staff cuts on patient care. The idea of staff restructuring—for example, by deprofessionalizing nursing duties and assigning some nursing tasks to nonprofessionals—also arguably worsens patient care.

6. *Reduce salaries.* Since labor costs are one of the highest cost centers in a hospital, the hospital may want to reduce its salaries. One can do so in a number of ways: by seeking a pay cut for all employees (which requires collective bargaining with any unions present), by reducing or eliminating bonuses or raises, or by establishing a differential pay scale (with which all new employees receive much lower compensation than current employees). Each possibility is morally difficult. These actions raise questions about the fairness of the compensation scheme—in other words, the correspondence between the labor offered and the payment rendered in return. They call attention to the moral culture of the institution in terms of how it respects and values its employees. Reduction in compensation also threatens the quality of patient care, because skilled staff will seek employment where they feel they are going to be fairly compensated.

This list of possibilities, though perhaps not exhaustive, is nonetheless reasonably comprehensive. These strategies all touch on important aspects of the mission. Yet if the financial goals of the board are to be met, what is the manager or management committee to do?

Obviously, the specific actions to be taken in a particular situation depend on the facts of the case. The challenge is to find those actions that can be justified as adhering to the mission, or to carry out the compromises demanded by a particular situation such that the multiplicity of values at stake in any significant moral conflict is recognized. Here are some suggestions.

First, PHC and St. Somewhere need to find ways to meet the duty to serve the health care needs of the community. Because Medicaid is a communitywide benefit, the needs of the Medicaid patient population ought to be addressed and planned for communitywide, either directly with the government or through a coordinated service plan among providers. The managers of St. Somewhere might meet their service duty to patients by negotiating with other providers to ensure that all share in meeting this need. If some institutions ignore the need and thereby increase pressure on others to take on more of this responsibility, then those institutions are failing to fulfill their mission as health care organizations.

As institutional citizens, PHC and St. Somewhere might also have obligations to negotiate with others to see that community needs are met. However, given antitrust and competition laws, a manager cannot take the initiative to resolve this conflict privately by sitting down with counterparts from another health care institution. Instead, it may be appropriate to meet with Medicaid or other governmental officials and ask them to mediate a comprehensive voluntary plan. This meets the duty to serve patients and is in accordance with the understanding of a health care organization as a mediating institution.

Second, most of the alternatives for addressing the income shortfall significantly affect St. Somewhere's employees and their work conditions. The organization must consider the service to others and relationships with its employees, two values that are supported by the overall mission of the organization.

In the context of employee relations, the widely acknowledged moral duty to respect the moral value of all human beings entails compensating employees fairly and treating them as valued participants in the shared tasks of the institution. Insofar as the institution requires sacrifice to survive, respecting employees suggests that they be consulted and participate in any important decision that affects their work and livelihood. Although this may not involve everyone, it should mean conferring with a widely representative sample of employees, giving them access to all available relevant information, and seeking their suggestions and input in important decision making.

Employees are partners in the mission of the organization, so they too have an obligation to maintain and support profitability. Their duties include not wasting the assets of the institution and furthering its mission. This is the moral rationale implicit in labor negotiations that result in a wage freeze or rollback, a justification that is often explicitly recognized when the organization involved is a charitable health care institution.

To be successful, there must be trust on both sides. Ideally, a health care institution seeks positive, collaborative relationships at all times—not just in a crisis situation. However, the traditional hierarchical understanding, in which a manager makes a decision and employees carry it out, has militated against such trust by inculcating an adversarial perspective on both sides. Involving employees in collaborative problem solving should be premised on the understanding that the institution is adopting employee participation as part of its mission. In the end, there may not be a perfect solution or one to which all can agree, but the more employees are involved and feel respected in the process, the more likely they are to buy into its results.

Integrating Mission Values: Systemic Concerns

As noted in Chapter Two, it is popular to think of an organization as a rational system governed by policy and the decisions of upper management. In fact, open systems theory and natural systems theory suggest that organizational behavior is powerfully shaped by such factors as external influence and internal culture(s) and structure(s). The PHC case illustrates how these forces can subtly influence decisions.

> Louise, an elderly woman, is a member of the St. Somewhere Medicaid health maintenance organization. Her doctor, who is an independent affiliate of the organization, is prepared to admit her to the hospital for a medical condition covered by Medicaid. Nurse Wilson, who is in charge of the St. Somewhere Medicaid HMO program, objects that the PHC *Best Practices Manual* indi-

cates that Louise's condition is better treated through provision of home care; PHC has a home care affiliate that can provide such services. Medicaid covers home care, but it does so at a lower rate of reimbursement than for hospital care. Moreover, to get home care coverage, additional paperwork must be completed. Louise's doctor claims not to have the resources to undertake such additional work without compensation; Wilson asserts that he does not have appropriate staff either. The hospital administrator, Wilson's boss, notes that the claim of best practice in this area is contested, with the doctor supporting the idea that Louise should be admitted to the hospital. The administrator also notes that having hospital staff complete the additional paperwork expends hospital resources while diverting income to the separate home care affiliate.

The problems in this case center on how the organization integrates elements of its mission and what individuals on staff should be expected to do in serving the mission. The difficulty lies both in the system of reimbursement and the structures of the organization, which (as discussed in Chapter Six) create conflict of interest between institutional and third-party financial interests and the mission of care for the patient. Although PHC can adopt policies asserting that financial concerns must be balanced with other important elements of mission, external influences and the organization's own practices and ways of organizing work can powerfully affect how this balance is handled in day-to-day decision making.

External Influences: The Medicaid Reimbursement Scheme

A health care institution does not operate in isolation. As the natural systems theory of organization teaches, it exists within an extensive, interconnected social community. The most dominant influences on organizational action come in the form of governmental regulation and financial relationships with external entities; but public opinion and even personal relationships among staff can also intrude on efforts to act in accordance with the identified mission.

In this case, the difficulty is caused by the discrepancy between reimbursement for home care versus hospital care. Both are covered, and there is no violation of Medicaid rules in whichever course of treatment is chosen. However, the difference in reimbursement rates makes it more profitable for St. Somewhere to admit Louise to the hospital than to provide home care. Moreover, to adopt policies and procedures supportive of home care (including necessary administrative support), the hospital and PHC would incur expenses that cannot be recouped from Medicaid. Medicaid policies and procedures thus create conflict between hospital and home care services within the integrated health care organization. The first task of an administrator is to identify this as a problem.

In its role as a mediating institution and advocate for good health care, St. Somewhere needs to lobby for change; it can offer a number of strong arguments. Medicaid is making an ethical mistake in its reimbursement scheme, which invites higher costs to the Medicaid program through hospitalization as opposed to home care. Obviously, the reimbursement rates for home care and hospital care differ so much because the legitimate costs are different. Hospital care is far more expensive. It is appropriate for Medicaid to cover both as they are legitimate forms of treatment, depending on the severity of the condition.

The difficulty is that Medicaid has failed to build in a mechanism to fairly determine the course of treatment. Regulations in themselves cannot and should not attempt to diagnose a patient or mandate the patient's appropriate course of treatment. At the same time, reimbursement policies should be monitored to ensure that there are neither incentive toward an inappropriate form of treatment nor disincentive away from appropriate treatment. In this case, there are both. Hospital treatment is more profitable, and the failure to reimburse administrative costs (the additional paperwork costs for entering home care) creates a disincentive for home care. At a minimum, Medicaid should cover these additional administrative expenses, either for the doctor or for the HMO, to remove this disincentive toward home care.

Internal Influences: Institutional Culture

The decision-making process can also be influenced by elements within the institution itself. For example, certain subcultures may exist, with their own norms and agendas. Financial administrators may become so involved with their efforts to manage the fiscal resources of the institution that they lose sight of other important goals. Medical professionals may become so involved in patient care that they fail to attend to the needs of the larger institution. Or the institution may be structured—consciously or unconsciously—in ways that motivate staff members to act inconsistently with the articulated goals.

Louise's case illustrates this last situation. PHC has publicly announced that it is committed to the best patient care. Its adoption of best practices guidelines is a constructive effort to create a mechanism by which to balance the mission goals of patient care and financial needs, where best practices represent a conscious effort to determine the fit of treatment and patient, and to achieve this balance for each individual diagnostic condition. But in this case, PHC has identified a balancing mechanism without considering the consequences of its internal financial organization (as well as Medicaid's impact on the independent physician) on the workings of that mechanism.

PHC institutionally mirrors the conflict created by the incentives and disincentives of this Medicaid scheme. Although PHC is a supposedly integrated health care delivery institution committed to providing appropriate care in a suitable facility, its various delivery functions are administratively separate—a common practice. The hospital administrator is evaluated according to the profitability of the hospital, the home care administrator by the financial performance of the home care service. The Medicaid HMO is administratively and financially under the auspices of the hospital.

Given the incentives for hospital admission and the disincentives for home care, one is naturally suspicious of the doctor's and the hospital's assertion that hospital admission is in fact the best plan of treatment. Admission to the hospital, after all, is not without risk: patients are exposed to various diseases at a time when, because of their admitting condition, they are particularly vulnerable to disease. There is always the risk that regardless of good intentions the judgment of doctor and administrator alike is being affected by these financial incentives.

To avoid not only the possibility of financial incentives impairing judgment on patient care but also the appearance of such contamination, PHC can administratively separate the HMO program and give it the resources to make fair and relatively impartial judgment about the best course of treatment for patients like Louise (say, by underwriting the additional paperwork costs for home care). This may mean that PHC makes less money overall (because of referral to home care as opposed to the hospital), but such an administrative change at least allows PHC to appropriately apportion administrative expenses between the hospital and the home care unit. Moreover, if this arrangement results in a loss, PHC is in the position to take this fact to Medicaid and negotiate changes. To the extent that this practice results in savings for Medicaid overall, Medicaid may be amenable to changing the reimbursement structure.

The Virtue of Courage

It is often easy to blame others for the problems one encounters, whether the government's Medicaid rules or the problems caused by "top management"; but an institution acts through the efforts of all its staff. For the institution to act morally, all staff personnel must act morally, and the institution must seek out and support morally sensitive employees.

Even if PHC is unwilling to change its administrative structure (or if there is no home care affiliate), it may be the hospital administrator's moral duty to develop and support a semi-independent HMO system to make referrals in cases like Louise's. An administrator at this level has some discretionary authority. In exercising that authority, he or she is also responsible for adhering to and enacting the mission of PHC. This includes finding a way to support PHC's commitment to best practices.

Admittedly, the hospital administrator faces some personal risk in this regard. The administrator is judged according to the performance of the St. Somewhere Hospital and HMO, and the loss of revenue and additional administrative expense of referral to home care can detract from the hospital's bottom line. The failure to maximize returns may have some impact on the administrator's career—it is easier, and possibly safer, for this person to focus efforts solely on improving the bottom line because he or she can then point to measurable results. Yet the administrator has the moral duty to seek to uphold St. Somewhere's commitment to patient care. In view of the potential personal disadvantages, fulfilling the duty to the overall mission of the organization requires a certain courage.

If employees who display such courage are not supported in ethical decision making, they will probably learn their lesson and not take such risks in the future. Their example will dissuade others from serving the institution's mission whenever doing so carries personal or professional risk. Individual employees cannot carry the full responsibility for the organization; they can only seek to contribute to its moral efforts in line with their place within the institution. Seeking out, hiring, and supporting individuals with moral courage offers the organization the opportunity to rethink its actions anytime a thoughtful, courageous individual questions or resists its action or decision. But it does not resolve the moral questions raised.

Integrating Mission Values: The Role of Nonexecutive Staff

With the rational systems theory focusing on hierarchy and formal control from the top down, it is very easy to conceptualize how the organization can integrate consideration of mission into its decision-making process. Senior management clearly defines the mission of the organization and, in general terms, determines how the various activities are to be balanced within the overall structure of the mission. The individual employee merely implements those decisions through applying those general principles to (often routinized) cases. In the event of uncertainty over a particular decision, referral to senior management is advisable; this should result in clarification of the general organizational rules.

In practice, even the most hierarchical organization does not and cannot operate according to this simple model. Interactions between the organization and its service community (internal or external) are so varied and ambiguous that senior management cannot anticipate and address all of the significant decisions that affect the mission. Employees at every level of management must have some discretionary authority. This discretion inevitably requires an employee to determine how the bottom line is to be integrated in carrying out the mission.

The marketing director for PHC has developed and implemented a marketing plan that includes public advertising. This advertising is a mix of public service informational announcements as well as explicit advertisements for PHC. At the end of the year, Medicaid sends PHC a form that allows it to bill Medicaid for certain public service informational announcements that do not include solicitations to contact PHC (such as a toll-free number for additional information).

The marketing director decides not to file for these reimbursements for five reasons. First, complying with the restrictions on content is difficult and somewhat controversial. The regulations are complex, and any enforcement effort against an inappropriate claim is treated as an action for fraud. Second, the amount of money at stake is relatively small, amounting to no more than $80,000. Third, the public health announcements benefit the entire organization because they help build public recognition of PHC within the community it serves. (They were, in fact, produced without considering whether Medicaid would pay for them.)

Fourth, these announcements are consistent with the mission of PHC to provide public health care through information. Finally, the marketing director believes that it would be unethical to seek reimbursement because she believes that Medicaid funds, which are limited, are intended to meet the clinical needs of Medicaid patients and should not be diverted to general activities supporting the institution.

This case offers a good illustration of how a nonexecutive staff person might act (internally) in service of the mission of the organization. Virtually every employee acts in ways that either advance or inhibit an organization's overall mission. Whether rendering patient care, handling billing, or working in environmental support, the work and how it is carried out publicly enact the mission.

For a person in advertising and marketing, this obviously requires carrying out his or her duties ethically. In accordance with the institutional mandate that it act with integrity and be honest and fair in its dealings with others, institutional advertising should also be honest and fair in what and how it communicates with the public. Moreover, in balancing financial interests against the interest in caring for both patients and members of the larger community, health care advertising should not encourage consumers to seek unnecessary health care.[13] What is different in this case is that we are expanding the moral compass beyond the marketing director's functional role in advertising to assess how her actions fit within the total mission of the organization, including consideration of profitability.

The marketing director's analysis of this situation is comprehensive and well considered. She demonstrates sensitivity to the need for honest behavior and regulatory compliance in confronting the murky nature of the Medicaid regulations. The advertisements are designed to benefit PHC in a way that advances the goals of the institution, which is not simply driven by the profit motive. The assessment that only a limited amount of money is involved represents sensitivity to the bottom-line needs of the institution, balanced against the risk of improper compliance.

One can question whether the marketing director properly weighs these factors in coming to her decision not to file for reimbursement. It may be argued that compliance is not that difficult, and that the money is sufficient to justify the attempt to do so. Moreover, that such advertising benefits PHC does not negate the fact that it also advances the interests of the Medicaid program, and the costs are justifiable charges against Medicaid to the same extent that providing clinical care advances the missions of PHC and Medicaid alike. Nor does this negate the fact that the marketing director has identified and considered the appropriate ethical issues. The only serious question, on these factors alone, is whether making this decision fits within the parameters of the marketing director's discretionary authority.

Every administrative employee has some discretion in answering individual questions about whether an act does or does not adhere to the mission. What the organization expects, however, is that the exercise of this discretion is within the limits of the employee's job description and the authority assigned to the employee. For example, an employee may have wide discretion over purchases having a value of less than a hundred dollars, provided that the total expenditures for the year do not exceed a set budget. For this employee to seek his or her superior's approval for all purchases, or to authorize purchases having a value greater than a hundred dollars, violates the employee's job responsibility, either through failing to exercise discretion or by exceeding the authorized parameters of that discretion.

Is the decision within the discretionary parameters of the marketing director's position? Although $80,000 is a significant amount of money, it may be only a small percentage of PHC's operating budget. The marketing director's financial discretion in relation to overall budget administration must be determined by considering her job description.

Even if the decision is within the parameters of the job description, she may nonetheless have an obligation to communicate her decision to her superiors. Because some people might question the propriety of this decision, the marketing director should probably communicate it to her manager and seek his or her opinion. Depending on the dollar amount involved, the normal authority of the individual employee, and the time constraints imposed on a given decision, such consultation can occur either at the time the decision must be made or afterward—for example, as the following year's budget is being planned. If there is no pressure for immediate action and a significant amount of money is involved, discussion at the time the decision is made is probably favored.

What is startling in this case is the marketing director's assertion that taking Medicaid reimbursement for advertising is unethical because it diverts money that should properly be directed toward clinical care. In effect, she is making an argument about public policy: because Medicaid funds are limited, those monies should be allocated to clinical care, not informational programs. Here there are two issues: whether an organization should consider social policy issues in its decision making and whether an employee—here, the marketing director—should make decisions on such a basis.

With respect to the first issue, the question is to what extent an organization has an ethical duty to act beyond the general requirements of public policy in conforming to its own understanding of the public good. Clearly, Medicaid has determined that health education is a public good it is willing to underwrite. The marketing director's assessment is that health education is a public good but the better public policy is to allocate these funds to direct patient care. The goal of public education can be and is being met as an incidental element within the marketing and mission of health care institutions like PHC and does not need the incentive of payment by Medicaid to be accomplished. But even if Medicaid allows financial claims to support this goal, is PHC morally obligated to seek reimbursement (which is to its advantage) or to adhere to its own interpretation of good public policy?

Given the fact that a health care organization has a moral responsibility transcending the bottom line, it is clearly within the moral prerogative of PHC to make decisions that adversely affect the bottom line. It can take a position that as a point of principle it will not make claims under a program with which it disagrees. Moreover, as a professional ideal and as part of the mission of a mediating institution, a health care institution should participate in developing sound public health care policy. Being a repository of important health care information and recognized as morally competent to advise on health care policies, PHC is clearly competent to act on that advice and elect to follow a moral course that results in not claiming the advertising reimbursement. Although there are strong arguments that to follow this course may not be wise, or may not best serve the mission of the organization in relation to its objectives of patient care, it is not morally wrong.

But what about the propriety of the marketing director grounding her decision in this way? It is, after all, far more likely that PHC (as an institution, and through its various professional associations) directly participates in public policy consultation than that the marketing director does. To the extent it is aware of this possible policy conflict, PHC can take the policy argument and seek to change policy. In simple terms, the marketing director's act passively avoids taking advantage of the policy that is in place.

The question hinges on her position within the organization. On the one hand, she may have an obligation to notify her manager about her approach to this conflict; if the problem is serious enough, it may need to be referred ultimately to the board. However, since upper management and the board cannot evaluate every detail and decision of institutional management, they must rely on individual managers to make some decisions on their own within the general parameters presented by the board. The greater the amount of money at stake in the decision, the greater the duty for the employee to involve his or her manager (and ultimately upper management and the board).

At the same time, a health care institution's moral culture depends not only on the actions and directions of the board but also on the actions and decisions of all its managers, and ultimately all the staff. Insofar as a decision properly lies within the discretion of individual managers and staff people, the institution's moral culture depends on their exercising moral judgment in the course of professional activities. One can commend the marketing director for attempting to live up to the moral duties she identifies as an employee of PHC, even if one is convinced that she is in error on this point. It is a sign of moral health that a manager includes moral concern within the matrix of principles by which he or she makes decisions.

Summary

These cases illustrate several conclusions that may be drawn regarding the relationship between mission and bottom line, and how the institution can address concerns that the need to make a profit inevitably tends to override its other moral obligations. They relate both to the institution and to its employees and managers.

First, the organization needs to explicitly and publicly articulate its purpose or mission. The bottom line is morally relevant and a proper element of mission. Nonetheless, profitability is not the only criterion of moral consideration. The institution has a variety of obligations that must be considered as well, among them direct patient care, serving the health care needs of the community, responsibility toward employees, and participating in developing public policy. The institution should seek to balance all of these considerations and clearly express its understanding of mission in the mission statement and all policies and published statements.

Second, the organization must consider how specific actions advance or impede efforts to meet its mission objectives. This requires information and reflection on the relationship between action and mission. The organization needs to develop informational systems that both identify the relationships between action and mission and track the effect of action on mission. This can be done either through formal systemization (such as developing an ethics auditing process) or through educational efforts directed toward employees and support for employee responses and initiatives. It may also adopt formal procedures that consider the moral dimensions of its actions by requiring that decision makers be prepared to identify how a proposed action may affect the overall mission (on the analogy of an environmental impact statement).

Third, the organization must develop mechanisms to balance or integrate seemingly incompatible mission goals. This requires developing rational decision-making patterns that consciously seek to achieve proper integration, and also systemic structures that facilitate making those judgments. It must be sensitive to structural incentives or disincentives (notably financial) that can affect decision making grounded on other organizational values (as with commitment to best practices) and must seek to avoid a situation in which conflict of interest obstructs good decision making. The organization also has to be sensitive to how its structure and external forces may affect judgment on the part of staff.

Fourth, because of the importance of organizational culture and the necessary diffusion of decision-making authority throughout an organization, an ethical organization needs to educate staff on the commitment to moral decision making, including the dimension of profitability and the moral duties that extend beyond profitability. In most cases, individual employees should not be directed to dedicate themselves to advancing any single goal (profitability, patient care, or other). To do so means that the decisions they make do not fulfill the overall mission of the institution or contribute to the overall moral wisdom of the institution. For instance, a manager who focuses exclusively on the bottom line and reporting requirements of financial procedures is not in a position to include information about the moral consequences of financial decisions, which is needed by upper management and the board in making comprehensive, morally sound decisions.

Finally, the institution is well advised to seek employees and managers who have certain basic characteristics or virtues necessary to furthering its mission. Staff should be perceptive of the moral world in which the institution operates and its moral obligations. They should be responsible in caring for the moral and financial assets of the institution. They need to be competent in performing the functions entrusted to them. They ought to have the courage to stand up for their convictions so as to help shape the institution's moral life. To achieve this, the institution must be sensitive to seeking this quality in the people it employs and in fostering an environment that is supportive of this virtue, in terms of its incentive programs and in providing an institutional example of living up to the values identified with the mission.

Notes

1. JCAHO standards require health care institutions to adopt particular codes of ethics (see, for example, RI.1 and RI.4) that can be used to inform creation of a mission statement. However, codes of ethics are directed at particular actions within an organization, while the idea of a mission is a more comprehensive identification of the values that underlie the particular topics identified in a code of ethics. Determining mission is, therefore, a predicate to creating a particular code.

2. See Darr, K. *Ethics in Health Services Management.* New York: Praeger, 1987.

3. See, for example, AMA Code of Medical Ethics, Principle I.

4. See, for example, Gray, B. H. *The Profit Motive and Patient Care.* Cambridge, Mass.: Harvard University, 1991; Daniels, N. "The Profit Motive and the Moral Assessment of Health Care Institutions." *Business and Professional Ethics Journal,* 1990, *10*(2), 3–30; Shelp, E. E. (ed.). *Philosophy and Medicine.* Vol. 8: *Justice and Health Care.* Dordrecht, Neth.: Reidel, 1981; and Claxton, G., Feder, J., Schatman, D., and Altman, S. "Public Policy in Nonprofit Conversions: An Overview." *Health Affairs,* 1997, *16*(2), 15–19.

5. Friedman, E. "Marginal Mission and Missionary Margins." *Healthcare Forum Journal,* Jan./Feb. 1990, pp. 8–12.

6. Toulmin, S. "Medical Institutions and Their Moral Constraints." In R. E. Bulger and S. J. Reiser, *Integrity in Healthcare Institutions.* Iowa City: University of Iowa, 1990.

7. Friedman, M. *Capitalism and Freedom.* Chicago: University of Chicago, 1962.

8. See, for example, Bird, F. *The Muted Conscience: Moral Silence and the Practice of Ethics in Business.* Westport, Conn.: Quorum, 1996; French, P. "Corporate Moral Agency." In W. M. Hoffman and J. M. Moore (eds.), *Business Ethics: Readings and Cases in Corporate Morality.* New York: McGraw-Hill, 1984.

9. Soelle, D. *To Love and to Work: A Theology of Creation.* Philadelphia: Fortress, 1984.

10. See Adams, J. L. *Voluntary Associations.* (J. R. Engel, ed.). Chicago: Exploration, 1986.

11. See, for example, AMA Code of Medical Ethics, Principles III, V, and VII.

12. See, for example, Peters, T., and Waterman, R. *In Search of Excellence.* New York: Harper and Row, 1981; Nash, L. L. *Good Intentions Aside.* Boston: Harvard Business School, 1990.

13. See, for example, Murphy, P. E. "Ethical Issues Facing Hospitals in Their Advertising." In Catholic Health Association of the United States. *Ethical Issues in Healthcare Marketing.* St. Louis: CHA, 1990; Arrington, R. L. "Advertising and Behavior Control." *Journal of Business Ethics,* 1982, *1*(1), 3–12.

Part Two

Cases

The Waiting Room

Eight years ago, Suburban Hospital built a new family waiting room by enlisting community philanthropic support widely from individuals, religious communities, and businesses. Clinical Manager Joan, a volunteer community leader for the campaign, has just overheard that, thanks to rapid hospital expansion, the new administration wants to eliminate the waiting room. She approaches her superiors, who confirm this. Her superiors request confidentiality because the administration is going to proceed without public announcement.

Joan is involved with church and civic groups that donated money for the room. She feels obliged to inform them and even galvanize community protest. What are her options?

When facing a clinical moral dilemma, Manager Joan, like most staff, turns to the ethics committee. In an organizational ethics case like this one, however, staff members are unsure how to voice concern. Before acting, it is best to understand both the range of, and the moral responsibility for, the dilemma. Among the issues in this case are conflict of interest, confidentiality, and promise keeping.

We regularly balance competing interests between family and work, but rarely does meeting a professional obligation simultaneously jeopardize civic obligations. How can Joan resolve the competing interests between obligations to her work and her community?

First, it is important to examine whether any clear moral directive informs either obligation. For instance, when physicians experience competing moral obligations between patient welfare and business, they often prioritize obligations by relying on a clear professional dictum to "do no harm." Joan has to ask herself if she has made any explicit commitments that might help prioritize the competing obligations—for instance, are there commitments in her work contract not to divulge management plans, or in her volunteer fundraising to be vigilant in the stewardship of the gift?

The issue of confidentiality is straightforward in this case. Joan's superiors have asked her to keep a confidence, and it is not immediately evident that the request is an immoral one. Simple fairness ("do unto others") dictates that we keep confidences held sacred. Even if Joan's superiors do not request silence on the matter, her job is most likely to require prudent use of sensitive management information. From an organizational ethics stance, it is important to examine whether the organization, in its job descriptions, policies, and training, explicitly reinforces its expectations about confidentiality.

Aside from the practical moral problem of alienating donors who support the mission of the hospital, what commitments has the hospital made to the donors? Moral evaluation of the hospital's promise keeping has to include examination of what the donors explicitly requested, what development professionals promised, and whether administration knew about its potential stewardship of the gift.

Plainly, the problems cut across the organization. Joan's challenges include how she can be a catalyst for the administration to rethink its decision. Other groups, such as administration and development, must rethink how the commitments of predecessors are to be honored. As this hospital, like many others, moves to address organizational ethics, it must not only identify and examine the problems but also imagine where they are best resolved, because no one locus is sufficient for all.

Nursing Strikes

Several years ago, before St. Somewhere merged with others to become Partnership Health Care, the nurses at this not-for-profit Catholic hospital agreed to a wage freeze for three years because the hospital was struggling financially. The financial problems were *not* caused by administrative mismanagement. Rather, St. Somewhere was one of the few hospitals in the county that provided care to the uninsured and contracted to provide health care services to Medicaid patients. The nurses agreed to the wage freeze to help stabilize the financial situation and maintain the hospital's mission of providing health care to the less fortunate.

Six months later, St. Somewhere still had financial problems. Thus it merged with Willow Hospital, a small, not-for-profit, secular institution. During the past three years, nurses at this hospital have received raises averaging 4 percent per year. These nurses are not unionized.

On October 5, the nurses' contract at St. Somewhere expired. They demanded a 12 percent increase, which would match nurses' wages at Willow. Of the 750 nurses at St. Somewhere, 480 are unionized. If the union is successful in obtaining the 12 percent increase, all St. Somewhere nurses, even those not in the union, will get raises. However, only the union members can vote to strike. Nurses at St. Somewhere have never gone on strike during the hospital's ninety years of existence.

St. Somewhere's administration was replaced when the two hospitals merged. St. Somewhere and Willow now have one corporate administration that oversees both hospitals. The administration would like to break the union.

The administration has counteroffered a proposal of a 7.5 percent wage increase spread over two years and investment in the hospital pension plan in the third year. If the nurses in St. Somewhere strike, the administration has indicated it will staff positions at St. Somewhere with nurses from Willow. St. Somewhere's site executive asks the ethics officer to review the situation and report back to him.

Treating unionized labor relations as a form of economic war has been an American norm for more than one hundred years. Employees, and especially their unions, are considered the enemies of management and the corporation. One of the things that distinguish organizational ethics from traditional business ethics is that the former rejects this approach, for at least two reasons. First, organizational ethics identifies the organization as having moral standing and obligations. As an ethical entity, the organization has moral duties toward all of the individuals with whom it interacts—including its employees. Second, on a pragmatic level, how an organization treats employees affects how it carries out ethical duties to all of the other individuals served. An organization acts through its employees. If it fails to attend to their needs, the organization is unable to develop the type of ethical culture that allows it to address other moral duties.

Of course, there are always points of tension between the organization and the employees. Clearly, balancing compensation levels against income and other expenses is one example. However, in making a compensation decision, the organization cannot fall back upon a simple adversarial model. It must instead weigh the ethical values at stake. The hospital's ethics officer should consider several points for her report.

First, there is the issue of the discrepancy between the salaries paid to nurses at the two hospitals. This creates a problem of possible discrimination and limits the organization's ability to create a unified culture and identity.

The ethics officer notes that a basic requirement of justice is that individuals be treated fairly and equitably with all other similarly situated individuals. An organization should not discriminate among its employees for reasons not related to job performance or other conditions that identify a legitimate difference between employees. This in turn requires assessment of whether there is a legitimate reason to categorize the two groups of nurses differently. If the two hospitals are operated as totally separate and distinct entities, this discrepancy may be justified. For example, St. Somewhere may not generate income sufficient to pay salaries comparable to those at Willow. However, if the two institutions have been merged into a single entity, it would appear to be discriminatory to treat the two groups of nurses differently unless some other morally relevant distinction can be identified.

In an organizational merger, many organizations seek to create a new, unified identity and culture. They may publicly advertise themselves as a single entity, creating an obligation that they live up to their professed standards. This type of salary discrimination limits the ability of the new organization to create such a unified organizational culture. The threat to use nurses from Willow to cover staffing needs at St. Somewhere in the event of a strike also acts against unity, creating a climate of suspicion and hostility among the nurses of the two hospitals.

A second area of concern for the ethics officer is the extent to which the merged organization has an obligation to uphold the moral commitments of a predecessor organization. Here the nurses at St. Somewhere voluntarily agreed to a wage freeze in consideration of the financial difficulties at the hospital and in support of its mission to the community. To what extent does this create an obligation for an organization to repay this charitable concession when financial circumstances change for the better? Significantly, if such an obligation existed for the original St. Somewhere, does the successor entity bear the same responsibility?

Third, there is the question of the administration's position with regard to its purported desire to break the union. One of the guiding principles of U.S. labor law is that employees have a right to organize, and employers have a duty to respect that right. Therefore, in opposing the union, the organization needs to offer moral justification for opposition. It is not enough to say that negotiating with a union is inconvenient. Rather, there must be some tangible justification for opposition. Perhaps the union is not representing the interests of the employees it claims to represent. Or the union may be so obstructionist in using work rules or in negotiation that it significantly impairs the ability of the organization to meet its other mission-based objectives.

On the facts given, it does not appear to the ethics officer that the union is being financially irresponsible. The administration's willingness to replace the nurses at St. Somewhere with the higher-salaried nurses from Willow Hospital (note that this threat is offered without any limitation on time) *may* suggest that the issue is one of administrative hostility to the union rather than a legitimate financial concern. Nonetheless, additional facts are needed to determine if there are other moral reasons for the organization's negotiating stance.

In summary, the ethics officer concludes that the hospital administration needs to recognize that the organization has a moral obligation to its employees to treat them fairly and equitably. As an extension of moral duties, the administration must also deal with the union as the representative of its employees.

| A Gift, or an Obligation?

Partnership Health Care is embarking on a major building program to support its research mission. As the capital campaign gets under way, one of the health care system's development officers contacts physicians who use the medical facility and asks them to contribute to the campaign. The officer tells a community primary care physician and her husband, a plastic surgeon, that their "fair-share" contribution is $200,000. The couple question the term *fair-share* and contact the medical staff president, who in turn refers them to the PHC's chief ethics officer.

Inasmuch as charity begins at home, health care institutions find ways to solicit gifts from the associates who work for the institution or are otherwise affiliated with it. This standard approach to fundraising generally raises few ethical concerns. Many institutions have an annual fund drive that solicits individual gifts from employees (often through payroll deduction) and from associates. Of course, not all staff members welcome this annual "opportunity" to give. Some actively resent solicitations by their employer, whether because they feel that they are paid too little for what they do, or too much is already asked of them on the job, or they previously "gave at the office" to other causes such as United Way. Physicians are not employees of PHC hospitals, and their support of programs such as this one is purely philanthropic.

Such reservations notwithstanding, asking institutional associates to participate in a major capital campaign is also a common and widely accepted practice. Would-be donors outside of the organization want to know whether its own people deem an institution worthy of support. Figures showing a high proportion of associate giving are a quintessential demonstration of such support. Moreover, many organizational associates appreciate the opportunity to give something back to their institution and support the worthy causes that it serves.

The capital campaign request in this case, however, raises not only the hackles of the physician couple involved but also significant ethical questions. For the most part, the questions seem to concern the conduct of the development officer, but they may extend to senior management (often in the person of the chief executive) who may give final clearance to the fundraising strategies employed in such a campaign. Given the evident need to finance the building program, what moral parameters should govern how the development function pursues the financial goals and targeted donor pool? What is senior management's moral responsibility in overseeing these development activities?

A health care organization's development function must raise funds that the organization needs for general or specific purposes, funds that are not readily available from other sources (such as the revenue streams generated by operations and investment). To fulfill their task, development personnel identify and cultivate potential donors and, sooner or later, solicit gifts from them. In this instance, a development officer tells the prospective donor physicians that their fair-share gift would be $200,000. The ethics officer might wonder what criteria were used to arrive at this amount. Why was this physician couple solicited on this occasion, and at this level?

Several plausible answers come to mind. First, perhaps the two physicians are donors already, either as individuals or as a couple. Second, they make part of their living through being credentialed to practice on the medical staff and are thus privileged to associate their practice with the reputation of the hospital. Third, because they are physicians, they are known or believed to make a very good living from the practice of medicine—two very good livings, in fact.

The fair-share label used in this instance, and common in such development efforts, can imply several things, all of which have moral overtones. It implies that a certain baseline expectation is being applied to all physicians on the medical staff. The development staff (and senior management) have determined that every physician should be readily capable of anteing up a certain amount—in this example, presumably $100,000 each. From this perspective the "share" is "fair" because the same expectation is applied to all physicians and all are deemed capable of meeting it. In this scenario, all physicians are treated as if their incomes and resources are roughly equivalent.

A second possibility is that the fair-share figure is actually a "stretch" figure, one that few, if any, physicians are actually expected to meet (even if no one from development voices this disclaimer in so many words). In practice, the $100,000 amount may then function as a beginning basis for the donor's "negotiation" with development personnel (or senior leaders, if they are personally involved in the effort), as well as the donor's negotiation with his or her inner sense of obligation or altruism. A development campaign may—intentionally or not—touch both donor gratitude and donor guilt. "Fair share" language can easily imply that a donor falls short if she does not (at least) give the stipulated amount; it may also imply that she will fail to keep up with her peers who (of course) are making the requisite contribution. Further gratitude and guilt may be elicited from yet another angle: fair-share language may suggest that the institution has given so much to the practitioner that she would want to give—or she owes—at least this much in return, as a kind of quid pro quo.

Another possibility is that the fair-share figure derives from calculating a percentage of this couple's estimated combined income from their medical practice—a calculation that they might (if they knew of it) find presumptuous, at best, if not also rather intrusive. Another possibility is that the development office has somehow obtained specific information about the incomes of some or all staff physicians (for example, alimony payments from a previous marriage) and has made a person-specific fair-share calculation on the basis of this income information. Obtaining this information from public records is legal, but privacy and confidentiality should be taken seriously. Such a direct investigation of resources is not unprecedented; in our age, people's credit histories are, after all, readily accessible. But employment of such means by an institution that presumably seeks not only an immediate contribution but also their long-term loyalty is likely, if discovered, to alienate them, not bind them to the institution.

This sketch of the moral possibilities implicit in the fair-share concept may help the ethics officer trace the moral landscape of some approaches to fundraising. The stark description in this case study of the development contact intimates that the fair-share amount and how it is presented to the two physicians come as something of a shock, and a rude one at that. Such a reaction serves as a reminder that the success of development efforts depends on, and must begin with, attitudes and practices of respect for the people being cultivated and solicited. As in so many matters of organizational ethics, respect for people is in part a matter of prudence, in this instance the enlightened self-interest of the institution as well as of the development function and its personnel. Assuming that senior management, perhaps even the medical center's chief executive, has signed off on the development strategy implemented here, the decision to adopt or at least approve this approach seems at best to have been unwise.

Moreover, if a productive development effort is crucial to the business of the medical center, its development practices also create another arena for the medical center to demonstrate its adherence to the humane values exemplified in health care. That is, medical staff members—like others working in health care—may legitimately expect a certain consistency between the organization's behavior toward patients and families and its behavior toward "its own," including physicians. Development efforts should therefore be conducted with the aim of embodying such consistency. Unfortunately, in this instance the hospital is in danger of undermining its credibility in the eyes of the medical staff on precisely this count.

This case is also a reminder that there are high-pressure and low-pressure ways of conducting development activities. Fair-share language can, if properly framed, serve as a motivating challenge to prospective donors, who may respond by raising the level of their giving. A fair share that sets the bar too high may be imprudent, and it may also be experienced as subtly coercive—even as a form of harassment. To be sure, fair-share language in itself carries neither connotation. But such language may trigger fears and suspicions in those physicians who are already ambivalent about the institution, and perhaps inclined to distrust it. They might wonder, *Will there be negative consequences if I fail to ante up my fair share? Can my privileges, or my contract with the PPO, be put at risk if I fail to donate at the requisite level?* Such perceptions can be toxic to the development campaign and to the organization as a whole—not to mention the needless distress they cause those who hold them. Failure to treat donors (especially those within one's organization) with respect may do far more damage than any mere failure to secure their financial contribution.

Obligations for Adequate Health Care Coverage

Long-Suffering Catholic Health System is an advocate for the right of all persons to basic health care services. The system board faces a dilemma. The director of contracting for the system strives to convince area employers to offer an adequate package of health care benefits to all their employees. However, despite seeking to be competitive with other insurers, its package requires such high deductibles and co-pays that lower-paid employees of these companies tend to opt out of health insurance benefits and elect other ones they find more affordable. In fact, the benefits director of Long-Suffering reports that most housekeeping and dietary employees at the system's own hospitals decline the health insurance benefits that are available. Managerial employees of Long-Suffering voluntarily contribute to a fund that minimum wage employees can access when they have emergency health care needs.

Several issues present themselves in this scenario. First, Long-Suffering's faith-based advocacy of a right to adequate health care finds rough sledding in the real world of competing insurers, a world in which Long-Suffering's own needs for organizational survival limit the system's freedom of action. How can this Catholic health care system honor its commitment to offer adequate health care benefits while maintaining—or, better, enhancing—the ability to support its overall health care mission financially?

Second, lower-paid employees (including Long-Suffering's own staff) are finding that the system's version of "adequate" health care coverage is, in fact, not adequate to their needs. What sort of benefits package would truly promote Long-Suffering's goal of offering adequate coverage? How can the organization craft health benefits that are adequate and affordable for those who would use them and, in part, pay for them?

Third, recognition of its own staff's limited resources has led Long-Suffering to institute a supplementary system in which managers, who earn more, can contribute voluntarily to the emergency health care of those who are paid less. How should we evaluate this approach as an institutional response to the problem?

In formulating its benefits package, Long-Suffering as a Catholic system has sought to act in accordance with the teachings and directives of its tradition. A key source of ethical guidance for Catholic health care organizations is the National Conference of Catholic Bishops' *Ethical and Religious Directives for Catholic Health Care Services*. The *Directives* recognize adequate health care as a human right, identify attention to the health care needs of the uninsured and underinsured as a special responsibility of Catholic institutions, and call on those institutions to promote healthy communities. Commendably, Long-Suffering seems to be acting in the spirit of the *Directives*. In this case, however, reality seems to be pressing Long-Suffering to rethink its vision of adequate health care supported by an adequate benefits package.

Perhaps the *Directives* can help Long-Suffering with the task of practically reenvisioning this commitment. For one thing, the *Directives* also call for "responsible stewardship" of available health care resources. It may be that Long-Suffering has embraced a somewhat idealistic interpretation of stewardship without fully considering the real world to which such stewardship must respond. If an adequate health benefits package is one that too few employees of client firms can afford, then the package becomes inaccessible to the very employees—those at the margin—whom the *Directives* single out for inclusion. To be sure, the area employers may be at fault for shifting more of the cost than is justifiable to their employees, especially those who are paid least. Indeed, the companies might be faulted for imposing the relatively expensive Long-Suffering plan on their employees in the first place.

In any event, prudent planners, marketers, and senior leaders at Long-Suffering might well have anticipated such a response to their benefits package. Employers typically shift some cost of coverage to associates; the costlier the coverage, the greater the likely shifting of expenses. Lower-paid employees are also consumers who can—and must—make choices about their use of limited personal and family resources. As free moral (and fiscal) agents, they are choosing to pursue goods other than health insurance, and they clearly do not feel obligated to make every possible sacrifice to ensure that they have adequate health care coverage. Perhaps most distressing is Long-Suffering's belated recognition of the impact the plan has on its own lower-paid staff members. Evidently they too are declining to enroll because Long-Suffering is shifting its costs at a level approaching that of the area employers.

Devising an organized means of charitable response to meet pressing health care needs of less-well-off Long-Suffering employees is a commendable step as far as it goes, but its dependence on individual generosity makes it appear to be a halfway measure in light of the *Directives'* norm of *institutional* justice in treatment of employees. Charity in a given instance is usually considered to be morally optional; justice is not.

Here again, the *Directives* may suggest a practical way of addressing the moral problems that a somewhat imprudent approach has created. The *Directives* suggest that responsible stewardship is most effectively implemented through "dialogue with people from all levels" of the community. In rethinking what adequate health care—being covered by an adequate benefits package that employees can afford—should look like, Long-Suffering can go to the source: through dialogue with both employers and employees, including lower-paid employees, especially at its own hospitals, Long-Suffering may discern how a right to adequate health care can become a practically reachable goal.

Knowing not only what benefits employers are able and willing to offer but also what contributions they require of employees who receive those benefits can help Long-Suffering design a benefits package that is competitive (thus serving the system's reasonable self-interest) and employee-affordable (thus supporting an achievable right to health care). Long-Suffering can ask lower-paid employees what adequate health care coverage means to them, given their financial situation and the context of their local community with its job marketplace. Perhaps their expectations of a fair and reasonable health care benefits package differ from the vision of Long-Suffering's benefits designers and leaders.

Equipped with the information gleaned from conversation with relevant stakeholders, Long-Suffering would be in a better position to act as a responsible steward of the health care resources at its disposal and better prepared to enact a practical vision of a right to adequate health care in its community. Long-Suffering's leaders may, however, also determine that what is achievable still falls short of what ought to be, in light of the *Directives* and their own conscientious assessment of responsibility. Then they can, and probably should, pursue the additional option of appropriate advocacy in the sphere of public policy.

A Manager's Dilemma in Hiring

Carol is the manager of the billing department at Deaconess Hospital. As an old associate of the site chief executive's, she was brought into the organization following a round of layoffs resulting from the hospital's merger into Partnership Health Care (PHC). After a lengthy search process, Carol finally has a candidate to fill a key vacancy in her department. An experienced employee who has been with the hospital for years possesses the unique skills needed to coordinate an important new project that carries additional responsibilities but no additional pay.

After working with human resources in the hiring process, and just prior to the final decision, Carol hears something that suggests the applicant falsified his monthly travel voucher. Word is that he claimed nearly $300 for travel reimbursement for various meetings at other sites of care, when in fact he was the passenger in another employee's car. Given PHC's clear policy on fraudulent behavior, she believes that if she reports this information to HR he will not be hired, and her project will suffer the loss of a valuable worker. If she does not report it, she is (at least technically) guilty of covering up his falsification of a travel voucher. And how can she treat the associate objectively, knowing what she does? Carol doesn't know what to do; she wonders if this is a matter for the hospital's ethics officer.

How Carol handles the situation is a signal to other employees. In the months since the merger that formed PHC, Carol has seen that many employees resent the turmoil and layoffs; they feel especially that fewer people are doing more work for no more money. Under such conditions, management and employees are seeking ways to influence one another's perceptions and actions about the conditions of work, or unilaterally renegotiate what they require of and provide to one another. Such renegotiations may occur, regrettably, in small instances, when an employee steals paper clips, or when someone pads an expense account in an effort to rectify what he perceives as unjust pay, or when management permits such behavior in order to defuse discontent. Under these conditions, appeals to teamwork, self-sacrifice, and the good of the organization fail to inform the working relationship and reinforce the tendency toward self-interest.

Carol meets with the ethics officer, who helps her analyze her dilemma. Should Carol ignore what she has heard? She has no proof that the applicant for the position in her department falsified his expense report. Perhaps she should choose not to pursue the matter. She was not oblivious to the resentment directed at her when she was brought in to head the billing department following the acquisition of Deaconess. This hire represents a chance to bring into an important position an employee from within Deaconess, thus sending a signal to other employees that their work is valued. If she investigates and the suspicion is corroborated, she will lose the opportunity to signal her staff in this way as well as a valuable contributor to her project. How she exercises her discretion in this matter is crucially important in relations with her employees.

Carol could choose to ignore her suspicions, let the hire go through, and develop a strategy to monitor this employee's expense reporting closely. However, if she does so for this one individual, her oversight is founded on suspicion and will color other facets of their relationship. If the strategy she develops is applied across the employee ranks, this technique of management control curtails or revokes the privilege of discretion for all employees.

Carol could take the individual in question aside and talk to him (out of court, so to speak). As the applicant's potential supervisor, it seems within the agent-principal relationship to negotiate understanding, without anyone else being aware of the concern. However, if he admits the incident, then despite assurance that such misrepresentation will not happen again Carol's trust in her employee is conditional. If he denies the charge, her suspicions may linger, and his trust in Carol is damaged. Either way, their relationship starts off on shaky ground. Further, if Carol adopts this approach and hires the applicant, others within the organization who are aware of the report might wonder about the true story. She also is concerned about the reputation of the applicant: if the matter is not directly addressed, his colleagues might always wonder about his integrity.

Finally, the ethics officer notes that indeed Carol's own reputation within the organization and her personal integrity are at stake. As a manager within PHC, she is a fiduciary entrusted with resources that belong to others. The principle of stewardship, a stated value of the organization, is intended to express and foster ethical commitment and internal restraint, to counter pressures of self-interest that can lead to inefficient use of organizational resources or to outright misappropriation. Carol herself is held accountable for stewardship in her own performance appraisal; she personally believes deeply that the resources she controls are not her property but rather are owned by others for whom she serves as steward.

After the conversation, Carol decides that she cannot condone expense-account padding and feels an obligation to report the applicant to HR so that a proper and confidential investigation can be followed. The argument that everyone does it, or that such padding represents some kind of compensation for unpaid work, is after all an excuse. Even if padding is taken for granted by the hospital culture, to PHC the action is legally and ethically unacceptable. Amid a lingering atmosphere of downsizing, she may lose a valuable employee. If the charge is groundless, and Carol's suspicions are laid to rest, perhaps the hire can go through.

This case is a good illustration of how an associate should exercise discretion and control within an organization to promote the values of fairness and openness. Despite the temptation to ameliorate employee tensions or to fill an important position to launch her project, her commitment to the organization's values and her personal conviction lend support to her decision to address the situation appropriately through channels. Although a very few individuals within Deaconess might know her decision, Carol's judgment fulfills the expectation of good management.

An additional frustration for Carol is that she has had little formal managerial training for situations such as this one. Because she came in with the new CEO, her managerial competence was taken for granted. Given the lack of an accepted forum within the hospital for discussion of ethical concerns, her inadequate training is an organizational ethics issue. It is unfair of the organization not to make available to its managers the resources to sort through this kind of problem. The ethics officer needs to address this "ethics resource" issue.

Conflict of Interest, or Just a Great Lunch?

During National Long-Term Care Week, staff on Outwest Hospital's respiratory care unit discover one day that the administration of a nearby long-term ventilatory care center has sent over a large and luscious—and obviously expensive—spread for lunch. The note that comes with the goodies reads, "With much appreciation for all that you do for your patients, and with many thanks for your referrals, both past and future, to VentCare." Unit staff are, in turn, pleased and grateful for the thoughtfulness that VentCare is displaying. Several remark that VentCare is one of the most pleasant organizations that they deal with. Both nurses and social workers comment that VentCare is an agency "well worth any referrals we can give them."

This case does not conjure up the specter of fraud or the problem of physician self-referral. Indeed, the situation described here may appear innocuous enough. Nevertheless, the case suggests issues with legal and ethical implications, and it may also be a matter addressed by existing institutional policy.

From an ethical perspective, the main concern is one of conflict of interest in receiving and accepting gifts. Will—or might—VentCare's seeming gesture of gratitude and goodwill influence referral decisions or referral recommendations given to patients and families? This question may not be easy to answer. The written words of the VentCare note suggest a possible intent to exercise influence over Outwest staff. Referral recommendations, and the spoken words of some of the employees, suggest that they are, in fact, influenced by the lavish lunch. On the other hand, VentCare's underlying intent could be innocent and the note imprudently worded. The staffers' comments could simply express their exuberant appreciation in the moment, without implying that their professional judgment in making referrals is affected in practice. The issue of the *appearance* of a conflict of interest remains, however: might someone who sees the lunch and reads the note or overhears the staff's response conclude that they will be influenced by this gift?

As a matter of law, this case raises issues about proper conduct with regard to referral. The government does not permit hospitals or their employees to accept payment for referrals. Accepting this lunch might look like acceptance of a form of *payment* for referrals previously made, and acceptance of an inducement to continue or accelerate the level of referral in the future. Moreover, Outwest Hospital may—and, from a compliance standpoint, should—have a policy limiting receipt of gifts from such sources as vendors and potential recipients of referrals. At the least, an institution normally requires disclosure of gifts exceeding a certain amount (for example, one hundred dollars) that are made to a supervisor or an internal auditor. Policy may also require that the gift be returned if it creates the appearance of conflict of interest.

So what should be done in this instance? The value of the gift may well exceed one hundred dollars, but it is shared among a number of staff people. In view of the source and the wording of the note, this gift probably should be reported to the appropriate party within Outwest. But must staff refrain from accepting the gift? That is, should they refuse to eat the lunch, or even return it if possible? Refusing it seems extreme, and returning it less than gracious. The staff should eat and enjoy.

But to show that Outwest and its staff appreciate the possible implications of a gift given in this way, perhaps a diplomatically worded letter can be sent to the VentCare administration, and a copy posted on the bulletin board at Outwest's respiratory care unit. The letter can express sincere appreciation for the gift, voice gently worded concern about the language of apparent inducement in the note, and conclude with genuine appreciation for the working relationship with VentCare, while stating clearly that referrals are—always—made on the basis of the staff's patient-centered professional judgment. In this way, Outwest communicates both to VentCare and to its own staff awareness of the issues at stake, commitment to put patients' interests first, and continuing resolve to work collaboratively with an evidently worthy partner in the caring community. Thus Outwest displays not only sensitivity to the law but also integration of its ethical (and indeed mission-based) commitments to patients and to excellence in care delivery.

Organizations and Spousal Equivalent Benefits

Sister Bernice Fletcher will long remember this day. At least, that's what she tells herself as she puts down the letter. The CEO of a Catholic health system with more than thirty-eight thousand employees and several hundred sites of care in cities and small towns across the Midwest, she finds herself thinking that things were much simpler in the old days before the Religious Sisters became a system, when it was just one hospital with a small staff. In the old days, all of the nurses and many of the supporting staff—the cafeteria personnel, the med techs, and even some of the aides—were nuns. Sister Bernice sighs and picks up the letter again. She reads:

> We, the gay and lesbian employees of three urban hospitals within the Religious Sisters Health System, seek fairness in benefits for our long-term partners. As employees, we have put many years of caring into expressing the values of the system's mission. Though we are small in number, we believe that our partners and our partners' children ought to be eligible for the same benefits for which married persons are eligible. And we believe that Church teaching mandates access to care for the disenfranchised and that therefore the Religious Sisters hospitals cannot, in good conscience, turn our partners away.

Putting the letter down for the second time, Sister Bernice picks up the phone and dials Dr. Louis O'Leary, the chair of the system's ethics committee.

"Good Lord!" says the chair. "We can't give these people benefits! What will the bishop say?"

There is a pause as the sister marshals her response: "I don't know the answer to that right now. All I know is, we can't afford to lose good employees. Not in this market."

"But same-sex marriages aren't even legal! How can we sanction a union that isn't recognized by state law? Let alone God's law."

"I don't know that we *are* going to sanction it."

"And what about the added financial burden on the system? If we do this, what's next? Where do we set the limits? What constitutes a committed relationship if there's no legal bond?"

"Louie, all I can say right now is, we're going to have to convene the committee to look into it."

"Fine. But the bishop isn't going to like this. And neither are a lot of Catholics out there."

Sister Bernice puts down the phone and sighs again. She will ask the system-wide ethics committee to review the situation, but she will also pursue her own study by using external professionals trained in health care ethics.

The gay employees' letter raises fundamental questions for this system and for religious health care ethics in general. Does a health care system with a specifically religious affiliation have a different set of moral obligations from that of an explicitly nonreligious system? How is the moral analysis different when conducted on the basis of religious ethics as opposed to explicitly nonreligious ethics?

It doesn't take long to summarize the moral arguments contained in the report from the organizational ethics consultant to Sister Bernice on the issues raised in the gay and lesbian employees' letter.

The first argument: "It's not legal."

The thrust is that if same-sex marriage is not legal, the system has no moral obligation to provide health benefits. Yet some corporations have taken the opposite tack and interpreted nonrecognition of same-sex partners under law as the reason for a moral obligation to provide benefits. The argument is that a same-sex couple has no legal remedy when the couple are denied benefits, and that discrimination based on sexual preference and sanctioned by the law creates the need for moral redress by the organization. Some organizations have used this pattern of reasoning to offer benefits to same-sex partners only, and to exclude opposite-sex partners who could avail themselves of marriage and benefits. To the chagrin of those ethics committee members who equate illegality with absence of moral obligation, the argument for moral redress supports the conclusion that if the law is unjust, illegality *grounds* the obligation.

The second argument made by the consultant: "It will cost too much."

The ethics committee at Religious Sisters agrees that this argument can only be settled by facts. A study by William Mercer, a benefit consulting group, indicated that more than six hundred major private U.S. corporations, including fifteen Fortune 100 companies and thirty-five in the Fortune 500, now offer some form of "spousal-equivalent" benefits, or in some cases more comprehensive "domestic partners benefits." The six hundred corporations saw a .01 percent increase in their health care costs. Bell Atlantic, which has more than 100,000 employees in the mid-Atlantic region, now offers the benefit to 233 employees; the resultant annual increase in spending is .07 percent.

To limit financial risk, an organization can establish eligibility criteria (such as living together for a set time in a permanent residence, and joint responsibility for each other's welfare and expenses). In general, the demand is not as great as anticipated, though there are indeed some additional costs.

The third argument in the consultant's report to Sister Bernice: "It would undercut, not promote, the organization's mission and philosophy."

Here the moral argument presses in one or another direction, depending on whether the perspective is nonreligious or religious. From the former, the argument in favor of same-sex partner benefits makes strong appeal to pragmatism, fairness, and diversity. Pragmatically, an organization needs workers to fulfill its mission, and offering partner health benefits is a means of attracting and retaining workers—the competition demands it. From an ethical perspective, the practice promotes the value of fairness, one much cherished in the world of business. A requirement of fairness is nondiscrimination—treating similarly situated persons equally. Same-sex partners can be similar in every aspect to married couples: loyal employees, in committed relationships, and encumbered with the financial burdens of the partner's medical care. Yet employees in a same-sex partnership are denied treatment equal to that provided to similarly situated married employees. Equal treatment offers a moral rationale for equal benefits.

A health care organization also promotes the value of diversity in the workforce, for several reasons. Creating an environment where diverse workers perceive they are treated fairly and with respect increases job satisfaction, which is thought to correlate highly with improved patient satisfaction and increased market share. An organization that expects employees to respect one another's differences (including sexual orientation) yet adopts a policy that discriminates against those who choose a same-sex partner can be perceived as hypocritical. Inconsistent policy erodes moral authority and lowers worker morale. So both a pragmatic and a moral case may be made in favor of same-sex partner benefits.

Religious considerations may turn this moral obligation upside down, depending on the tradition. In this case, where the tradition is Catholic, the teaching authority speaks against homosexual acts and out-of-wedlock relations. Appeals by gay and lesbian workers to Catholic social teaching or to equal and fair treatment meet the counterargument that a Catholic institution has no moral obligation to respect interpersonal relationships (in other words, homosexual partnerships). No right to relations means no moral obligation, including benefits. Other religious traditions with positions ranging from mild accommodation to all-out acceptance of same-sex or domestic-partner relationships might support a conclusion similar to that arrived at by common human morality.

The ethics committee at a religiously based institution has to answer for the extent to which it promotes the moral reasoning of the institution that employs it. The real question in this case may be, Can one ethics committee, or even one system, act in outright defiance of institutional teaching—for example, if the committee arrives at a position that is contrary to Roman Catholic authority? Against a values system that is well defined, all arguments are likely to be moot.

Organizational Teflon
Making Sure the Case Doesn't Stick

After the suspicious respiratory arrest of a patient, a group of investigators from the Ohio State University hospitals met to review the performance of the patient's resident physician, Dr. Michael Swango.* Along with administrators, doctors, and lawyers, the group included a supervisory nurse, who had requested the review based on her suspicions that Swango had injected something into the patient's IV tube. The hospital's medical director reviewed the case record and additional information and told the group that he believed the patient had suffered a grand mal seizure, becoming paralyzed immediately afterward.

Denying a nurse's recollection that he had injected something into the patient's IV, Swango offered different explanations of his actions to the doctors who interviewed him. He was never asked about these inconsistencies. The OSU investigators concluded that Swango could return to patient care, but with greater supervision.

The university did not renew Swango's appointment for the following year, but the chairman of the department of surgery recommended, with reservations, that Swango be licensed to practice medicine in the state of Ohio. When the State Medical Board asked for details, the physician told the board that Swango

---

*For more information, see the article in the Cleveland *Plain Dealer,* "How Dr. Michael Swango Became a Poisoner and Outwitted Two Medical Schools," Dec. 19, 1993, sec. A, pp. 1, 18. Also see Stewart, J. B. "Professional Courtesy." *New Yorker,* Nov. 24, 1997, pp. 90–105; and *Blind Eye: How the Medical Establishment Let a Doctor Get Away with Murder.* New York: Simon & Schuster, 1999.

had been exonerated upon investigation of the incident. Ohio State doctors subsequently recommended that he be licensed to practice medicine in Illinois.

Later, when evidence began to mount connecting Swango to a number of possible homicides of patients under his care, one member of the inquiry group strongly denied that a cover-up had occurred.

At first glance, Michael Swango's case may look more like a health care provider turned serial killer than a problem in organizational ethics. It's easy to interpret the moral story as one man's malevolence toward his patients and coworkers, not bureaucratic bumbling. Further moral analysis might seem pointless, in part because other moral issues are oblique and difficult to identify—there are many moral actors (doctors, nurses, administrators, and lawyers) and choices here. Compared to poisoning and murder, other moral issues in this story seem like peccadilloes, hardly deserving serious critical attention and unrelated to the tragic outcomes.

The tragic events in the Swango case may well be extreme, but they are as much the consequence of organizational failure as they are the actions of a deranged individual. The social interactions, most of them predictable and seemingly benign, set the stage for Swango's subsequent misdeeds.

In fact, this story highlights many of the problems of organizational ethics. The first everyday mistake: fear of litigation becomes the excuse for inaction. Appropriately placed decision makers in the organization had enough evidence to move against Swango but believed that legal inaction was the prudent course. Although many organizational ethics problems do not have such untoward results,the fact that this case went to the brink of criminal investigation should have suggested to organization leaders that alternative grounds for action were mandated. Instead, after the internal investigation two other suspicious but less well-documented incidents occurred, and the chairman of the department nonetheless recommended that Swango be licensed to practice medicine in Ohio.

The second everyday mistake: subtle obstruction. The physicians and administrators resented the checks and balances provided by law enforcement, and they told investigators what they thought the investigators wanted to hear. Passive opposition and misleading information became deadly obstruction. An all-too-common problem of organizational ethics is the lack, evasion, or even obstruction of checks and balances. The division of labor required in a complex organization and the professional discretion afforded health care workers require every organization to have checks and balances. The internal professional regulation that served this function in this case were insufficient for a complex organization; in fact, the hospital group investigating Swango failed to call the actual witnesses before them for statements. As health care organizations rapidly transform into an even more complex set of interactions, professional oversight offers only one part of the needed checks and balances.

A third commonplace mistake: moral blindness. One lawyer who reviewed the case noted that one does not expect a meeting participant—in this case, a physician—to be a killer. Is this comment evidence of the personal trait of always wanting to presume the best about people? Is it a professional courtesy of expected reciprocity among professionals? Or is it an understandable desire to avoid negative publicity for the organization? Certainly the simplest explanation of this blindness is to place the responsibility on individual weakness or on the common practice of protection that professionals afford one another. Yet about this blindness, an investigator concluded that university officials did not want to take responsibility for Swango. They just wanted him out of the hospital. Pinning the blindness on the organization seems futile, except that it has a great responsibility to exercise oversight of its staff. By necessity, a health care organization must have oversight and be vigilant, especially where patient welfare is at stake.

It is easy to miss the organizational ethics problems in this case. Those other than Swango can be exonerated; there was little or nothing they could do from their distance, and why should they be held responsible for the aggregation of infractions committed by a deranged individual? But distance among moral actors and choices as well as an approach of nonstick moral responsibility are organizational aspects that must be addressed if there is to be movement in organizational ethics.

| **Investment Policy**

Partnership Health Care's board of directors is ethically concerned about its investment policy regarding employee pension plans and corporate investments. The board has asked the ethics officer to make recommendations (including social investment guidelines) about PHC's current and future investments in tobacco, liquor, and gaming companies; weapon manufacturing; abortion and birth control; firms engaged in environmentally unsound practices; nuclear power producers; extractive industries such as mining and lumber; and those that exploit or discriminate against women, children, minorities, and religions.

Given how specific the question is, the system's ethics officer decides against using the standing organizational ethics committee and assembles an ad hoc committee that includes the chief financial officer, employees who actively manage the organization's pension policy and corporate investments, and an external investment consultant.

In several short meetings, the ad hoc committee examines all the questions that are adequate for a moral analysis of this organizational ethics problem. First, the group identifies the moral problems. Some frame the issue by asking whether the organization has any moral obligation based on the assumption that only individuals, not organizations, are moral agents. The question is reframed when a consensus emerges that PHC is a moral agent by way of its policy. When PHC invests, its choices affect the corporate income stream, employees' retirement, and the wider community, which may experience some consequences through good and bad investing.

Other committee members frame the moral issue as how to balance resource stewardship with not cooperating with industries that undermine the mission of health. By *stewardship* the committee means maintaining a healthy rate of return on investment, which is necessary to keep the organization solvent, fund capitalization, and provide for adequate retirement for employees. The committee identifies other moral questions but agrees their mandate requires only a formulation that adequately captures the values at risk: financial health and promoting activities consistent with the organization's mission for health.

The committee decides it will first list alternatives and then examine which alternative provides the greatest moral advantage and least disadvantage. One of the alternatives is a total hands-off approach, which ignores obligations of responsible investment because they are not the primary mission of the organization. Committee members reject this alternative, assuming the organization has a moral obligation to the community. Another investment approach is to avoid companies that violate the social guidelines that the committee is going to develop. A third investment option is to proactively invest by supporting only investments that are consistent with the social guidelines. This proactive approach might entail not only careful scrutiny of investments but also letter writing, picketing, and organizing other investors.

The committee decides that the third investment approach could interfere with the primary mission of the organization to provide health services. They reason that the proactive approach requires substantial funds to manage. Consequently the organization might have to shift funds from its core mission.

Even though the committee adopts the middle investment approach, from a sense that it is the least unpalatable option, it still faces the difficult task of developing criteria to select or avoid particular investments. If the organization is to become involved in selecting or eliminating investments, this active management might cost the same as the proactive approach that they veto. Alternatively, they can avoid active management of the investments, simply offering fund managers guidelines for investment and presenting employees with options for socially responsible investment. By shifting the decision making to the employees for their own investment decisions, the committee's obligations are lessened, but the members still have to offer guidelines to corporate investment fund managers.

The committee is at an impasse about social guidelines. Should the system avoid all investments that are morally suspect, or only those that directly affect people's physical health? No committee member questions avoiding tobacco and liquor because they directly affect physical health, but there is less consensus about companies that indirectly affect health, such as the ones in gaming, nuclear power, and mining and lumber. Moreover they are undecided about whether they should avoid investment where the primary business(to take an example) is tobacco, or avoid companies that have any involvement with tobacco. The difficult options lead the committee to recommend that the finance committee continue to discuss and scrutinize these ambiguous options and report regularly to the board. This is an integrity-preserving compromise.

Compassionate Sedation, or Euthanasia?

Compassionate Communication, or Deceit?

Mr. A., a fifty-six-year-old Euro-American male, is suffering from amyotrophic lateral sclerosis (ALS) and was ventilator-dependent. He consented to ventilation with the proviso that he might want to discontinue the ventilator at some future point.

The attending pulmonologist wants a consultation from the ethics committee because "that day has come": the patient has requested removal of the ventilator. The physician indicates that the patient's medical condition has deteriorated, that Mr. A. can barely communicate, and that discontinuing the vent will result in death. Mr. A's family supports the patient's wish to have the ventilator removed.

The physician is concerned. Unlike other patients for whom he has discontinued ventilation, Mr. A. is conscious and alert. Does honoring his request amount to euthanasia? Further, in withdrawing the ventilator, can pain or discomfort be minimized by using sedation, even though the medication itself might possibly hasten death?

After considerable discussion, the ethics committee advises the physician that it is ethically acceptable to discontinue the ventilator. The committee gives the physician journal articles describing use of sedatives in a process of compassionate ventilator withdrawal.

Arrangements are made to discontinue the ventilator on a particular day, and an ICU nurse who is willing to participate in the process is scheduled to care for the patient. The family is alerted to various contingencies, such as the possibility that the patient does not die immediately after the ventilator is withdrawn.

Unfortunately, events betray the best-laid plans. First, the family requests that the withdrawal occur on an earlier date, and the attending physician agrees. But he is on vacation then, so he asks his partner to be present in his stead. The change also means that another nurse is caring for the patient on the actual withdrawal date. Further, the patient is in better shape than the ethics committee has been led to expect; he is communicative and in fact is entertaining himself and others by whispering risqué stories.

When the ventilator is discontinued, with the family and their clergy person in the room, the physician soon pronounces the patient dead. In fact, Mr. A. is still alive; after the family and pastor leave, another twelve hours elapse before the patient stops breathing. In the meantime, by physician order, the dosage of morphine is titrated upward until death actually occurs. (The physician leaves after giving the order; the nurse, though uneasy about implementing it, administers the morphine after conferring briefly with her manager.) The family is not informed of the sequel in their loved one's "death." The primary nurse and the nurse manager do not report the course of events through their chain of command, but some other staff members observe—or surmise—what has taken place.

Soon word of these events reaches the hospital's patient care executive, who is responsible for administrative oversight of nursing. She in turn informs the CEO.

This case poses questions for clinical and organizational ethics. Thus it affords an opportunity to examine the interaction of both sets of issues, while keeping a primary focus on the organizational concerns.

Clinically, the case has already raised questions for the ethics committee: Is withdrawing the ventilator tantamount to euthanasia in disguise? Does using sedation, even for the stated purpose of avoiding discomfort in ventilator withdrawal, tip the scales toward the euthanasia interpretation—especially if the morphine itself carries a known risk of precipitating death? In a retrospective review of the situation, it might be tempting to focus on the ethics committee's advice on these issues. However, although some might disagree with the committee's conclusions, a plausible defense of those conclusions can be made. (For example, it remains true that a patient with decisional capacity retains the legal right to refuse treatment, including mechanical ventilation, even if death will result.) In any case, there is no necessary connection between the committee's advice and the clinical mismanagement that follows. It appears, rather, that several changes in the initially agreed plan of care set the stage for the debacle that follows.

Certainly the clinical management of Mr. A's care during his last hours is highly questionable. There are questions about misinforming or lying to a family about a patient's death, the possibility that something resembling active euthanasia has occurred, the reluctant involvement of a second person and profession in carrying out a physician's dubious order, and the apparent failure of a nurse who is in a management role to question the order or support a staff person in doing so.

"Clinical" though they are, the actions precipitating these questions follow a series of problematic decisions made prior to Mr. A's last hours; the entire process of clinical and managerial decision making seems to deserve retrospective review. Moreover, the clinical questions are now a matter of administrative concern because they also pose legal and public-image risks for the hospital. Irate family members might sue if they get wind of—or figure out—the physician's ineptitude or deception in pronouncing death prematurely. Perhaps worse, if word of this situation reaches the community and is reported by the local media, or even investigated by a district attorney, the hospital will have a public relations nightmare on its hands. Its reputation can be damaged and the community's trust diminished.

Thus the organizational context becomes the primary focus of administrative—and ethical—concern. This context contributed to developing the clinical ethical questions in the first place, and it is the context from which responses to the clinical, legal, and public-relations issues must emerge. Now that word of the situation has reached the institution's senior leadership, there are immediate questions about who (if anyone) else should be informed;

whether the situation should be investigated further, and if so by whom; and what, if anything, should be done (and by whom) following such an investigation.

But what values, virtues, and principles should guide administrative review of the situation? Senior clinical and administrative leaders have a fiduciary responsibility for the good of the organization, which may be understood as the ability to carry out its health care mission. Thus they should exercise the virtue of prudence in support of organizational good; they should act wisely and with discernment to uphold its reputation, financial well-being, and ability to provide excellent patient care in the future. At the same time, they should act in accordance with principles of justice (informed by virtues of integrity and compassion) insofar as they must review the conduct of individual clinicians, make judgments, and perhaps impose sanctions in light of evidence and applicable procedures.

The moral discernment that the leaders undertake interacts with analyses from clinical, legal, and public-relations perspectives. Legal and public-relations questions concern external entities: the civil legal system or law enforcement (or both), and print and broadcast media. The question of whether to inform Mr. A's family of the error or deceit is also a genuine concern. Internal questions are likely to involve hospital governance, the medical staff and its leadership, nursing and patient care functions, the human resource function, and staff morale.

A besetting inclination (or temptation) in such a situation is to keep the lid on. If word of the situation has not yet spread widely, many would advise against doing so. Some might counsel not to let on how much the administration knows, unless it becomes apparent that the lid is already off and passive containment is not possible.

Others might suggest a more active, though still muted, course of action: identify the principal parties involved, investigate the incident discreetly, and have a trusted administrator or medical staff leader (or both) take appropriate parties aside and counsel (in other words, reprimand and admonish) them concerning appropriate professional behavior in such circumstances. If it is possible to obtain a quiet resignation or two, perhaps even that of the responsible physician partner, so much the better. As for the law, the press, and Mr. A's family, the less said the better, unless circumstances necessitate dealing with concerns that emerge from those quarters. There is something to be said for such a discreet approach, but it may evade some of the harder questions—for example, what in the hospital's internal processes or culture could make such a situation possible. Further, it is unlikely to facilitate optimal individual and organizational learning from this unfortunate occurrence.

A quiet yet thorough investigation of the situation seems to be in order, for the sake of quality assurance and process improvement and because of legitimate concern about possible violation of criminal law. In the process, unpleasant questions have to be asked and unwelcome judgments made—facts of administrative life that all concerned might prefer to avoid. But the situation described in the case amounts to a sentinel event, if not exactly by the Joint Commission's definition of the term, nevertheless a disturbing event that leaves a blemish on organizational integrity if left unexamined.

If in the judgment of hospital counsel (or a criminal attorney) the internal investigation yields possible grounds for criminal investigation, appropriate authorities should be contacted. In the process, care should be taken to preserve materials that might later serve as potential evidence (see Case Eight in this regard). The administration and medical staff leadership are also legally bound (and probably ethically obligated, as well) to follow applicable guidelines about reporting information relevant to the licensure of professionals involved, including nurses.

Justice understood as equitable treatment seems to impose a caveat when it comes to possible internal sanctions applying to the nurses and the physician involved. If an investigation shows that errors in care that are subject to disciplinary action have been committed, and if human resource policies require a more stringent disciplinary response to a nurse's conduct than medical staff bylaws or credentialing processes stipulate in response to the physician's actions, a question of fair treatment then arises. For one thing, it is the physician who wrote the order in the first place. Further, in light of the power differential between physicians and nurses, and also from related cultural factors that perhaps contributed to the nurse's acquiescence in carrying out the order, there might be justifiable grounds for some lessening of sanctions that human resource procedures otherwise require.

In any event, it appears the medical staff's elected leaders (and not just the medical director or vice president for medical affairs) should be brought into the loop in such a case. They have a responsibility for medical staff issues, including but not limited to credentialing, and the quality assurance process operates through the medical staff structure. In addition, it is probably better that medical staff leaders hear of the situation directly from senior management than from unofficial sources such as the grapevine.

What about disclosing to the family that they were given inaccurate information about the timing and manner of their loved one's death? Choosing to inform the family of what really happened could be a product of genuine integrity, but such an act might also be intended to preempt the possibility that the family finds out through other channels and then sues the hospital. There is, however, no guarantee that the family will refrain from suing just because the hospital is open with them, and the risk of the family going public to either the media or the police is substantial. On the other hand, compassion for the family suggests not telling them what happened, because such information will only cloud their mourning for their loved one; at the same time, this expression of administrative compassion can also be self-serving by justifying the common inclination to duck the issue and avoid telling.

What about partial disclosure—in other words, informing the family that their loved one died later than they were originally told, while withholding the information about the upward titration of the morphine dosage? Even if the administrative intent is to spare the family additional emotional distress, it is easy to imagine the family wondering what happened to their loved one after he was pronounced dead, demanding to see the medical record, and approaching an attorney and the authorities in any case. The disclosure question may not really be an all-or-nothing proposition. It is not easy to decide how the administrators should proceed on the matter of disclosure to the family, but it is nevertheless important that they think through as clearly as they can, for each course of action, the practical and moral implications for all parties concerned.

Ethical Considerations in Charting

The administration at Outwest Hospital wants to implement a computerized approach to patient medical records. The guiding committee recommends a date-and-time stamp that automatically logs the time of an entry into the patient's chart. An option with this feature is the possibility of setting the clock back, as much as eight hours, to permit late entries. A nurse contacts the hospital's ethics officer with a concern about the backdating feature.

The possibility of backdating raises a number of concerns for the ethics officer, about the purpose of data entry into a patient record, current practices among caregivers, and the best practice to demonstrate desired institutional values. The purpose of data entry in patient records is to document, accurately and honestly, the treatment and the context in which it takes place. The chart is the basis for confirmation of care and medical billing. The patient, caregivers, the hospital, and third-party payers are vitally concerned with the information the chart contains.

The ethics officer knows that during a shift, however, time may not permit immediate and complete data entry. How, she wonders, can we document care in a timely manner that offers all caregivers, supervisors, and the billing office an accurate, honest picture of the patient's care?

If the hospital values accuracy, entries must be factually correct; the chart must contain all pertinent information, entered on a designated form and in proper order for the right patient. Among the questions for the committee to consider are: What data entry

behaviors produce common mix-ups in charting? How is error related to the time of entry?

Honesty requires that the context of care be stated truthfully.
Unanticipated consequences result from a less-than-factual entry.
An oral report is insufficient.

Best practices aim to increase patient safety through prompt
charting of accurate data. In this way, the document is the foundation for making further decisions without delay. The integrity of
the chart is not compromised when used in treatment decisions,
in assigning costs in billing, and in continuous quality improvement review by supervisors.

What about the late-entry window for the date-and-time stamp?
Rather than institute a system that does not promote the values
and virtues of best practice, the ethics officer recommends that the
hospital consider a standard that a patient's chart be considered
incomplete until one hour following the end of a shift, thus recognizing that data entry does not supersede actual patient care.
The standard removes individual discretion to self-determine the
parameters of postshift charting. It gives supervisors a consistent
management approach, and it does not withhold the document
from review for billing.

Executive Use of Discretionary Funds
The Bonus Pool

Martin is the director of development for Partnership Health Care's Charitable Foundation. Jim, a major gifts officer who reports to him, has recently brought in a $25 million gift for the system's new research facility. It is Martin's style to publicly congratulate everyone who secures a gift of $20,000 or more, but in this instance he feels that the size of the commitment warrants extra attention. He makes plans to acknowledge Jim's work at his annual performance review, scheduled in two months.

One Tuesday, Martin gets a phone call from the PHC chief executive, who says Jim has asked for a $10,000 bonus for his recent success. The CEO is pleased at the large gift, since she is acquainted with the donor and the gift is a basis on which to build the capital campaign. She feels that Jim deserves some tangible recognition. Although the health care system's associate bonus plan does not apply in an occasion of this kind, the CEO says she might consider giving such a bonus. However, she tells Martin that he needs to deal with the situation himself.

Martin is furious. He has access to a bonus pool that historically has been used to give merit rewards to associates within the development program, but he has always defined *merit* as work above and beyond satisfactory job performance and never gives large cash bonuses. Martin has used the pool over the years in a discretionary manner to take an associate to dinner, to hold a party rewarding an individual or work team for a job well done, and occasionally to make a salary adjustment for an associate depending on the number of solicitations successfully closed. Although the size of the gift is significant, Martin feels that Jim has merely been doing his job—the very large gift is due more to the generosity of the donor than Jim's extra hard work.

Although the pool can cover Jim's request for $10,000, Martin is reluctant to give it under these circumstances for several reasons. Jim is already the most highly compensated major gifts officer. Martin does not want to signal to other associates that there are "commissions" attached to gift size. Such a bonus would set a precedent and might cause ill will and jealousy among his staff. Finally, he feels manipulated and placed in an awkward position with the CEO because of the action of his subordinate. Should Martin give Jim the bonus he wants?

This case poses a problem for the director of PHC's charitable foundation. Even though organizations are noted for hierarchy, rules, and procedures, many decisions are left to a particular person's discretion. In a general sense, the higher one's position within an organization, the more the discretionary latitude the person possesses, and checks and balances are not always clearly or publicly enumerated. An executive—indeed, any associate—should exercise responsible judgment to minimize the potential for abuse of discretion. In this case, Martin wants to encourage the associates to promote good work and extra effort, but fairness to other associates precludes favoritism to one.

Martin stands to lose a valuable employee. Jim feels unappreciated; he is restless and has been thinking about leaving the foundation. Martin is reluctant to lose Jim, who has been at the foundation for years and has cultivated good relations with a number of potential donors whose support is crucial to the success of the building campaign.

Discretionary decision making always occurs in the broader context of the formal and informal needs and values of the organization. PHC's policies and procedures, covering the many aspects of its operations, guide the individual employee's immediate decisions and actions. The informal culture of the PHC foundation circumscribes Martin's discretionary latitude. Everyone knows that there is a bonus pool, separate from the health care system's formal bonus program, but there has been no established standard by which bonuses are given. By having no set guidelines for dispensing money from this pool, Martin is now worried about the appearance to other associates of giving Jim what he wants. Does this set a precedent, so that the next officer who solicits and secures a large gift will also expect a bonus?

Martin is free to grant the bonus: the money is there, and he has implied permission from the CEO to use it. A couple of options occur to him. To keep Jim on staff, Martin can give him half of his request now and half if he stays for some set period of time (for example, the end of the next calendar year). If he feels that this option also seems like a commission, he can offer Jim a pay raise retroactive to his last performance review and on the condition that if he stays a full year, he will receive the $10,000.

Second, his concern about other associates' perceptions is sound. Other major gifts officers have brought in significant gifts, several at the $10 million dollar level, but none of them have received special bonuses. Others involved in the fundraising program have been successful with corporate donations, too, but the opportunity for very large money is remote in this sector. If other development officers think that Jim is receiving special treatment, Martin may be accused of showing favoritism, thus undermining associate morale.

Finally, Martin personally believes that in philanthropy there is an unwritten rule that commissions are not a part of not-for-profit fundraising. He must decide what values message he wants his staff to hear. If granting Jim's bonus compromises this view, he can tell Jim that his work will be recognized at the next review. At the same time, Martin needs to establish a more carefully prescribed policy about the bonus pool. Delineating and distributing a clear understanding of how the bonus pool is used sets a limit on the director's discretionary authority, but such guidelines should work against actual or perceived abuse of discretion.

Integrating Spirituality in the Health Care Setting

The Partnership Health Care system is under pressure from its board to make spirituality more tangible within its institutions. The motivation arises out of competitive marketing as much as the mission of the founding hospitals to provide health care that respects the faith of the individual seeking help.

Through all its acquisitions, the system has become secular. The board, the chief operating officer, and senior management are unsure what spirituality is, let alone how to make it tangible. Nor are they sure about the long-term implications of emphasizing spirituality in day-to-day operations. What are the organizational ethics issues, and what mechanism is most capable of addressing them?

"I'm not religious, but I am spiritual" is a remark that one hears with increasing frequency. What the speaker means by the word *spirituality* is not particularly clear. What does health care look like when spirituality is explicitly part of it? Is attention to spirituality an appropriate arena of concern for an ethics officer or ethics committee?

Aside from the puzzle of what the term *spirituality* has meant, what it means now, and what motivates expanding interest in it, the recent rush to integrate spirituality into health care threatens to reduce spirituality to one more instrumental good supporting improved health outcomes. For instance, some studies suggest that religious activity can lower blood pressure and fortify the immune system. The danger of such studies is that they may oversimplify the value of spirituality by treating it strictly in terms of its usefulness to health. In contrast, other studies argue that although spirituality promotes outcomes such as inner resiliency, detachment, and theological creativity, it does not necessarily cure physical disease.

It is a useful experiment to imagine integrating spirituality through the perspective of the moral actors who inhabit modern health care. Is a health care professional who has little interest in spirituality but is faced with patients seeking spiritual help expected to offer a prayer or ritual even though he or she does not have a spiritual belief? Is personal integrity diminished if he or she merely goes through the motions? On the other hand, if a health care provider has an interest in spirituality, should he or she engage a patient in some spiritual practice if the provider does not have sufficient time or ability to deal with it? How far should the health care provider go if the spiritual practice does not contribute to positive health outcomes, or if the patient has a different spiritual practice? Whether a health care worker engages in a spiritual practice or not, what are his or her professional obligations to be a source of (and be able to provide the diversity of possible) spiritual beliefs and practices?

From a health care leader's perspective, such as that of an executive or trustee, what should motivate the organization to spend resources on spirituality: being sensitive to the market, improving employee and patient satisfaction, or fulfilling its mission? Is an executive off the hook if the organization is secular and nonreligious? Should professionals other than pastoral care staff attend to spirituality? How adept should each group be at spirituality, and how should the organization go about teaching spirituality to these groups—if it can be done at all? Finally, what institutional safeguards are necessary to avoid coercive practices?

Even if one does not work within health care, as a citizen one might want to imagine what the posture of society should be toward spirituality through publicly funded organizations, government regulations, and incentives. Suppose that spirituality is a basic human good because it helps individuals and societies flourish. What is society's obligation to promote the good of spirituality (what philosophers term the "good of religion")? If spirituality is a basic human good like health and education, who ought to promote it?

These are only first steps into this murky area, but for a health care organization the initial lesson is clear. To responsibly integrate spirituality into the health care setting, diverse personal beliefs about religion and spirituality require those concerned with the ethics mechanism to reflect on it from a variety of perspectives. Whatever direction is taken should honor the value of *primum non nocere:* above all, do no harm.

Alternative and Complementary Medicine

A nonprofit health care system, PHC is interested in opening a for-profit complementary and alternative medicine (CAM) clinic. Under current planning, the new clinic will offer services ranging from acupuncture, massage, and chiropractic care to nutritional supplements. The system will grant medical staff credentials to some of the clinic's specialized service providers and reimburse them on a discounted fee-for-service basis. PHC will aggressively advertise its CAM clinic to the public.

At a recent meeting of the planning group for the new CAM clinic, several members have raised issues that threaten the initiative. Struggling to convince area employers to contract with PHC's package of health care benefits, the director of contracting for the system is excited about the appeal of the new clinic's services. "There's a lot of interest in alternative therapies out there," he exclaims, "It's really popular. This could be a real moneymaker."

The human resource director of PHC wonders if the system's own health benefit package will include coverage for this alternative medicine as an option. Otherwise, system employees will have to pay full fee for the CAM services. A board member wonders about the match of this for-profit enterprise with the system's nonprofit mission. "We're not only in this for the money," she states. "Besides, I understand that its very popularity carries a risk to our bottom line. Since we would contract directly with employers on a discounted fee-for-service basis, the risk of financial loss is carried by us. We benefit from low utilization. We suffer if utilization is higher than we planned."

At this point, the medical director explodes: "A lot of physicians don't accept this decision to provide these alternative services. They see the move as motivated by money. And you're granting privileges to acupuncturists and chiropractors? What about issues of safety, effectiveness, and benefit to patients?"

Partnership Health Care's desire to set up a CAM clinic is an example of a rapidly growing trend in the United States: integrating alternative medicine into a conventional health care system. The director of contracting has reason to be excited about the trend. In 1997, Americans paid $27 billion out of pocket for 629 million visits to practitioners of complementary and alternative medicine (exceeding visits to primary care physicians). Growing popularity, however, does not decide the matter of whether or how complementary and alternative therapies should be made available as covered benefits.

There are a number of ethical concerns the planning group must consider before issuing a recommendation. A large group of affiliated physicians has not endorsed the decision to provide CAM services. Understandable ethical concerns about the clinic's for-profit status have been raised by these physicians (and halfheartedly by a board member), fearing that the move is purely economic in motivation. Conferring privileges on CAM practitioners, apparently without assessing the array of services in terms of evidence of safety, effectiveness, and benefit to patients, strengthens these physicians' ethical concerns. At the very least, the system's communication with its own medical staff has been inadequate. The system needs to be careful, too, about the message it may be sending to the communities it serves.

Because opening a CAM clinic certainly represents endorsement of alternative medical practices, PHC must be satisfied about the qualifications of the clinical practitioner and the safety of services for the patient. Discussion about standards of efficacy and effectiveness of CAM is vigorous. The methodological problems in designing research studies to measure effectiveness of alternative treatments are real, but they are consistent with those in the literature attempting to evaluate medical procedure interventions. Studies do show that acupuncture and chiropractic medicine benefit many patients, especially those with chronic pain. Most CAM therapies are relatively inexpensive, in comparison to the costs of conventional medications and surgical procedures. No societal or professional consensus on criteria for including CAM therapies exists, but it seems reasonable that they be evaluated individually, as with conventional medical therapy, in terms of safety; practitioner qualification; and evidence of efficacy, benefit, and cost-effectiveness. The evaluation must be rigorous and the standards high.

The concern about PHC's motivation in this case raises the issue of its not-for-profit identity. A for-profit and a not-for-profit health care organization alike require capital resources to provide and improve quality services, and they compete in the marketplace on the basis of quality and cost. However, the for-profit's motive is to make money, but the not-for-profit company exists to serve community interests and sees community benefit as the principal mission. A for-profit company's primary question in any policy decision is how to ensure a reasonable return on investment. For a not-for-profit health care organization, the question is how to benefit patients and community, using resources prudently in service of the mission. A higher percentage of profit for this organization is invested into the community served, to improve facilities and programs, purchase community services, and provide uncompensated care to the poor.

PHC's current stance sends a confusing message to the community. By opening a CAM clinic, the system conveys endorsement of the safety, effectiveness, and benefit of those patient services. If the system is confident about these concerns and aggressively markets the services as a health benefit to companies and individuals, it should not restrict covered access by its own employees. Otherwise, PHC seems to devalue its stated commitment to holistic health and to maximizing quality by promoting safe and cost-effective treatment.

Partnership Health Care needs to formulate methods and mechanisms to assess the quality of its services and their patient outcomes. It also has an opportunity to develop and publicize the ethical principles and economic values that guide decisions in entering into contracts with employers, health plans, and its own medical staff.

Overstepping the Bounds of Expertise

A thirty-year-old woman undergoes surgery for removal of a benign fibroid tumor in her uterus—a routine outpatient procedure, during which she dies. Two doctors perform the surgery, using equipment they are neither familiar with nor authorized to use. In addition, a salesperson from the medical device manufacturer that makes the equipment used in the surgery operates the controls while the doctors perform the procedure on the woman. Nurses in the operating room express concern that they are not trained in assisting with the equipment, but the doctors tell them not to worry because the salesperson is operating the controls—a violation of hospital policy.

Later, a hospital spokesman states, "The hospital is saddened by the patient's death. Those who acted inappropriately violated hospital rules and procedures and will be severely disciplined." Behind the scenes, after much bickering between the medical staff and hospital administrators, the medical staff president asks the ethics officer to investigate the case and make recommendations.

On one level, this case presents no difficulties: there has been clear violation of several standards of patient care and professional responsibility. Although the salesperson was not implicated in the death, clearly the medical staff disregarded concerns for patient safety by allowing an uncertified person to participate in a surgical procedure. The actions also violated the ethical standard of informed consent regarding use of a new piece of equipment and the salesperson's presence. Everyone involved exercised poor judgment; the tragic outcome involved the death of a patient who entrusted the physicians and the hospital with her safety. The state health department, the hospital, the medical staff, and other regulatory groups should investigate and issue appropriate sanctions.

Yet the ethics officer still wonders how something like this can happen. The case reveals attitudes within a health care organization that affect how associates exercise their judgment (see Chapter Seven). It reflects the risk to the organization that arises when people who have specific expertise or leadership roles overstep the bounds of their authority and competence. Sometimes these actions have adverse consequences—in the worst case, causing injury or death. Such risk can be reduced through regulation (a system of reward and punishment), through terms of the employment contract, by insisting on ethical commitment on the part of workers (for example, to a professional code of ethics, or loyalty to the organization or to fellow employees), or a combination of these controls. Routine insensitivity or competing obligations, however, may lead health care workers to question and disregard the appropriate boundaries placed on their discretion.

Among health care workers, the ethics officer notes, physicians have the greatest discretionary latitude in decision making, but even a doctor makes a decision within certain boundaries. Moral and legal controls exist in the form of regulation, standards of practice, and professional ethics. Professionalism suggests that a physician should do more than merely comply with controls of this type. The physician should also have a sense of what is right for a particular occasion. The two physicians in this case did not just violate standards; they also appeared to think that what they were doing was in no way wrong. By performing an invasive procedure on a patient, using equipment on which they were not trained (operated by a person not medically certified), the physicians showed disregard for their patient's safety and well-being.

The fact that physicians can so easily—unthinkingly—violate professional and organizational norms and values reinforces the importance of the informed consent process, not as perfunctory patient acceptance of a proposed procedure but as a review and commitment to the patient regarding actions to be undertaken on his or her behalf. By means of informed consent, the patient authorizes and trusts the physician to act within agreed-upon bounds.

Under those conditions, overstepping the bounds of authority means the doctor must accept accountability and critical scrutiny for his or her decision.

This episode raises a significant question for the hospital: If the patient had not died, would this practice have been reported? Formal standards of care and regulations are designed to prevent such an occurrence, but if the physician violates them more or less routinely it seems that the informal organizational culture is not supporting exposure of this behavior.

A big problem in organizational ethics is identifying inappropriate practice. Nurses are responsible for raising concerns when they perceive dangers to patient well-being. In this case, the operating room nurses expressed concern that they were not trained in using the technology, but they apparently did not question the salesperson's presence in the operating theater. In this hospital culture, as with health care generally, a nurse may be reluctant to directly question a physician's action. Usually, an inappropriate, or even illegal, practice is not exposed thanks to lack of protection for employees (nurses in this case) who ask questions. Along with clear standards of practice, the organization must establish a means for expressing concern about the standard of care to be addressed, along with adequate safeguards for people who bring violation to light.

Beyond appropriate investigation and disciplinary action of the particular professional groups, the first step for the ethics officer at this hospital is to delineate clear boundaries to the authority attached to a position and ensure adequate understanding of the responsibility and accountability that accompany discretion. The second step is that, working with the medical and nursing staff, administrators should design a system of checks and balances to routinely evaluate a health care provider's use of discretion. Building on this case, the hospital should review existing policy and develop new management systems to prevent future tragedy. The staff needs to be educated about appropriate roles and professional responsibility. Finally, the organization should establish a forum to address staff concern with violation of authority, and design safeguards for those who expose them.

Marketing Products and Practicing Medicine

A West Coast managed care organization offers a variety of HMO and PPO products. At the last several board meetings, the medical board report has indicated great dissatisfaction among affiliated physicians. It is most apparent in the organization's inability to retain regional medical directors and physicians. Such dissatisfaction on the part of physician-employees can translate into lower patient satisfaction and potentially lower volume.

In particular, physicians have voiced the problem as a values conflict arising out of the marketing department, which is developing and selling products to employers. The products are limiting physician discretion in providing care—what physicians can do within their offices and under what circumstances they can refer. Physicians mutter that those who develop the products for sale to PPOs are "practicing medicine" because the decisions affect professional discretion. Those responsible for developing products within the managed care organization point out that they are making decisions about "centers of excellence"—which physicians to keep on the panel, where services are assessed, etc.—on the same statistical or epidemiological criteria that evidence-based medicine now practices.

If the managed care organization relinquishes decision making to the physicians, the predictability (and benefits) of improved cost and outcomes might be lost. The physicians' concerns are part of a larger, growing debate in the state—evidenced by the vocal nurses' association that claims managed care is "de-skilling" nursing and treating the nurses as fungible widgets, replaceable by any number of less professionally trained workers.

The board is concerned about what to do with this growing conflict. The value of professional autonomy and discretion is in conflict with the value of producing a cost-effective product that serves the needs of the community in the midst of an aggressive market. Some board members suggest that this is not an ethics issue, but rather a political one for professions wanting to regain authority. Other board members, though sympathetic to physicians' professional authority, believe there is no reason to initiate a discussion of this volatile issue because the movement of the external environment is largely out of their control. In short, the issue will be played out elsewhere. Still others intuit that not answering the values conflict forces it to flash out in subversive ways. Yet board members holding this last opinion are unclear on how to engage the growing conflict: Should the board examine this issue? If so, what questions should it ask? What method of analysis should be applied? What outcomes are to be expected from the analysis?

As those responsible for governing care and services, the board members recognize that how they deal with this conflict is important. They are responsible for containing costs and providing quality care. In an aggressive market, they have to make decisions and set policy that affects the viability of the organization and the quality of its services. Therefore, the board should examine the situation for systemic problems, of which there are several: employee dissatisfaction and turnover, patient dissatisfaction and loss of volume, challenges to professional autonomy and discretion, control of decision making and of the health care marketplace, cost containment, and risk to patient well-being.

Ignoring the situation, as some members advocate, sets the stage for potential abuse that can sabotage developing a responsible managed care organization. For example, if the schism continues, physicians may attempt to fix a systemic problem by gaming the system (trying to subvert the reimbursement system to get care that they believe is necessary for patients). This action defeats the managed care organization's mission and undermines its services.

The board recognizes that the product developers are charged with creating reasonably priced but nonetheless excellent and highly competitive products—that is, charged with combining cost containment strategies with the more elusive task of achieving real and measurable quality and accountability. They must balance patient good with the good of other patients served by the plans, the good of the plan and the organization expressed in the limits they place on care, and the self-interest and professional interest of caregivers. Increasingly, these goals have drawn them into uncomfortably detailed involvement in health care delivery. It is no longer unusual to find developers engaging in activity that only recently would have been considered the private and inviolable business of patients and physicians.

In this case, the board should identify individual participant concerns and seek to understand the values that underlie them. First, affiliated physicians are concerned that their loyalty and commitment to patient well-being is being undermined, leading to loss of freedom of choice for clients and providers and inappropriate denial and reduction of necessary services. This perception reflects a common dislike for managerial dominance of medical practice, which is expressed in various ways: crucial decisions made by a minimally informed reviewer; undue delay in authorizing covered treatment; and reliance on practice guidelines and protocols that threaten individualized care. Those on the board with a managerial bent see these concerns as complaining on the part of professionals who are losing traditional control of their work.

The accusation that their concern is a political one dealing with limits on authority may have merit, but to give physicians sympathetic credit, the pressure in managed care to contain cost conflicts with the physician's duty to act in each patient's best interest. This issue of divided loyalty seems especially sharp when a physician's compensation arrangement, as devised by the organization, sharply pits the physician's own finances against patient health needs.

The product developers (and some board members) may believe that traditional notions of physician discretion amount to wasteful use of resources and inconsistent outcomes. They feel that reducing expenditures and use of services by means of increasing efficiency and coordinating client care benefits the patient by eliminating unnecessary and potentially harmful treatment. According to the theory of managed care, good case management founded on evidence-based medicine yields better or more desirable treatment for patients than treatment based on individual physician performance and can expand the range of services offered, improving quality of care and quality of life. Physician autonomy may be redefined according to new criteria. Also, by controlling costs, managers increase shareholder return.

Although not mentioned in this case, the patient clearly has a stake in this controversy. Patients desire quality care that minimizes harm and takes their best interest to heart. They want to be treated justly. Finally, patient trust in the physician is an important value affecting compliance and follow-through.

The board can then define the ethical issues: How can all members of the organization balance loyalty to the patient with just and prudent gatekeeping of social resources in an intensely competitive health care environment?

For the organization to be an ethical provider, the board must cultivate a process, not a set of rules, in which all associates must share. To the extent that institutional policy and structure are central to the complex causality that produces patient benefit and minimizes patient harm, administrators and managers must understand that they have a moral obligation (a prospective responsibility) traditionally reserved for clinicians. The clinician must also recognize the new health care playing field of managed care, with its tension between cost containment and quality of care. The physician must balance traditional patient advocacy with new gatekeeping roles. All associates, therefore, must work together to provide efficient, quality care.

The board might recommend some antidotes to ethical concerns. First, it should reinforce the organization's quality assurance programs. It should design effective procedures to monitor and evaluate denial and accessible mechanisms for appeal. The board should strengthen protection against unauthorized access to confidential information and encourage caution in developing and refining practice guidelines or protocols, balancing evidence-based data with physician input.

If the board does nothing, it runs the risk of being perceived by physicians, and eventually patients, as putting financial considerations ahead of patient care. A managed care organization puts appropriate concern about cost containment alongside patient and physician values in pursuing ethical practice.

Following the Rules, or Using Them as a Smokescreen?

For many years, the administration and the personnel department of St. Somewhere have openly sought to establish a "humane" work environment. Believing that a rule-driven atmosphere undermines such a goal, the director of personnel instead developed a set of broad principles to guide employer-employee relations. He explained at managerial meetings that most employee relations problems are too complex to be solved by rigidly applying "the rules": "In most employee practice disputes," he would say, "we give you the principles that are derived from our mission and values, and we believe that you can listen impartially to all sides and render a fair decision."

This director is now ready to retire. The personnel department has become human resources (HR), and it is clear that other changes are needed as well. Federal and state regulations have multiplied geometrically, enforcement is more exacting than ever, and accrediting bodies now insist on seeing detailed human resource manuals as evidence that standards are being met. It is time for "less idealism and more practicality," as the CEO puts it.

The new director of human resources has an MBA from a prominent business school and knows what has to be done in the new climate. Although she solicits input for a new HR handbook from managers and line staff, the finished product bears the unmistakable stamp of her training and efficiency.

Among other things, the new handbook features clear and rather detailed rules for employer-employee relations. The new director explains that the changes, though necessary, benefit managers and employees alike. Clear guidelines, rules, and procedures mean that employees know precisely what is expected, what is not tolerated, and what procedures they and their supervisors should follow when questions or problems arise.

In general, the new system works well enough. Some managers complain about having to do things by the book, and many lament the apparent need to document *every* employee performance problem. But having clear rules to guide practice proves to be a time-saver in most instances.

However, some HR staff think they see a problem as St. Somewhere begins to downsize its workforce in certain departments. The handbook promises the terminated employees that they will be automatically placed on a wait list for new openings, with the proviso that "the terminated employee will have the requisite skills to perform the open position at an acceptable level."

Many employees with an unblemished work record at the hospital quickly find new jobs under this procedure. Even if they do not have all the skills listed in the job description, good employees are given an edge over external applicants. But it is different for any employee whose work record is marred by a warning for tardiness, a note that the employee registered a complaint against her supervisor, or excessive absence due to "care of sick children." It seems that the recruitment function seldom passes on these names to hiring managers, or does so without recommending them—even when an employee appears to have the requisite skills.

The question that HR staff not involved in recruitment begin to ask one another is whether the rules are really being followed, or whether purporting to follow the new rules is serving as a kind of a smokescreen for actually breaking them.

It is easy for old-guard staff to blame the apparent problem in this case on the new rules. After all, the practice uncovered here was evidently unknown before the detailed rules (and accompanying documentation practices) were established. But discrepancies between actual practice and presumed or espoused practice surely existed in the old regime as well. The real question is whether the new rules and the use to which they are put serve the values they are meant to uphold. The human resource procedures governing treatment of downsized employees presumably aim to serve the organizational good—which primarily means the ability to carry out the health care mission—while treating terminated staff members fairly and humanely.

It is unlikely that any organizational promises to employees who are terminated because of staff reduction are made solely out of compassion, loyalty, or a sense of fairness. Promises of favorable consideration for future employment can also reflect recognition that good new employees are hard to come by (especially in a seller's job market), and perhaps further realization that employee morale will benefit if St. Somewhere finds a place for its own who lose their jobs.

On its face, the handbook language cited here is somewhat ambiguous. The promise of being put on a waiting list, even if one has the requisite skills, does not necessarily entail an additional promise of favorable consideration. At the least, St. Somewhere should clarify whether being on the wait list implies favored consideration for those who have the skills. Employees who already feel vulnerable because of the reductions need clarity and forthrightness from the organization; potentially misleading promises do not help.

Indeed, it appears that the recruitment staff have not interpreted this so-called rule as a blanket promise, whether their interpretation reflects their own reading of the rule or the dictum of some higher authority within HR. That some terminated employees—those whose HR files are clean—receive favorable consideration even though they lack required job skills makes this case troubling. By waiving the requisite-skills condition, the HR function is not following its own rules. Moreover, by apparently withholding recommendations from other employees on the basis of work record rather than job skills, the recruiters seem to be following another set of (unwritten) rules. This possibility in turn raises questions of basic fairness, and even discrimination, insofar as some of the unwritten criteria involve minor or one-time problems, denigrate the situation of a working parent, or even retaliate against employees who have simply exercised their right to complain or file grievances through proper channels.

Covertly using such tacit recruitment and selection criteria is also troubling because it is reminiscent of the dubious organizational practice of eliminating positions whose incumbents just happen to be marginal performers or otherwise deficient in someone's eyes— even if there is little or no paper trail documenting performance problems. In the present case, it does not seem that a position is selected for elimination on this basis; rather, it is an employee's chance for reemployment that appears to be affected by unwritten, indeed unspoken, criteria. As a result, staff belatedly discover (if they get wind of the exclusionary practice) that their former work record *can* be used against them—with no explicit warning that such use might occur in a time of downsizing and rehiring.

It is not unreasonable for an organization to consider overall work performance in deciding to transfer or rehire a downsized employee. But the criteria used should not be arbitrary or picky—let alone downright discriminatory—and they should be stated in advance, as clearly as possible. Moreover, in addition to violating such considerations of fairness and humane treatment, failing to deal honestly with downsized staff members is likely to become known by other employees (the "layoff survivors"), who pay special attention to the employment fate of former colleagues and friends. If real or perceived promises are not kept, if the organization falls short of integrity in dealing with those who have served it with some measure of competence and loyalty, then in the long run it is also a loser—and, whether directly or indirectly, so are patients and clients.

Organizational Advancement and Corporate Compliance

A decade and a half ago, Deaconess Hospital enjoyed a reputation for a superb pathology department. Those glory days were almost solely attributable to the long and distinguished career of the department chair, Dr. Alfred Markham. In addition to his own careful lab work and widely heralded articles in respected journals, Markham attracted to his staff a number of talented young clinician-researchers who shared his strong commitment to service in the hospital and wider community.

When Markham retired fifteen years ago, the hospital leadership knew it could not replace him with someone of equal stature. They selected one of his most promising associates to head pathology, but the new chair did not work out. By the time he left, Deaconess's reputation in pathology was badly damaged. The hospital then chose as chair a solid, if unspectacular, external candidate, Dr. Frank Joste. During his tenure, the department held its own, albeit without that former prominence.

Joste's retirement is now six months away. The search for a successor is in full swing. But should the hospital again settle for his brand of "good, standard professionalism," as one search team member put it, or should it seek a return to the glory days in pathology by trying to land a sterling candidate?

At this juncture, Dr. Elva Brighton suddenly enters the picture. She is a well-known, midcareer pathologist who likes the Deaconess opportunity for two reasons: it would allow her to pursue both a clinical practice and research and to live within driving distance of her aging parents. The search committee is soon convinced that she is their candidate. They want to make every effort to bring her on board.

Unfortunately, some of Brighton's expectations seem extravagant. Salary and benefits are not the problem. The hospital has developed a range of compensation packages that give Deaconess flexibility in attracting and retaining outstanding physicians. The worry is Brighton's programmatic demands in research: she says she needs a lab furnished with the latest equipment, two full-time research assistants, and funds to attend three professional meetings a year, one of which requires travel abroad.

Actually, Brighton's expectations are not so unusual in a hospital with a strong research component. But Deaconess has let that dimension of its identity wane. No one on staff has a lab of his or her own, and research assistants are appointed only if a grant includes them in the approved budget. Furthermore, in an effort to cut costs, the hospital gives staff the funds to attend only one professional meeting a year.

Although meeting Brighton's demands would create an exception to existing procedure, the search committee argues that this is precisely what is required if Deaconess is to rebuild a reputation as a center where the outstanding clinician-researcher can find a home. As everyone recalls from the Markham years, that kind of reputation can have transforming consequences both within and outside the hospital.

The Deaconess administrators listen attentively to the search committee's arguments. But they are also keenly aware of the hospital's new corporate compliance policy. How can they approve exceptional benefits for Brighton when they fear that discovery through a government audit could endanger the hospital's tax-exempt status and key funding streams? How can they find a way, within the bounds of good-faith compliance, to fulfill the desire to return Deaconess to its glory days?

Corporate compliance is concerned with the law. One requirement of the law is that a nonprofit organization avoid paying inappropriate compensation, benefits, or other remuneration to individuals, including benefits designed to function as recruitment incentives. Insofar as corporate compliance is a concern here, the heart of the issue is the administrative team's perception that they are being asked to approve exceptional benefits for Dr. Brighton. They fear that a federal audit will discover and question such benefits, with potentially devastating consequences for Deaconess's tax-exempt status and government revenue sources. The administrators evidently believe that meeting Brighton's costly expectations for program support may be seen as an improper incentive.

They may be more fearful on this point than is necessary. Making inappropriate payments or offering other improper incentives is called "private" inurement because an individual profits or otherwise benefits by receiving a payment or benefit *for personal use*. In this instance, Brighton appears to be asking for *program* support, however extravagant her request may seem. The benefits in question appear unlikely to line the physician's pockets (or find their way there by some devious route).

Nevertheless, in its compliance program the hospital should be—and probably is—monitoring all physician compensation plans to ensure compliance with applicable laws and regulations. The appropriate person(s) or department(s) within Deaconess should evaluate all proposed compensation and benefit packages. Brighton's package is no exception. In addition, even though the program money she requests is not to be paid to her, the proposed expenditures will also be reviewed because they are to be part of her employment contract.

Could Deaconess still commit inadvertent violations in meeting Brighton's demands for program support? After all, fulfilling her expectations means favoring her pathology program over all other research programs at the hospital. Is there a "business" justification for doing so? This case indicates that in the labor market, which includes teaching and research hospitals, what Brighton asks is often granted. She is neither asking for, nor likely to receive, support that exceeds what the market already supports.

Moreover, the search team has articulated a business rationale for honoring her demands: the desire to rebuild a vibrant research program and regain the reputation that goes with it. Such results can be parlayed to the hospital's advantage through sound advertising and marketing strategies. Funds given to Brighton's research program thus serve to promote the well-being of the hospital, as well as that of its research programs. Given the evidence at hand, it does not appear that the administration needs to fret about violation here, so long as it maintains adequate vigilance through the normal monitoring processes. If the language of Deaconess's corporate charter makes room within the hospital's mission for research, then generously supporting Brighton's research efforts is not problematic from a compliance standpoint.

The proposed course of action seems to raise another organizational ethics issue, however. Many at Deaconess wax nostalgic for the glory days when outstanding research won recognition for the hospital. At the same time, the current de facto reality is that funding for research has been cut back significantly since the Markham era. If Brighton is brought on board on her terms, a precedent is set and will be hard to break. She will have been promised research support in grand style. Is the hospital really prepared to pay—and keep paying—for the privilege of her presence over the long haul?

Further, what about those who already engage in medical research at Deaconess? They have learned to do without over the years, but they have probably not forgotten how to ask for more if an opportunity presents itself. They might of course be envious if Brighton is blessed with research perks that they do not receive—a morale issue that might well need to be addressed. But her success in negotiation might also embolden them to ask for budget increases. If they invoke a fairness argument in making their case ("You're doing it for her; why not for us too?"), what would the administration say to their requests for more support? Is the hospital willing to ante up to establish a semblance of proportionate, if not equal, research support? Or is it instead prepared to give a thoughtful rationale for instituting and maintaining a significant disparity in the level of support it gives to other research programs and their leaders?

These are some of the challenges that Deaconess must meet if it chooses to embrace a research agenda as a means of building a reputation in its community and beyond. In stewarding resources, the senior leaders—and perhaps the governing body as well—must determine whether such gains are worth the inevitable price to be paid. Do (and, over the long haul, will) administration and governance value prominence in research enough to channel substantial resources to it—in direct contrast to the belt-tightening approach that the hospital has long pursued? Indeed, how much should Deaconess's mission not simply include but emphasize research? Answering these questions means clarifying the nature of the organization and measuring the resolve of its leaders.

The Compliance Officer and the Ethics Committee

Outwest Hospital has recently hired a corporate compliance officer, attorney Phillida Trant. It has been suggested that she be invited to join the hospital ethics committee.

Deciding whom to invite to be a member of an ethics committee is a challenging and important task. Members must have certain interpersonal skills, such as the ability to articulate their opinions clearly and openness to discussing difficult and sometimes controversial moral positions. The committee should also be representative of the whole community. It should have members from a variety of professions within the hospital, and perhaps even members of the surrounding community. Broad membership brings additional perspective to the issues discussed by the committee and avoids the perception that it may be manipulated to conform with the professional interests of the committee, which could be the case if membership is limited to certain professions.

The question of whether or not Trant should be invited to join the ethics committee, however, goes beyond the simple matter of personal qualification. It raises fundamental questions about the nature and identity of the ethics committee and the corporate compliance effort within Outwest. What is the function and purpose of the ethics committee? Is it limited to consideration of clinical ethics, or is it intended to address a wider range of institutional issues? If the latter, is it to be the coordinating locus of institutional ethics, or merely one element of it?

Some prominent bioethicists believe that a clinical ethics committee should be kept separate from any consideration of institutional ethics. They argue that the committee lacks the necessary expertise to address institutional ethics issues and that consideration of institutional values and interests can hamper the committee's ability to maintain the primacy of patient interest. They view institutional ethics as just another form of business ethics, which should be addressed in another forum. If this is the approach taken at Outwest, Trant may not have the appropriate skills to serve on the ethics committee. Her professional focus upon legal liability and corporate compliance issues may introduce those issues into the committee's deliberations and inhibit the effort to make patient interests paramount.

Other bioethicists disagree with this position on limiting the scope of the committee. In an age in which questions about justice and allocation of institutional resources have become a pervasive issue in connection with patient care, they wonder how a clinical ethics committee can avoid confronting these concerns about institutional ethics. For a committee that accepts the necessity of considering institutional issues, Trant can offer some important insights drawn from her training and position within the organization. The question then becomes whether her contributions might unduly influence the committee.

People often have difficulty understanding the difference between ethics and law. They fail to recognize that ethics can and generally does call for adherence to standards more exacting than the minimalist morality imposed by the law. Equally, Trant could be so professionally concerned with protecting the organization that she overemphasizes caution in protecting the interests of the organization in every situation. This could impair the committee's consideration of patient interests if they challenge this cautious approach. This potential role dynamic may argue against inviting Trant (or any member of the corporate legal department) to join the committee.

There is also a question about the structural relation of the ethics program(s) and the corporate compliance program. If issues of legal compliance are the sole concern of the corporate compliance program, then there is some risk that the institution's employees and its patients may view the compliance officer as the organizational police. Inviting Trant to join the ethics committee may lead some to consider the ethics committee as an extension of the compliance program. They may not feel comfortable raising controversial issues in front of the ethics committee for fear that it will lead to an investigation by the compliance office, or they may feel that the only appropriate subjects for the ethics committee are those that touch on problems of law and health care regulation. Because of this apprehension, important questions might not be brought to the committee. This would limit its ability to bring moral guidance and leadership to the institution.

On the other hand, if the compliance program is formulated as a more expansive integrity program, intended to support broad moral values as well as strict legal compliance, this threat of confusion may not arise. Indeed, in such a case, inviting Trant to join may confirm the organization's commitment to linking compliance with ethics. It may facilitate coordination between these two programmatic efforts. Trant could provide the committee with insights on regulatory concerns while, at the same time, she is exposed to some of the larger mission and ethics concerns of the organization outside the area of strict legal compliance.

In summary, the decision about inviting the corporate compliance officer to join the ethics committee rests, first of all, upon determining the purpose and function of the committee and the compliance program, and second, upon weighing issues relating to the personal dynamics of the committee and the individual involved.

Case Twenty

Aggressive Accounting

Three years ago, when Suburban Hospital found itself in financial trouble, it hired Allan Hale as a senior administrator on the basis of his experience in revitalizing a large health care corporation not in health care. In reviewing hospital billing practices, Hale immediately noticed that the coding of a given medical condition significantly affected reimbursement. He instituted new policy such that, whenever there was an ambiguity in a patient's diagnosis, clerks would enter the most remunerative code possible.

Hale has also found the billing department too cautious in its reimbursement claims for expenses such as interest charges for the facilities under Medicaid and Medicare programs. He has directed that whenever there is any doubt, staff should claim the maximum amount. As a realist, however, he has instructed accounting personnel to develop two financial plans: one to incorporate the reimbursements claimed under the aggressive approach, and the second to assume that many of those claims will be disallowed.

This case raises questions of law and corporate compliance. Perhaps Hale is thinking *This is how the health care reimbursement game is played,* but his approach is likely to result in numerous violations of federal law. Routine "upcoding," or seeking the most remunerative way to code a procedure, is an easily detectable practice that is often targeted by government investigators. Since distinctions between codes are based on the severity of a medical problem, coding a condition under a more severe heading constitutes fraud.

Further, federal health care laws uphold a strict standard of honesty in making claims. If a claimant seriously doubts the legitimacy of a claim, it should not be submitted. Moreover, although making best-case and worst-case financial plans can have some legitimacy, the existence of two plans and two sets of supporting records has been seen by prosecutors as evidence of bad faith. If Suburban's records betray doubt about reimbursable claims, regulators might infer that senior management knows certain claims are inaccurate. If government investigators discover billing irregularities, Suburban could face substantial fines *and* possible exclusion from all federal health care programs.

The legal and financial jeopardy created by this conduct might be avoided by attention to ethical as well as legal dimensions. Ethically, the essential duplicity of the aggressive approach should be an immediate sign of trouble. Practices that require a pattern of duplicity to succeed are always questionable and should be avoided.

Part Three

Appendixes

Appendix One
Joint Commission on
Accreditation of Healthcare
Organizations

The following standards, intents, and examples are excerpted from the Joint Commission on Accreditation of Healthcare Organizations' *Comprehensive Accreditation Manual for Hospitals: The Official Handbook* (Oakbrook, Ill.: JCAHO, 1999), RI-1 through RI-34.

[1.1] Patients' Rights and Organization Ethics

Overview

The goal of the patient rights and organization ethics function is to help improve patient outcomes by respecting each patient's rights and conducting business relationships with patients and the public in an ethical manner.

Patients have a fundamental right to considerate care that safeguards their personal dignity and respects their cultural, psychosocial, and spiritual values. These values often influence patients' perception of care and illness. Understanding and respecting these values guides the provider in meeting the patients' care needs and preferences.

A hospital's behavior towards its patients and its business practices has a significant impact on the patient's experience of and response to care. Thus, access, treatment, respect, and conduct affect

Reprinted with permission from the Joint Commission on Accreditation of Healthcare Organizations. *Comprehensive Accreditation Manual for Hospitals: The Official Handbook.* Oakbrook, Ill.: JCAHO, 1999.

patient rights. The standards in this chapter address the following processes and activities:

- Promoting consideration of patient values and preferences, including the decision to discontinue treatment;
- Recognizing the hospital's responsibilities under law;
- Informing patients of their responsibilities in the care process; and
- Managing the hospital's relationships with patients and the public in an ethical manner.

Practical Application

The following example illustrates all components of the flowchart for Patient Rights and Organization Ethics, including the rights that the hospital protects on behalf of the patient, and the hospital's ethical practices. First, the patient's rights to access, treatment, and respect.

A four-year-old girl is severely injured by an automobile. En route to the hospital, she is managed by the emergency physician staff via radio-telephone. Hospital staff are aware that she will be taken directly to a trauma room, so her access to care and treatment will not be hindered by check-in procedures; her parents will take care of these later.

As soon as the emergency medical technicians arrive at the hospital, they report the child's condition and care since the accident, her current physiological status, and the results of efforts to determine her name and her parents' names and addresses. The child's hospital treatment team takes over, and is responsible for continuously assessing the patient's critical vital functions and treating all life-threatening conditions.

When the child's parents arrive, they are informed of their daughter's condition; according to the trauma room protocol, a member of the child's treatment team speaks with them as soon as possible after the patient's arrival and every thirty minutes thereafter. The protocol is designed to meet the patient's treatment needs and to respect the right of the family to be involved in the care process.

The hospital also has in place procedures that address the organization's ethical practices.

Since the family belongs to a health maintenance organization (HMO), the hospital follows the HMO's procedures for notifying the child's primary care physician. The child's stay in the hospital, from her arrival at emergency service to her discharge from the pediatric unit, is evaluated as part of the hospital's utilization management program, and her length of stay in each unit is compared with data from an external utilization management service.

The child's condition does not respond to the prescribed medication, but the physician staff believes she can be helped by one of the hospital's medication clinical trials. Before placing the child in the trial, however, they fully inform her parents and obtain their consent. If the child had no hopes of recovery, staff members would ask her parents if they wish to donate her organs or tissues.

As the child approaches discharge, it appears she will need a specially made prosthetic device. Although the device is not available in the hospital, it is available from a wholly owned subsidiary of the hospital. The staff informs the parents of this relationship while the referral is being planned and asks if there is any other prosthetic group practice they wish to use. They also check to see if the HMO requires them to use a particular practice.

Standards

The following is a list of all standards for this function. They are presented here for your convenience without footnotes or other explanatory text. If you have a question about a term used here, please check the Glossary, pages GL-1 through GL-24. [*Note:* the glossary is not included in this Appendix to *Organizational Ethics in Health Care.*] Terms that are critical to the understanding of the standard are defined in the margin adjacent to the term as it appears in the next section of this chapter, "Standards, Scoring, and Aggregation Rules."

RI.1 The hospital addresses ethical issues in providing patient care.
    RI.1.1 The patient's right to treatment or service is respected and supported.
    RI.1.2 Patients are involved in all aspects of their care.
        RI.1.2.1 Informed consent is obtained.

RI.1.2.1.1 All patients asked to participate in a research project are given a description of the expected benefits.

RI.1.2.1.2 All patients asked to participate in a research project are given a description of the potential discomforts and risks.

RI.1.2.1.3 All patients asked to participate in a research project are given a description of alternative services that might also prove advantageous to them.

RI.1.2.1.4 All patients asked to participate in a research project are given a full explanation of the procedures to be followed, especially those that are experimental in nature.

RI.1.2.1.5 All patients asked to participate in a research project are told that they may refuse to participate, and that their refusal will not compromise their access to services.

RI.1.2.2 The family participates in care decisions.

RI.1.2.3 Patients are involved in resolving dilemmas about care decisions.

RI.1.2.4 The hospital addresses advance directives.

RI.1.2.5 The hospital addresses withholding resuscitative services.

RI.1.2.6 The hospital addresses forgoing or withdrawing life-sustaining treatment.

RI.1.2.7 The hospital addresses care at the end of life.

RI.1.2.8 Patients have a right to appropriate assessment and management of pain.

RI.1.3 The hospital demonstrates respect for the following patient needs:

RI.1.3.1 Confidentiality;

RI.1.3.2 Privacy;

RI.1.3.3 Security;

RI.1.3.4 Resolution of complaints;

RI.1.3.5 Pastoral care and other spiritual services;

RI.1.3.6 Communication.

> RI.1.3.6.1 When the hospital restricts a patient's visitors, mail, telephone calls, or other forms of communication, the restrictions are evaluated for their therapeutic effectiveness.
>
> > RI.1.3.6.1.1 Any restrictions on communication are fully explained to the patient and family, and are determined with their participation.

RI.1.4 Each patient receives a written statement of his or her rights.

RI.1.5 The hospital supports the patient's right to access protective services.

RI.2 The hospital implements policies and procedures, developed with the medical staff's participation, for the procuring and donation of organs and other tissues.

RI.3 The hospital protects patients and respects their rights during research, investigation, and clinical trials involving human subjects.

RI.3.1 All consent forms address the information specified in RI.1.2.1.1 through RI.1.2.1.5; indicate the name of the person who provided the information and the date the form was signed; and address the participant's right to privacy, confidentiality, and safety.

RI.4 The hospital operates according to a code of ethical behavior.

RI.4.1 The code addresses marketing, admission, transfer and discharge, and billing practices.

RI.4.2 The code addresses the relationship of the hospital and its staff members to other healthcare providers, educational institutions, and payers.

RI.4.3 In hospitals with longer lengths of stay, the code addresses a patient's right to perform or refuse to perform tasks in or for the hospital.

RI.4.4 The hospital's code of ethical business and professional behavior protects the integrity of clinical decision making, regardless of how the hospital compensates or shares financial risk with its leaders, managers, clinical staff, and licensed independent practitioners.

Standards, Intents, and Examples for Organization Ethics

Standards

RI.4 The hospital operates according to a code of ethical behavior.

RI.4.1 The code addresses marketing, admission, transfer and discharge, and billing practices.

RI.4.2 The code addresses the relationship of the hospital and its staff members to other healthcare providers, educational institutions, and payers.

Intent of RI.4 Through RI.4.2

A hospital has an ethical responsibility to the patients and community it serves. Guiding documents, such as the hospital's mission statement and strategic plan, provide a consistent, ethical framework for its patient care and business practices.

But a framework alone is not sufficient. To support ethical operations and fair treatment of patients, a hospital has and operates according to a code of ethical behavior. The code addresses ethical practices regarding:

- Marketing;
- Admission;
- Transfer;
- Discharge; and
- Billing, and resolution of conflicts associated with patient billing.

The code ensures that the hospital conducts its business and patient care practices in an honest, decent, and proper manner.

Example of Implementation for RI.4 Through RI.4.2

A hospital's governing body reviews a proposed relationship before entering a contractual agreement with a provider of service. The proposed contract is approved or rejected based on best-bid practices and the potential for conflict of interest. Marketing materials only reflect the services available and the level of licensure and accreditation. All initial patient billing is itemized and includes dates of service. The hospital has a formal process to review patient or other payer questions about charges expeditiously and resolve a conflict or discuss a question without real or perceived harassment.

Admission and transfer policies are not based on patient or hospital economics. Only patients whose specific condition or disease cannot be safely treated at the hospital are diverted, refused admission, or transferred to another hospital.

Examples of Evidence of Performance for RI.4 Through RI.4.2
- Interviews with hospital leaders
- Conflict of interest statements
- Governing body bylaws
- Governing body minutes
- Code of ethical behavior
- Patient billing procedures

Standard

RI.4.3 In hospitals with longer lengths of stay, the code addresses a patient's rights to perform or refuse to perform tasks in or for the hospital.

Intent of RI.4.3

Patients are encouraged to take responsibility for their own living quarters. In addition, patients may be offered the opportunity to perform work for the organization (for example, patient work therapy programs in grounds keeping or the library) that does not endanger the patient, other patients, or staff. If the hospital asks longer-stay patients to perform such tasks (work), the patient has the right to refuse. If the patient agrees to perform tasks for the organization:

- The work is appropriate to the patient's needs and therapeutic goals;

- The organization documents the patient's desire for work in the plan of care;
- The plan specifies the nature of the services performed and whether the services are nonpaid or paid;
- Compensation for paid services is determined based on the work performed, whether the work would be otherwise done by a paid employee, and the applicable wage and hourly standards in the community for the work; and
- The patient agrees to the work arrangement described in the plan of care.

  The intent of this standard does not extend to the patient's care of his or her body, maintenance of his or her room or space, or the patient's preparation of his or her own meals.

Standard

RI.4.4 The hospital's code of ethical business and professional behavior protects the integrity of clinical decision making, regardless of how the hospital compensates or shares financial risk with its leaders, managers, clinical staff, and licensed independent practitioners.

Intent of RI.4.4

To avoid compromising the quality of care, clinical decisions (including tests, treatments, and other interventions) are based on identified patient health care needs. The hospital's code of ethical business and professional behavior specifies that the hospital implements policies and procedures that address the relationship between the use of services and financial incentives. Policies and procedures addressing (and information on) this issue are available on request to all patients, clinical staff, licensed independent practitioners, and hospital personnel.

Examples for RI.4

A network component hospital is directed to base its code of ethical behavior on its mission and to document in the hospital's annual budget and strategic planning process how the code is used as a framework for ethical business practices.

Examples for RI.4 Through RI.4.2

1. A small hospital develops a plan to identify and implement a code of ethical behavior. An ad hoc committee—composed of two

members each from governance, senior executive leadership, the medical staff, nursing, social services, and the business office—is appointed and given the responsibility for developing a code.

The first step in the committee's work plan is to ask the local university's resource center to do a literature search for existing codes of ethics for the health care professions, organization development literature, and business literature. The committee reviews the articles found and identifies codes that include activities appropriate to the hospital's services and business practices.

The committee then develops an outline for its own code by identifying key phrases common to each of the codes that can be reasonably related to business ethical practices. Several meetings are devoted to developing the structure of the hospital's code of ethical behavior. Once the structure or draft outline is in place, it is reviewed by staff from the various groups represented by members of the ad hoc committee over a one-month time period.

The results of this review are then considered by the ad hoc committee, whose members write a full draft of the code. This draft is passed before all involved groups—governance, senior management, medical staff, nursing, social services, and business—and department heads.

Department heads are asked to discuss the draft code with their staff and to provide feedback to the ad hoc committee within a month. The discussions result in further revisions. Once complete, the hospital's governing body adopts and approves the code, and publishes it in the hospital newsletter. An article about the code is also published in the local newspaper. Because of widespread community support, the hospital's leaders decide to share their experience in developing such a code by submitting articles for publication in professional journals.

2. The hospital's code of ethics was developed in consultation with its legal counsel and addresses:

- A general policy statement;
- References to documents such as the Board-approved Mission, Vision, Strategic Plan, Performance Improvement Plan;
- A list of patient rights and responsibilities;
- An implementation policy that listed, among other items, employee orientation, the employee handbook and newsletter, a

medical staff newsletter, community education about advance directives, and the Values and Ethics Committee [as educational and supportive resources];

- Other references to manuals and policies and procedures, such as those on DNR (Patient Care Manual), protective services (Social Service Department Manual), confidentiality (Administrative Manual), and staff conflict of values (Human Resources Manual);
- Patient billing and associated conflict resolution procedures;
- Marketing and public relations processes;
- Admission, transfer, and discharge processes that list various policies addressing these issues; and
- A section on conflicts of interest pertaining to contractual relationships that referenced Board policy in the Administrative Manual, a requirement for an annual conflict of interest statement signed each year by each board member, an Administrative Manual policy on contracts and agreements, gratuities/vendor relationships, anti-trust policy, prudent buyer concept policy (Materials Management Policy), and conflict of interest (Human Resources Manual).

Examples of Implementation for RI.4.1

1. Fee and payment policies are posted or provided to the ambulatory patient or responsible party upon entry into the hospital's outpatient services system. Patients are made aware of the hospital's procedures for resolving billing issues. These procedures are included in a patient brochure, posted in waiting rooms, or verbally provided by staff.

2. Staff in hospital physician offices are able to identify policies related to marketing and billing practices that address such issues as accuracy of billing, resolution of disputes over billing, and accuracy of printed marketing materials. These policies may be contained in a brief ethical code of conduct statement, or they may be incorporated within the policies of the hospital's financial and marketing departments.

Examples of Implementation for RI.4.2

1. Staff must respect the rights of patients across the entire continuum of care and services when their diagnosis and treatment plans involve multiple referrals. Ambulatory clinics or physician of-

fice practices owned by the hospital share the full health services continuum with the hospital and must provide full disclosure of their relationships with all other health care organizations, providers, and educational institutions. The requirement for full disclosure should be framed in the context of the hospital's code of ethics.

2. All hospital-owned and -operated ambulatory care clinics and centers have an ethical code of conduct of individual policies that address such issues as the disclosure of ownership and contracting policies for individuals or groups who may benefit from their business relationships with the community-based ambulatory health centers.

3. Co-owners of the ambulatory care facility and members of the hospital's governing body annually complete conflict-of-interest statements or comparable documents. Any potential conflicts of interest identified in these statements are addressed by the governing body.

4. Ambulatory surgery managers conduct quality review activities that provide an analysis of:

- Cost factors, when appropriate, such as the costs of specific categories of medications (for example, antibiotics) or the costs associated with lab test ordering patterns when specific disease-related quality activities are performed;
- Variances in the number or type of preoperative diagnostic tests that are ordered to determine their appropriateness; and
- Standing protocols or orders for care to determine if unnecessary testing or procedures are included.

Purchasing records demonstrate cost pricing for large-volume items, major purchases, and high-cost items.

Example for RI4.4

The organization reviews and updates its code of ethics to protect clinical decision making. It then ensures all staff, including those in hospital-owned and operated ambulatory settings, are aware of the revisions. Ethical statements define the ways all health care professionals in an ambulatory setting care for patients. For example, the owners and other leaders of a hospital-owned ambulatory facility met with the professional staff to discuss revising the clinic's code of ethical practice to describe how practitioners work with each of their patients in an "ethical manner." Facility leaders decided to use a combination of statements from the state's medical and nursing practice acts that outline the legal duty of the practitioner to assess the needs of patients and then inform and educate patients about the array of interventions, care, or treatment options that meet those assessed needs.

The following standards are excerpted from the Joint Commission on Accreditation of Healthcare Organizations' *Comprehensive Accreditation Manual for Hospitals: The Official Handbook* (Oakbrook, Ill.: JCAHO, 1999), HR-21.

[1.2] Managing Staff Requests

HR.6 The hospital addresses a staff member's request not to participate in any aspect of patient care.

HR.6.1 The hospital ensures that a patient's care will not be negatively affected if the hospital grants a staff member's request not to participate in an aspect of patient care.

HR.6.2 Policies and procedures specify those aspects of patient care that might conflict with staff members' cultural values or religious beliefs.

Appendix Two
Sample Ethics Statements

[2.1] American College of Healthcare Executives Ethical Policy Statement

Organizational Ethical Mechanisms

Statement of the Issue

A number of factors have contributed to the growing concern in health care organizations with ethical and bioethical issues: pressures to lower costs, scarcer financial resources, advances in medical technology, decisions near the end of life, and increased patient demands, to name just a few. Increasingly, executives of health care organizations are being called upon to resolve these serious ethical conflicts, but they cannot and should not make these decisions alone. Health care organizations should have vehicles, such as an ethics committee, a set of written policies, and/or a staff ethicist, to assist in the decision-making process. In this way, demands from patients or their families, physicians, the government, special interest groups, and the community can all be weighed and balanced, and the decision making process can reflect these multiple interests.

The Joint Commission on Accreditation of Healthcare Organizations has also recognized the ethical issues present in the health care setting. The commission's *Comprehensive Accreditation*

American College of Healthcare Executives Ethical Policy Statement reprinted with permission of the American College of Healthcare Executives, copyright 1993.

Manual for Hospitals now requires accredited hospitals to have in place "mechanism(s) for the consideration of ethical issues arising in the care of patients and to provide the education to caregivers and patients on ethical issues in heath care."

Simply stated, ethics can be defined as the application of a person's values in decision making situations. These values are derived from a number of sources—family background, religious training, social interaction, education, and employment experiences. In addition, an individual's ethics are often impacted by societal boundaries such as state and federal laws and business practices. And, of course, any value system is always subject to change.

Policy Position

The American College of Healthcare Executives supports the development in health care organizations of mechanisms to deal with general ethical and bioethical issues and decisions. Further, the College supports and encourages its affiliates, as executives of health care organizations and as leaders in their communities, to play an active role in developing organizational ethical guidelines, policies, and/or committees.

Decision making mechanisms should also be ones that can deal with a variety of ethical concerns—medical, social, and financial. The most obvious examples include providing assistance and counsel on care for the terminally ill, care for the critically ill and/or handicapped newborns, organ transplantation, patients' right to refuse treatment, and providing support for patients and family members. However, more abstract issues should also be addressed, such as the allocation of scarce resources, the fair distribution of benefits and burdens, and the rights of individual patients in relation to other patients and to society. These mechanisms, ideally, should allow for the just distribution of power, the protection of human rights, and security for the weak and the vulnerable.

As leaders in their respective organizations, health care executives have a primary role in the development and operation of these organizational ethical mechanisms. The effectiveness of such a process should be of personal as well as professional concern to the manager since it is his or her responsibility to act as facilitator and advocate in upholding the values of the organization, safeguarding the rights of patients, and promoting a full and fair discussion of the issues. In addition, it is the health care executive who assists others in the organization in reaching a consensus on value-laden questions.

While other health care personnel, such as physicians, nurses, social workers, etc., often consider ethical decisions individually on a case-by-case basis, it is the executive's task to also consider the implications for the community in general and society at large in any ethical decision-making situation. To effectively perform this task, the health care executive must work with the trustees of the organization to establish clear ethical standards that will serve as guidelines in their decision making.

The exact form of decision-making mechanisms may vary. For example, if it is an ethics committee, it might include some or all of the following types of persons: physicians, nurses, managers, trustees of the health care organization, social workers, attorneys, patient and/or community representatives, and the clergy. All of these individuals have a unique perspective in discussing current and anticipated ethical problems, as well as in considering possible solutions and outcomes. It is the task of the executive to facilitate this discussion, and it is also his or her responsibility to ensure that no one person or group controls the process.

Other mechanisms to advance ethical decision making include the establishment of agreed upon ethical standards, education of trustees, staff, physicians, and suppliers regarding these standards, and the provision of forums for open discussion of ethical issues.

As technology advances and as financial resources shrink, ethical and bioethical dilemmas will likely become an increasing element in the decision-making process in health care organizations. No one policy will be effective in every organization. Each organization, under the leadership of its executives, must develop its own processes and procedures for discussing and dealing with these sensitive issues.

Approved by the Board of Governors of the American College of Healthcare Executives, August 6, 1993.

Source: American College of Healthcare Executives, Suite 1700, One North Franklin St., Chicago, IL 60606-3491.

[2.2] Moral Commitments Guiding Organizational Conduct

St. Somewhere Medical Center strives to conduct its affairs in accord with the words and deeds of Jesus as handed on in the Catholic faith tradition. All organizational activities contribute to offering health care services to persons with physical, spiritual, and emotional needs, especially for those who are poor. Medical Center activities are based upon St. Somewhere's Five Key Values:

1. Compassion, care, concern
2. Respect for the dignity of each individual
3. Quality care of the whole person
4. Care of the poor
5. Teamwork

Each member of the St. Somewhere community—governing board members, medical staff, employees and volunteers—is responsible to act in a manner consistent with the Medical Center's ethical principles and moral commitments.

All persons associated with St. Somewhere Medical Center are obligated to exercise good faith and honesty in all dealings and transactions touching upon his or her duties to the Medical Center.

St. Somewhere Medical Center creates a workplace that respects the dignity of every person, promotes employee participation, and ensures safety and well-being.

St. Somewhere Medical Center will act honestly and justly in its financial transactions with patients, payers, and vendors.

St. Somewhere Medical Center will provide accurate and truthful information in its public relations, media, and marketing communications.

St. Somewhere Medical Center will maintain a high level of knowledge and skill among its employees and volunteers in the delivery of quality care for the whole person with compassionate concern.

We Will	*We Will Not*
Conform to all applicable state and federal laws when not in conflict with St. Somewhere Medical Center ethical standards.	Profit from relationship to St. Somewhere Medical Center in personal, entrepreneurial endeavors.
Maintain compliance with all standards and regulations pertaining to health care and employment.	Profit from participation on hospital committees or from hospital sponsored events, for example, formulary committee or medical education.
Obtain legal consultation when appropriate.	Fail to establish internal control in any area of business cycle.
Educate employees, members of medical staff, and board members as to potential conflicts of interest.	Hire on basis of nepotism or political considerations rather than on need and competence.
Require that an annual Conflict of Interest Statement be signed by all who have access to confidential organizational information, including employees, members of the medical staff and board members in leadership positions.	Receive inappropriate gifts of value or monetary compensation, i.e., kickbacks.
	Use or divert Medical Center property for private benefit.
Request and review all potential conflicts and take appropriate action.	

[2.3] Advocate Health Care Ethics Statement

Preamble

Advocate Health Care's five values—equality, compassion, excellence, partnership, and stewardship—are an expression of organizational, as well as personal, beliefs and convictions. In this statement, we publicly profess how our values will guide our organization's behavior in four areas of organizational activity: patient

Advocate Health Care Ethics Statement reprinted with permission of Advocate Health Care.

We Will	*We Will Not*
Treat patients and staff in a manner that accommodates their beliefs, customs, and values whenever it does not conflict with St. Somewhere Medical Center ethical standards.	Provide personnel information to individuals without authorized access
Create a work environment that is free from verbal, physical and sexual harassment, as well as free from discrimination and favoritism.	Gossip about patients, their family members, or coworkers.
Demonstrate dignity and respect in all interactions.	Use profanity.
Prevent unauthorized sharing of patient or personnel information, with particular sensitivity to the increased accessibility to such information through advanced technology	Tell off-color or ethnic jokes.
	Disregard cultural or religious sensibilities of others.

care, billing, marketing, and external relations. (Future versions may address additional areas of organizational behavior.) This statement will assist us in weighing our values and choosing among alternative courses of action in decision and policy making. As a living expression of Advocate's values, the statement is a work in progress. The Advocate community is asked to study and examine the statement and to participate in the process of continuing review and revision.

Ethics in Patient Care

Guided by our value of Compassion, we will care for patients throughout the continuum of care on the basis of medical judgment and with due consideration for their personal preferences.

Guided by our value of Stewardship, we will care for patients throughout the continuum of care in the context of our commitment to responsibly manage available resources.

We Will	*We Will Not*
Maintain accurate, fair, and prompt billing practices.	Overbill by adding services that are provided.
Resolve all billing issues consistently according to established organizational policies	Create hardships for those truly unable to pay by use of collection agencies.
Assist patients in understanding how they are charged for the health care services they receive.	Fail to adequately orient collection agencies to the mission, philosophy, and values of St. Somewhere Medical Center.
Work toward resolving patient questions, concerns, and disputes in a way that is mutually satisfying to both the patient and the institution.	Communicate charges in an unclear, deceptive or misleading manner.
Administer the charity care program fairly.	
Deal honestly and fairly with all customers, suppliers, competitors, and financial partners.	

Guided by our value of Equality, we will formulate timely and appropriate patient care plans in conjunction with the patient, the family and/or significant others, and members of the health care team.

Guided by our value of Partnership, we will provide to our associates and other caregivers appropriate information—including the patient's follow-up treatment plan, explanation of medication and medical equipment, and advance directives as patients are transferred within the continuum of care.

Ethics in Billing

Guided by our value of Excellence, we will issue accurate, understandable, and timely bills to patients and payers and charge only for services rendered. We will interact with our customers through associates who are well informed about the billing process and responsive to inquiries and requests for assistance in this process.

We Will	*We Will Not*
Consider the needs of the community when planning programs, services, and health promotion activities.	Recommend hospital-based services when cheaper, quality services are available elsewhere.
Provide clear, truthful, fair, and accurate information in all advertising, communications, and disclosures of information and data.	Market types of care that the provider cannot deliver completely or well.
	Create services that are not aligned with the community health needs, or plan services without community involvement.
Advocate for the health of all citizens and members of our community.	Market simply to please particular physicians or vendors.
	Favor programs that are profitable but not essential to meet community needs.
	Make extravagant claims or provide inaccurate information in public communications.

Guided by our value of Partnership, we will assist patients in the resolution of billing conflicts involving third parties.

Guided by our value of Compassion, we will respect the patient and his or her family throughout the billing and collection process.

Ethics in Marketing

Guided by our value of Excellence, we will protect the confidentiality of our customers and associates who participate in research or other information-gathering forums.

Guided by our value of Partnership, we will exercise responsibility in communications with external and internal audiences and avoid misleading or exaggerated statements.

Guided by our value of Equality, we will create communications that are responsive and sensitive to our diverse audiences and seek the opinions of our customers and associates in developing our communications.

We Will	*We Will Not*
Ensure access to health care for all patients, regardless of their ability to pay.	Fail to provide interpreters or educational material as necessary.
Provide services to meet the identified needs of our patients.	Admit based on ability to pay rather than medical need.
Provide only services that are necessary and considered to be effective.	Admit based on facility's need rather than the need of the client/patient.
Adhere to a uniform standard of care throughout the organization.	Fail to respect the dignity of people in the admissions process because of economic status, race, religion, or sexual orientation.
Provide services only to those patients for whom we can safely care within this organization.	Fail to disclose to patients their financial responsibility for services.
Address patients' psychological, social, spiritual, and physical needs.	Fail to provide pertinent information related to transfer.
Provide care that is appropriate and needed for each patient's condition, following well-designed standards of care.	Fail to acknowledge patient's right to be involved in the decision process.
Provide to patients and significant others information regarding rights and responsibilities, as well as complaint processing procedures.	Transfer solely for convenience or economic advantage of the medical center or physician.
Provide information as needed about services, costs, admission, transfer, and discharge practices.	Transfer triggered by DRG reimbursement to exclusion of considering patient-specific clinical and social circumstances, for example, comorbidities or capacity of family for caregiving.
Initiate search for third-party funding for indigent patients, when appropriate.	Transfer on basis of ability to pay (dumping).
Educate uninsured patients and families about possible low-cost state-initiated programs.	Prioritize nursing home transfers by payer source rather than by patient need.
	Discharge prematurely on basis of financial rather than medical considerations.
	Discharge to home without adequate care capabilities because long-term care facility is not readily available.
	Fail to involve patients and families in plan for after-hospital care.
	Fail to investigate the discharge situation from the perspective of health and safety of the patient.
	Fail to network with community services.

Ethics in External Relationships

Guided by our value of Partnership, we will select partners who promote values and business practices consistent with ours. We will promote partnerships with community-based organizations in an effort to benefit our local communities.

Guided by our value of Equality, we will conduct our relations with partners in a way that promotes diversity and avoids discrimination and unfair treatment.

Guided by our value of Excellence, we will strive to contain costs while continuously improving the quality of our services. We will expect all our associates to avoid foreseeable conflicts of interest in external relationships, and we will work collaboratively with them to remove actual or potential conflicts of interest.

Guided by our value of Stewardship, we will manage the resources entrusted to us and our partners in a responsible, accountable, and environmentally sound manner.

[2.4] Sample Catholic Hospital Organizational Ethics Statement

I. Purpose

This policy articulates the overarching values (Section II) and general procedures (Section III) that apply to Sample Catholic Hospital's organizational ethics. Values and risks specific to organizational units within Sample Catholic Hospital and the procedures necessary to address these risks are developed on an as-needed basis and at the discretion of the Organizational Ethics subcommittee.

II. Values

A. *Sources of Values.* Sample Catholic Hospital is committed to an integrated institutional ethics program; this is accomplished by the establishment of an ethics committee. One subcommittee of the ethics committee addresses patient care. A second subcommittee, considered in this document, addresses organizational ethics, including all business aspects of the institution.

Sample Catholic Hospital's institutional ethics are grounded in its Mission Statement and its Roman Catholic heritage. This grounding is uniquely articulated in the National Conference of Catholic Bishops' *Ethical and Religious Directives for Catholic Health Care Services* and further augmented by principles of business ethics. Sample Catholic Hospital stands behind these values on the belief that actions directed by these values contribute to a high standard of patient care and promote excellence of practice of all those who work within or with the institution.

Among the values that inform excellence in practice are those found in the Mission Statement: Dignity, Compassion, Commitment, Nonabandonment, and Caring. The *Ethical and Religious Directives* also highlight values that should promote excellence in practice, including stewardship and subsidiarity (promoting subunits within the hospital to make choices before being sent to higher administrative levels). Finally, principles of business ethics augment these values. Some values are the very precondition for doing business, for example, truth telling and promise keeping. Without these moral virtues, business itself would be impossible.

This organizational ethics statement acknowledges that each member of the clinical and administrative staff possesses obligations that are articulated in professional codes of ethics and are not repeated in this policy. In addition, conflicts arising between professional and personal/family values are omitted from this policy. Conflicts arising from working within an organization are spelled out in this policy.

B. *Common Risks to Cherished Values.* Any employee of any institution could place the institution at risk, not because they fulfill a specific role such as physician, nurse, or administrator, but simply because they work in the institution. These organizational risks are not limited to those employees whose work concentrates on the business side of the hospital; these risks affect all agents of the hospital, including the Board of Trustees, administrators, and all clinical and nonclinical employees.

These common risks to cherished values are offered here as tools for personal reflection to assist individuals in striving for excellence in the workplace. Common examples that agents could fall victim to include inefficiently using resources, either through sheer waste, failure to use the most cost-effective means for achieving ends, hiring extra personnel, or using organizational resources to provide perks for companions. Equally important to be aware of are goal substitution (covertly pursuing one's personal or professional goals rather than those of the hospital) and basing clinical decisions (including tests, treatments, and other interventions) on financial incentives rather than on patient health care needs. Another risk would be the misappropriation of resources: improper requests for reimbursement for travel, equipment, and other expenses, as well as the diversion of resources from projects for which they were intended to other legitimate projects.

Assuming tasks that do not fall within the employee's domain of expertise in order to appropriate the resources available for pursuing them is overstepping professional authority, another organizational risk. Additionally, passive opposition, such as stalling on implementation, requesting further studies, more data, etc., as a deliberate though unacknowledged attempt to impede implementation can also thwart the goals of the organization. Finally, the more commonly recognized risks to cherished values are shirking (pursuing leisure or other unauthorized activities during compensated work time) and partiality (basing personnel placement and advancement decisions on personal loyalties rather than on performance).

C. *Promoting an Ethics of Excellence.* Employees who are motivated by a sense of excellence can avoid risks common to all employees. Some of the central principles organizations use to respond to these problems are:

- Stewardship to counter self-interest or misappropriation;
- Separation of powers to avoid substitution of one's own goals (whether laudable or not) for those of the institution;
- Promoting impartiality to insure unprejudiced treatment of employees and patient/families;
- Truth telling and promise keeping to establish and promote trust and fidelity;
- Fairness to ensure equal treatment of similar cases;
- Subsidiarity to foster the assumption of responsibility by even the smallest group;
- Due diligence to avoid shirking.

III. Procedures That Promote Excellence

A. *Means to Identify, Study and Address Risks and Values of the Organization.* The institution realizes that the risks to values it cherishes are difficult to identify and that it is also difficult to find easy solutions when values are compromised. Sample Catholic Hospital is therefore committed to the establishment of an ongoing organizational ethics subcommittee whose responsibility it is to identify, study, and address issues of organizational ethics.

The organizational ethics subcommittee is part of the institutional ethics functional committee; its membership and scope of authority is described in that committee's guidelines. The first responsibility of this subcommittee is to educate itself and the hospital community to issues of organizational ethics. Its second responsibility is to provide consultation to members of the hospital community who have questions about organizational ethics. The method of the consultation and the availability of consultation follow the procedures outlined by the patient rights subcommittee procedure on consultation. . . .

B. *Checks and Balances.* The risk most common to all employees of all organizations is in not pursuing the mission of the institution. It is essential therefore at every level of the organization to have in place checks and balances to ensure that the goals of the organization are pursued. For example, the Board of Trustees must have oversight of strategic plans and alliances to ensure the organization is pursuing its goals. Likewise, administration must ensure that every subunit's functioning is consistent with the mission of the institution. It accomplishes this by establishing clear lines of authority and clear scopes of authority for employees. Policies and procedures are in place to ensure fair business practices, address potential conflicts of interest, and protect quality of care through clinical decisions based on the identified needs of patients rather than on financial incentives. These policies and procedures are available, on request, to all patients, clinical staff, licensed independent practitioners, and hospital personnel.

C. *Appeals Processes.* Employees and patients/families must have a means to resolve disputes when questions arise over organizational ethics. This obligation to provide an appeals mechanism arises out of the hospital's commitment to a central value of business ethics: the value of due process. Due process requires powerful bodies to act according to established rules, to provide notice, render an opportunity to be heard, provide access to a reasonable appeals process, and return timely responses. Due process generally requires that like cases be treated alike. It calls for consistency in the treatment of employees.

Some subunits of the hospital that negotiate a high number of questions must consider formal mechanisms for appeals, for example, patients/families with billing questions, or employees who seek reasonable accommodation in the work setting. Not all subunits of the hospital will require their own appeals process, and when questions arise they should consider seeking information from the organizational ethics committee.

[2.5] The Hospital Medical Center Statement of Organizational Ethics

I. Purpose

This policy articulates the ethical obligations of the hospital to patients, the community, staff, employees, medical staff members, and in our professional and business relationships.

II. Policy

As a health care provider, employer, and professional organization, the hospital is responsible to maintain exemplary ethical standards and practices and to safeguard its social responsibility.

This organization is responsible to behave toward its external and internal communities in a humane and respectful manner consistent with its mission. Consistent with the holding corporation vision and values, the hospital will honor and behave with integrity to its commitments and principles.

III. General Principles

A. The hospital is accountable, as a health care organization and for its empowered representatives. The hospital has established and implemented a code of ethical behavior and procedures that respect the rights and duties of the organization, its employees and staff, the patients we serve, and the community to whom we are accountable.

B. The hospital commits to fair business practices in its relations with patients, payers, physicians, other professionals, employees, and the general public. It will seek, where feasible, long-range relationships built on trust and honoring of commitments.

C. The hospital acknowledges the critical importance of shared values, including trust and teamwork, and it commits to provide an environment in which those values are optimized.

D. The hospital is committed to provide beneficial services to the population for which it is responsible. It will seek opportunities to maintain or improve the health of its community.

E. The hospital is accountable to its community. To the extent that some members of the community do not have access to necessary health care, the hospital will attempt to meet the needs as a provider, in partnership with other organizations, or as a leader in developing and implementing appropriate programs.

F. Ethical conduct has strong implications for quality of care, which is a valued goal of the hospital. We will behave to promote quality, and we will measure the impact of these behaviors on health status and organizational performance.

G. The hospital recognizes the cultural diversity of its community. It will strive to implement patient care and personnel policies that respect the individual rights that arise out of that diversity. Concurrently, the hospital actively promotes community consensus that grows out of the commonality of mankind, common goals, and the need to live and work together.

H. The hospital accepts and values its responsibilities to educating its patients, staff, and community. It supports education programs and encourages continuing education of its personnel, leadership, and medical staff.

I. The hospital has an active research program. Essential components of research include protection of human subjects, informed consent, adherence to highest professional norms of scientific and ethical truth, and fair access to the research and its findings or products. These values will be respected and protected in this institution.

J. The hospital has established an ethical policy and procedures for the procurement of organs that respect the confidentiality, dignity, and rights of patients and their families. Procedures are conducted with sensitivity to the feeling, values, and beliefs of the family, its culture, and religious beliefs.

K. In addition to its commitment to fair business practices, the hospital acknowledges the importance of, and adheres to, truth in marketing to all, including the public, other providers, and patients. We strive to assure that information at admission, transfer, and in billing will be accurate and specific. Conflicts will be managed with respect, and the dignity of the patient will be supported at all times.

L. The hospital is committed to maintain confidentiality of medical information, and to recognize patients' rights to access their own record.

M. Conflicts about patients' or families' rights in treatment and medical decisions that cannot be resolved among caregivers may be referred to the Ethics Committee by any of the involved parties. These requests will be responded to promptly, professionally, consistent with the hospital guidelines, and in a manner that respects the dignity and rights of all involved. Representatives will be sensitive to the emotional, cultural, and spiritual needs of the patients, families, and staff.

Appendix Three
American College of
Healthcare Executives:
Code of Ethics

Preface

The code of Ethics is administered by the Ethics Committee, which is appointed by the Board of Governors upon nomination by the Chairman. It is composed of a least nine Fellows of the College, each of whom serves a three-year term on a staggered basis, with three members retiring each year.

The Ethics Committee shall:

- Review and evaluate annually the Code of Ethics, and make any necessary recommendations for updating the Code.
- Review and recommend action to the Board of Governors on allegations brought forth regarding breaches of the Code of Ethics.
- Develop ethical policy statements to serve as guidelines of ethical conduct for healthcare executives and their professional relationships.
- Prepare an annual report of observations, accomplishments, and recommendations to the Board of Governors, and such other periodic reports as required.

The Ethics Committee invokes the Code of Ethics under authority of the ACHE Bylaws, Article II, Membership, Section 6, Resignation and Termination of Membership; Transfer to Inactive Status, subsection (b), as follows:

> Membership may be terminated or rendered inactive by action of the Board of Governors as a result of violation of the Code of Ethics, nonconformity with the Bylaws or Regulations Governing Admission, Advancement, Recertification, and Reappointment; conviction of a felony; or conviction of a crime or moral turpitude or a crime relating to the healthcare management profession. No such termination of membership or imposition of inactive status shall be effected without affording a reasonable opportunity for the member to consider the charges and to appear in his or her own defense before the Board of Governors or its designated hearing committee, as outlined in the "Grievance Procedure," Appendix I of the College's Code of Ethics.

Preamble

The purpose of the Code of Ethics of the American College of Healthcare Executives is to serve as a guide to conduct for members. It contains standards of ethical behavior for healthcare executives in their professional relationships. These relationships include members of the healthcare executive's organization and other organizations. Also included are patients or others served, colleagues, the community and society as a whole. The Code of Ethics also incorporates standards of ethical behavior governing personal behavior, particularly when that conduct directly relates to the role and identity of the healthcare executive.

The fundamental objectives of the healthcare management profession are to enhance overall quality of life, dignity and well-being of every individual needing healthcare services; and to create a more equitable, accessible, effective, and efficient healthcare system.

Healthcare executives have an obligation to act in ways that will merit the trust, confidence and respect of healthcare professionals and the general public. Therefore, healthcare executives should lead lives that embody an exemplary system of values and ethics.

In fulfilling their commitments and obligations to patients or others served, healthcare executives function as moral advocates. Since every management decision affects the health and well-being of both individuals and communities, healthcare executives must carefully evaluate the possible outcomes of their decisions. In organizations that deliver healthcare services, they must work to safeguard and foster the rights, interests and prerogatives of patients or others served. The role of moral advocate requires that healthcare executives speak out and take actions necessary to promote such rights, interests and prerogatives if they are threatened.

I. The Healthcare Executive's Responsibilities to the Profession of Healthcare Management

The healthcare executive shall:

A. Uphold the values, ethics, and mission of the healthcare management profession;
B. Conduct all personal and professional activities with honesty, integrity, respect, fairness, and good faith in a manner that will reflect well upon the profession;
C. Comply with all laws pertaining to healthcare management in the jurisdictions in which the healthcare executive is located, or conducts professional activities;
D. Maintain competence and proficiency in healthcare management by implementing a personal program of assessment and continuing professional education;
E. Avoid the exploitation of professional relationships for personal gain;
F. Use this Code to further the interests of the profession and not for selfish reasons;
G. Respect professional confidence;
H. Enhance the dignity and image of the healthcare management profession through positive public information programs; and
I. Refrain from participating in any activity that demeans the credibility and dignity of the healthcare management profession.

II. The Healthcare Executive's Responsibilities to Patients or Others Served, to the Organization and to Employees

A. Responsibilities to Patients or Others Served

The healthcare executive shall, within the scope of his or her authority:

1. Work to ensure the existence of a process to evaluate the quality of care or service rendered;
2. Avoid practicing or facilitating discrimination and institute safeguards to prevent discriminatory organizational practices;
3. Work to ensure the existence of a process that will advise patients or others served of the rights, opportunities, responsibilities, and risks regarding available healthcare services;
4. Work to provide a process that ensures the autonomy and self-determination of patients or others served; and
5. Work to ensure the existence of procedures that will safeguard the confidentiality and privacy of patients or others served.

B. Responsibilities to the Organization

The healthcare executive shall, within the scope of his or her authority:

1. Provide healthcare services consistent with available resources and work to ensure the existence of a resource allocation process that considers ethical ramifications;
2. Conduct both competitive and cooperative activities in ways that improve community healthcare services;
3. Lead the organization in the use and improvement of standards of management and sound business practices;
4. Respect the customs and practices of patients or others served, consistent with the organization's philosophy; and
5. Be truthful in all forms of professional and organizational communication, and avoid disseminating information that is false, misleading, or deceptive.

C. Responsibilities to Employees

Healthcare executives have an ethical and professional obligation to employees of the organizations they manage, which encompasses but is not limited to:

1. Working to create a working environment conducive for underscoring employee ethical conduct and behavior.
2. Working to ensure that individuals may freely express ethical concerns and providing mechanisms for discussing and addressing such concerns.
3. Working to ensure a working environment that is free from harassment, sexual and other; coercion of any kind, especially to perform illegal or unethical acts; and discrimination on the basis of race, creed, color, sex, ethnic origin, age, or disability.
4. Working to ensure a working environment that is conducive to proper utilization of employee's skills and abilities.
5. Paying particular attention to the employee's work environment and job safety.
6. Working to establish appropriate grievance and appeals mechanisms.

III. Conflicts of Interest

A conflict of interest may be only a matter of degree, but exists when the healthcare executive:

A. Acts to benefit directly or indirectly by using authority or inside information, or allows a friend, relative, or associate to benefit from such authority or information.
B. Uses authority or information to make a decision to intentionally affect the organization in an adverse manner.

The healthcare executive shall:

A. Conduct all personal and professional relationships in such a way that all those affected are assured that management decisions are made in the best interests of the organization and the individuals served by it;
B. Disclose to the appropriate authority any direct or indirect financial or personal interests that pose potential or actual conflicts of interest;
C. Accept no gifts or benefits offered with the express or implied expectation of influencing a management decision; and
D. Inform the appropriate authority and other involved parties of potential or actual conflicts of interest related to appointments

or elections to boards or committees inside or outside the healthcare executive's organization.

IV. The Healthcare Executive's Responsibilities to Community and Society

The healthcare executive shall:

A. Work to identify and meet the healthcare needs of the community;
B. Work to ensure that all people have reasonable access to healthcare services;
C. Participate in public dialogue on healthcare policy issues and advocate solutions that will improve health status and promote quality healthcare;
D. Consider the short-term and long-term impact of management decisions on both the community and on society; and
E. Provide prospective consumers with adequate and accurate information, enabling them to make enlightened judgments and decisions regarding services.

V. The Healthcare Executive's Responsibility to Report Violations of the Code

A member of the College who has reasonable grounds to believe that another member has violated this Code has a duty to communicate such facts to the Ethics Committee.

American College of Healthcare Executives Grievance Procedure

1. In order to be processed by the College, a complaint must be filed in writing to the Ethics Committee of the College within three years of the date of discovery of the alleged violation; and the Committee has the responsibility to look into incidents brought to its attention regardless of the informality of the information, provided the information can be documented or supported or may be a matter of public record. The three-year period within which a complaint must be filed shall temporarily cease to run during intervals

when the accused member is in inactive status, or when the accused member resigns from the College.

2. The Committee chairman initially will determine whether the complaint falls within the purview of the Ethics Committee and whether immediate investigation is necessary. However, all letters of complaint that are filed with the Ethics Committee will appear on the agenda of the next committee meeting. The Ethics Committee shall have the final discretion to determine whether a complaint falls within the purview of the Ethics Committee.

3. If a grievance proceeding is initiated by the Ethics Committee:

A. Specifics of the complaint will be sent to the respondent by certified mail. In such mailing, committee staff will inform the respondent that the grievance proceeding has been initiated and that the respondent may respond directly to the Ethics Committee; the respondent also will be asked to cooperate with the Regent investigating the complaint.

B. The Ethics Committee shall refer the matter to the appropriate Regent who is deemed best able to investigate the alleged infraction. The Regent shall make inquiry into the matter, and in the process the respondent shall be given an opportunity to be heard.

C. Upon completion of the inquiry, the Regent shall present a complete report and recommended disposition of the matter in writing to the Ethics Committee. Absent unusual circumstances, the Regent is expected to complete his or her report and recommended disposition, and provide them to the committee, within sixty days.

4. Upon the Committee's receipt of the Regent's report and recommended disposition, the Committee shall review them and make its written recommendation to the Board of Governors as to what action shall be taken and the reason or reasons therefore. A copy of the Committee's recommended decision along with the Regent's report and recommended disposition to the Board will be mailed to the respondent by certified mail. In such mailing, the respondent will be notified that within thirty days after his or her

receipt of the Ethics Committee's recommended decision, the respondent may file a written appeal of the recommended decision with the Board of Governors.

5. Any written appeal submitted by the respondent must be received by the Board of Governors within thirty days after the recommended decision of the Ethics Committee is received by the respondent. The Board of Governors shall not take action on the Ethics Committee's recommended decision until the thirty-day appeal period has elapsed. If no appeal to the Board of Governors is filed in a timely fashion, the Board shall review the recommended decision and determine action to be taken.

6. If an appeal to the Board of Governors is filed in a timely manner, the College Chairman shall appoint an ad hoc committee consisting of three Fellows to hear the matter. At least thirty days' notice of the formation of this committee, and of the hearing date, time, and place, with an opportunity for representation, shall be mailed to the respondent. Reasonable requests for postponement shall be given consideration.

7. This ad hoc committee shall give the respondent adequate opportunity to present his or her case at the hearing, including the opportunity to submit a written statement and other documents deemed relevant by the respondent, and to be represented if so desired. Within a reasonable period of time following the hearing, the ad hoc committee shall write a detailed report with recommendations to the Board of Governors.

8. The Board of Governors shall decide what action to take after reviewing the report of the ad hoc committee. The Board shall provide the respondent with a copy of its decision. The decision of the Board of Governors shall be final. The Board of Governors shall have the authority to accept or reject any of the findings or recommended decisions of the Regent, the Ethics Committee or the ad hoc committee, and to order whatever level of discipline it feels is justified.

9. At each level of the grievance proceeding, the Board of Governors shall have the sole discretion to notify or contact the com-

plainant relating to the grievance proceeding, provided, however, that the complainant shall be notified as to whether the complaint was reviewed by the Ethics Committee and whether the Ethics Committee or the Board of Governors has taken final action with respect to the complaint.

10. No individual shall serve on the ad hoc committee described above, or otherwise participate in these grievance proceedings on behalf of the College, if he or she is in direct economic competition with the respondent or otherwise has a financial conflict of interest in the matter, unless such conflict is disclosed to and waived in writing by the respondent.

11. All information obtained, reviewed, discussed, and otherwise used or developed in a grievance proceeding that is not otherwise publicly known, publicly available, or part of the public domain is considered to be privileged and strictly confidential information of the College, and is not to be disclosed to anyone outside of the grievance proceeding except as determined by the Board of Governors or as required by law; provided, however, that an individual's membership status is not confidential and may be made available to the pubic upon request.

Ethics Committee Action

Once the grievance proceeding has been initiated, the Ethics Committee may take any of the following actions based upon its findings:

1. Determine the grievance complaint to be invalid.
2. Dismiss the grievance complaint.
3. Recommend censure.
4. Recommend transfer to inactive status for a specified minimum period of time.
5. Recommend expulsion.

As amended by the Council of Regents at its annual meeting on August 22, 1995.

Source: American College of Healthcare Executives, Suite 1700, One North Franklin St., Chicago, IL 60606-3491.

Appendix Four
Partnership Health Care:
Conflict of Interest Policy

I. Policy

Maintaining the integrity of Partnership Health Care (PHC) as a provider of quality health care requires the dedication and commitment of a quality workforce. Accordingly, the PHC Board of Directors has established standards of conduct which require the Board of Directors, members of facility Boards and their committees, administrative officers and staff members, volunteers, medical staff members having administrative responsibilities, and certain other associates to disclose all interests that could result in either a duality of interest or a possible conflict of interest. The PHC Corporate Compliance Officer is responsible for obtaining the Conflict of Interest compliance statements annually and reporting questionable or unacceptable disclosures to the Compliance Committee of the PHC Board of Directors.

A. PHC's associates must avoid any personal interest or association that may be inconsistent or even appear to be inconsistent with their dedication to the best interests of the organization. PHC's ability to compete with others and its choice of suppliers or others with whom it may do business must not be affected by a personal interest of any PHC associate.

B. Conflicts may arise in many forms. Some typical examples are the following:

- A facility Board member has a financial interest in a competitor, supplier, or customer of the organization.
- An associate who purchases services for her area conducts business on behalf of the organization with a supplier that employs one of her relatives.
- A department director accepts gifts, favors, services, entertainment, or other things of value from competitors or suppliers.
- An associate has an outside business interest that gains some special advantage from his employment by PHC.

C. Many interests and relationships that at first glance seem to involve conflicts may, because of their minor nature, be considered acceptable when disclosed. Others may require only periodic review to determine whether a conflict exists. The first rule for any PHC associate is to make prompt and full disclosure of any interest or relationship that could be interpreted as involving an actual or potential conflict.

D. PHC maintains a system of internal controls to ensure that transactions are executed in accordance with appropriate authorizations; that transactions are recorded and financial statements that conform to generally accepted accounting principles or other applicable criteria can be prepared; that accountability for assets is maintained; and that access to assets is permitted only as authorized. All PHC associates deal personally with the assets of the organization in one way or another. This is a relationship of trust and must not be abused.

Reimbursement for personal expenses must be limited to those expenses legitimately authorized and incurred for the benefit of PHC. No personal use may be made of organization property or resources.

E. The relationships of the President, administrative staff members, other selected associates, volunteers, and medical staff members having administrative responsibilities with PHC and its subsidiaries carry with them a requirement of loyalty. It is the responsibility of such persons to administer the organization's affairs honestly and to exercise economically their best care, skill, and judgment for the benefit of PHC.

It is also the responsibility of the President to make full disclosure of any interest that might result in a conflict on his or her part. The Board of Directors makes a like requirement of administrative staff members, certain associates, and medical staff members with administrative responsibilities and forbids any material conflict of interest on the part of such persons.

1. All parties for whom this policy applies shall exercise the utmost good faith in all transactions touching upon their duties to PHC and its property. In their dealings with and on behalf of PHC, they shall be held to a strict rule of honest and fair dealing between themselves and the organization. They shall not use their positions, or knowledge gained therefrom, in a way that may generate a conflict between the interest of the organization and that of the individual. They shall keep confidential all matters in which PHC and its subsidiaries have proprietary interests.

2. Such persons shall not accept any gifts, favors, services, or entertainment to the extent that decision making or actions affecting PHC might be influenced. Gifts over $100 must be reported to an individual's supervisor and the Corporate Compliance Officer.

3. Although it is recognized that a degree of duality of interest may exist from time to time, such duality shall not be permitted to influence adversely any decision-making process of PHC. To this end, any person subject to this policy and procedure shall promptly report the possible existence of a conflict of interest for himself or herself or for any other person subject to this policy. The report shall be made to the Corporate Compliance Officer.

4. If a transaction is subject to any doubt because of a possible conflict of interest, a full disclosure of all facts pertaining to the transaction shall be made before it is consummated.

5. Compliance with the foregoing shall not serve to excuse or condone any undue gain or advantage obtained by virtue of position, any violation of law, or any other irregularity or prohibited practice.

II. Procedure

A. Annually, the President of PHC sends to all officers, administrative staff, selected associates, volunteers, and medical staff members having administrative responsibilities a copy of the Conflict of Interest policy and the annual Conflict of Interest certification to be returned to the Corporate Compliance Officer. The Statements are reviewed by the Corporate Compliance Officer and questionable or unacceptable disclosures are reported to the Compliance Committee of the PHC Board of Directors.

B. All new administrative staff members and medical staff members with administrative responsibilities are required to submit the Conflict of Interest certification to the Corporate Compliance Officer within thirty calendar days of assuming their responsibilities.

C. To comply with the Conflict of Interest policy, persons included in the annual mailing are asked to complete and return their Conflict of Interest certification to the Corporate Compliance Officer within two weeks. The disclosure requirements are intended to provide a systematic and ongoing method for disclosing and ethically resolving potential conflicts of interest.

D. Although it is impossible to list every circumstance giving rise to a possible conflict of or duality of interest, the following will serve as a guide to the types of activities that cause conflicts and that should be fully disclosed.

1. Outside interests
    A. Holding, directly or indirectly, a position or a material financial interest in any outside concern from which the individual has reason to believe that PHC secures goods or services (including the services of buying and selling securities) or that provides services competitive with PHC.
    B. Competing, directly or indirectly, with PHC in the purchase or sale of property rights, interests, or services.
2. Outside activities
    Rendering directive, managerial, or consultative services to any outside concern that does business with, or competes with, the services of PHC or rendering other services in competition with PHC.
3. Gifts, favors, services, and entertainment

Accepting gifts, favors, services, or entertainment from any outside concern that does or is seeking to do business with, or is a competitor of, PHC under circumstances from which it might be inferred that such an offer was intended to influence, or possibly would influence, the individual in the performance of his or her duties.

4. Inside information

Disclosing or using information relating to PHC's business for the personal profit or advantage of the individual or his or her immediate family. The term *immediate family* includes a spouse, child, parent, grandparent, brother, sister, cousin, uncle, aunt, niece, nephew, grandchild, or in-law.

5. System software

A. Using for personal benefit, selling, or distributing system software developed for any project, task, or production support of owned, leased, or developed systems to any other facility, organization, or person.

B. Altering or inserting code into any software used by PHC or performing any other act which by its nature modifies a system willfully and intentionally to the associate's advantage and/or to the detriment of PHC.

C. Using one's position or knowledge gained from PHC to develop software for sale to the health care market or becoming involved in consulting agreements for the same purpose or to compete against PHC in the marketplace.

E. Full disclosure of any situation that raises doubt about a possible conflict of interest should be made so as to permit an impartial and objective determination. It should be particularly noted that disclosure relates not only to the associate but also to the associate's immediate family as defined above.

Recommended Reading

General

Business Ethics

Childs, J. M., Jr. *Ethics in Business: Faith at Work.* Minneapolis: Fortress Press, 1995.

Dosick, W. *The Business Bible: Ten New Commandments for Creating an Ethical Workplace.* New York: William Morrow, 1993.

Ewing, D. W. "The Corporation as a Just Society." *Business Ethics,* Mar.–Apr. 1990, p. 21.

French, P. A. "Corporate Moral Agency." In W. M. Hoffman and J. M. Moore (eds.), *Business Ethics: Readings and Cases in Corporate Morality.* New York: McGraw-Hill, 1984.

Goodpaster, K. E. "Business Ethics, Ideology, and the Naturalistic Fallacy." *Journal of Business Ethics,* 1985, *4,* 227–232.

Goodpaster, K. E., and Matthews, J. B., Jr. "Can a Corporation Have a Conscience?" *Harvard Business Review,* 1982, *60*(1), 132–141.

Hasnas, J. "The Normative Theories of Business Ethics: A Guide for the Perplexed." *Business Ethics Quarterly,* 1998, *8*(1), 19–42.

Nash, L. *Good Intentions Aside: A Manager's Guide to Resolving Ethical Problems.* Boston: Harvard Business School Press, 1990.

Solomon, R. C. *Ethics and Excellence: Cooperation and Integrity in Business.* New York: Oxford University Press, 1993.

Organizational Ethics

Brodeur, D. "Health Care Institutional Ethics: Broader Than Clinical Ethics." In D. Thomasma and J. Monagle (eds.), *Health Care Ethics: Critical Issues for the 21st Century.* (3rd ed.) Gaithersburg, Md.: Aspen, 1998.

Carlson, D. S., and Perrewe, P. L. "Institutionalization of Organizational Ethics Through Transformational Leadership." *Journal of Business Ethics,* 1995, *14,* 832.

McCurdy, D. B. "Organizations and Individuals Need Each Other to Be Ethical." *Park Ridge Center Bulletin* (Feb./Mar. 1998), pp. 14–15.

Reiser, S. J. "Administrative Case Rounds: Institutional Policies and Leaders Cast in a Different Light." *Journal of the American Medical Association,* 1991, *266*(15), 2127.

Reiser, S. J. "The Ethical Life of Health Care Organizations." *Hastings Center Report* 1994, *24*(6), 28–35.

Organizational Ethics in Non–Health Care Organizations

Moskowitz, E. H., and Nassef, D. T. "Integrating Medical and Business Values in Health Benefits Management." *California Management Review,* 1997, *40*(1), 117–139.

Organizational Culture

Arndt, M., and Bigelow, B. "Reengineering: Deja Vu All Over Again." *Health Care Management Review,* 1998, *23*(3), 64.

Catholic Health Association Culture Project Team. "Understanding Culture: Key Messages for Leadership." *Health Progress,* 1995, *76*(2), 20–48.

Friedman, E. "Ethics and Corporate Culture: Finding a Fit." *Healthcare Executive,* Mar./Apr. 1990, pp. 18–20.

Giganti, E., and "Think Tank Participants." "A New Social Contract: Catholic Healthcare Leaders Rethink Their Relationship with Employees." *Health Progress,* 1995, *76*(5), Special Section, pp. 1–5.

Gordon, G. "Industry Determinants of Organizational Culture." *Academy of Management Review,* Apr. 1991, pp. 396–415.

Hammer, M., and Champey, J. *Reengineering the Corporation: A Manifesto for Business Revolution.* New York: HarperCollins, 1993.

Jackall, R. *Moral Mazes: The World of Corporate Managers.* New York: Oxford University Press, 1989.

Martin, J. *Cultures in Organizations: Three Perspectives.* New York: Oxford University Press, 1992.

Ryan, K. D., and Oestreich, D. K. *Driving Fear out of the Workplace: How to Overcome the Invisible Barriers to Quality, Productivity, and Innovation.* San Francisco: Jossey-Bass, 1991.

Schein, E. H. *Organizational Culture and Leadership.* (2nd ed.) San Francisco: Jossey-Bass, 1992.

Stevens, R. *In Sickness and In Wealth.* New York: Basic Books, 1989.

Voglewede, R. "The Application of Faith-Based Principles: Mission Leaders Can Facilitate an Organization's Cultural Transformation." *Health Progress,* 1996, *77*(1), 46ff.

Wiener, Y. "Forms of Value Systems: A Focus on Organizational Effectiveness and Cultural Change and Maintenance." *Academy of Management Review,* 1988, *13*(4), 534–545.

Organizational Support

Abramson, M. "Reflections on Knowing Oneself Ethically: Toward a Working Framework for Social Work Practice." *Families in Society: The Journal of Contemporary Human Services*, 1996, 77(4), 195–201.

Baron, R. *What Type Am I? Discover Who You Really Are.* New York: Penguin, 1998.

Brown, M. T. *Working Ethics: Strategies for Decision Making and Organizational Responsibility.* San Francisco: Jossey-Bass, 1990.

Donabedian, A. "Quality Assurance: Corporate Responsibility for Multihospital Systems." *Quality Review Bulletin*, 1986, 12(1), 3–7.

Harvey, J. *The Abilene Paradox and Other Meditations on Management.* San Francisco: Jossey-Bass, 1996.

James, G. G. "In Defense of Whistle Blowing." In J. C. Callahan (ed.), *Ethical Issues in Professional Life.* New York: Oxford University Press, 1988.

March, J. G., and Olsen, J. P. "Organizational Choice under Ambiguity." In O. Grusky and G. A. Miller (eds.), *The Sociology of Organizations: Basic Studies.* (2nd ed.) New York: Free Press, 1981.

Maslach, C., and Leiter, M. P. *The Truth About Burn-Out: How Organizations Cause Personal Stress and What to Do About It.* San Francisco: Jossey-Bass, 1997.

McCurdy, D. B. "Clinical Bioethics Education in Clinical Pastoral Education." *Journal of Supervision and Training in Ministry*, 1992–93, 14, 3–20.

McCurdy, D. B. "Creating an Ethical Organization." *Generations*, 1998, 22(3), 26–31.

Murphy, P. E. *Eighty Exemplary Ethics Statements.* Notre Dame, Ind.: University of Notre Dame Press, 1998.

O'Connell, L. J. "Healthcare Management Ethics." *Healthcare Executive*, 1996, 11(3), 48.

Smith, D. H. *Entrusted: The Moral Responsibilities of Trusteeship.* Bloomington: Indiana University Press, 1995.

Verhey, A. "Integrity, Humility, and Heroism: May Patients Refuse Medical Treatment?" In S. E. Lammers and A. Verhey (eds.), *On Moral Medicine: Theological Perspectives in Medical Ethics.* Grand Rapids, Mich.: Eerdmans, 1987.

Organizational Theory

March, J. G., and Simon, H. A. *Organizations.* New York: Wiley, 1958.

Morgan, G. *Images of Organization.* (2nd ed.) Thousand Oaks, Calif.: Sage, 1997.

Scott, W. R. *Organizations: Rational, Natural, and Open Systems.* (4th ed.) Upper Saddle River, N.J.: Prentice Hall, 1998.

Organizational Virtues

Paine, L. S. "Managing for Organizational Integrity." *Harvard Business Review.* Mar.–Apr. 1994, pp. 106–117.

Psychology, Moral

Messick, D. M., and Bazerman, M. H. "Ethical Leadership and the Psychology of Decision Making." *Sloan Management Review.* Winter 1996, pp. 9–22.

Petrick, J. A., and Manning, G. "Developing an Ethics Climate for Excellence." *Journal for Quality and Participation,* Mar. 1990, pp. 84–90.

Psychology, Organizational

Bird, F. B. *The Muted Conscience: Moral Silence and the Practice of Ethics in Business.* Westport, Conn.: Quorum, 1996.

Bird, F. B., and Waters, J. A. "The Moral Muteness of Managers." In T. Donaldson and P. H. Werhane (eds.), *Ethical Issues in Business.* (5th ed.) Upper Saddle River, N.J.: Prentice Hall, 1996 [1983].

March, J. G., and Olsen, J. P. (eds.). *Ambiguity and Choice in Organizations.* Bergen, Norway: Universitetsforlaget, 1976.

Petrick, J. A., and Manning, G. E. "Developing an Ethical Climate for Excellence." *Journal of Quality and Participation,* Mar. 1990, p. 84.

Spirituality in Organizations

Briskin, A. *The Stirring of Soul in the Workplace.* San Francisco: Jossey-Bass, 1996.

Special Topics

Advertising

Arrington, R. L. "Advertising and Behavior Control." *Journal of Business Ethics,* 1982, *1*(1), 3–12.

Murphy, P. E. *Ethical Issues Facing Hospitals in Their Advertising.* Notre Dame, Ind.: University of Notre Dame Press, 1990.

Allocation of Resources

ATS Bioethics Task Force. "Fair Allocation of Intensive Care Unit Resources." *American Journal of Respiratory and Critical Care Medicine,* 1997, *156*, 1282–1301.

Bloche, M. G. "Clinical Loyalties and the Social Purposes of Medicine." *Journal of the American Medical Association,* 1999, *281*(3), 268–274.

Conflicts of Interest

Greene, J. "Appearance of Conflicts of Interest Can Damage, Too." *Modern Healthcare,* Jan. 20, 1992, p. 32.

Rodwin, M. *Medicine, Money, and Morals: Physicians' Conflicts of Interest.* New York: Oxford, 1993.

Conscientious Objections
Weber, L. "When to Excuse Employees from Work Responsibilities." *Health Progress,* Dec. 1995, pp. 50–51.

Corporate Compliance
Gunn, J. F., Goldfarb, E. R., and Showalter, J. S. "Creating a Corporate Compliance Program." *Health Progress,* 1998, *79*(3), 60–63.
Tuohey, J. F. "Covenant Model of Corporate Compliance: 'Corporate Integrity' Program Meets Mission, Not Just Legal, Requirements." *Health Progress,* 1998, *79*(4), 70–75.

Discretion and Control
Darr, K. *Ethics in Health Services Management.* New York: Praeger, 1987.
Herman, S. *Durable Goods: A Covenantal Ethics for Management and Employees.* Notre Dame, Ind.: University of Notre Dame Press, 1997.
Herman, S. "The Modern Business Corporation and an Ethics of Trust." *Journal of Religious Ethics,* 1992, *20,* 111–148.
May, W. F. "Moral Leadership in the Corporate Setting." In W. L. Robison, M. S. Pritchard, and J. Ellin (eds.), *Profits and Professions: Essays in Business and Professional Ethics.* Clifton, N.J.: Humana Press, 1983.
Niebuhr, H. Richard. *The Responsible Self: An Essay in Christian Moral Philosophy.* New York: Harper and Row, 1963.
Stackhouse, M., and McCann, D. "A Post-Communist Manifesto." *Christian Century,* 1991, *108,* 44–47.
Sturm, D. "Corporations, Constitutions, and Covenants: On Forms of Human Relation and the Problem of Legitimacy." *Journal of the American Academy of Religion,* 1973, *41,* 331–54.

Ethics Mechanisms
Felder, M. "Can Ethics Committees Work in Managed Care Plans?" *Bioethics Forum,* Spring 1996, pp. 10–15.
McCurdy, D. B. "Creating an Ethical Organization." *Generations,* Fall 1998, pp. 26–31.
Metzger, M., Dalton, D. R., and Hill, J. W. "The Organization of Ethics and the Ethics of Organizations: The Case for Expanded Organizational Ethics Audits." *Business Ethics Quarterly,* 1993, *3*(1), 27–43.
Potter, V. R. "Individuals Bear Responsibility." *Bioethics Forum,* 1996, *12*(2), 27–28.

Spencer, E. M. "A New Role for Institutional Ethics Committees: Organizational Ethics." *Journal of Clinical Ethics*, 1997, *8*(4), 372–376.

Human Resources

Coye, R., and Belohlav, J. "Disciplining: A Question of Ethics?" *Employee Responsibilities and Rights Journal*, 1989, *2*(3), 155–162.

Glazer, M. "Ten Whistleblowers and How They Fared." In J. C. Callahan (ed.), *Ethical Issues in Professional Life*. New York: Oxford University Press, 1988.

Heisler, W. J., Jones, W. D., and Benham, P. O., Jr. *Managing Human Resource Issues: Confronting Challenges and Choosing Options*. San Francisco: Jossey-Bass, 1988.

Herman, S. W. *Durable Goods: A Covenantal Ethic for Management and Employees*. Notre Dame, Ind.: University of Notre Dame Press, 1997.

Hinderer, D. E. " Hospital Downsizing Ethics and Employees." *Journal of Nursing Administration*, 1997, *27*(4), 9–11.

James, G. G. "In Defense of Whistle Blowing." In J. C. Callahan (ed.), *Ethical Issues in Professional Life*. New York: Oxford University Press, 1988.

Maslach, C., and Leiter, M. P. *The Truth About Burnout: How Organizations Cause Personal Stress and What to Do About It*. San Francisco: Jossey-Bass, 1997.

Noer, D. M. *Healing the Wounds: Overcoming the Trauma of Layoffs and Revitalizing Downsized Organizations*. San Francisco: Jossey-Bass, 1993.

Rosen, S. D., and Juris, H. A. "Ethical Issues in Human Resource Management." In G. R. Ferris, S. D. Rosen, and D. T. Barnum (eds.), *Handbook of Human Resource Management*. Blackwell Human Resource Management Series. Cambridge, Mass.: Blackwell, 1995.

Thomas, R. R., Jr. "From Affirmative Action to Affirming Diversity." *Harvard Business Review*, 1990, *68*(2), 113.

JCAHO

Joint Commission on Accreditation of Healthcare Organizations. "Organization Ethics." In *Ethical Issues and Patients Rights in the Continuum of Care*. Oakbrook Terrace, Ill.: Joint Commission on Accreditation of Healthcare Organizations, 1998.

Schyve, P. M. "Patients Rights and Organization Ethics: The Joint Commission Perspective." *Bioethics Forum*, 1996, *12*(2), 13–20.

Managed Care

Christensen, K. T. "Ethically Important Distinctions Among Managed Care Organizations." *Journal of Law, Medicine and Ethics*, 1995, *23*(3), 223–229.

Mission and the Bottom Line

Block, P. *Stewardship: Choosing Service Over Self-Interest.* San Francisco: Berrett-Koehler, 1996.

Daniels, N. "The Profit Motive and the Moral Assessment of Health Care Institutions." *Business and Professional Ethics Journal,* 1990, *10*(2), 3–30.

Friedman, E. "Marginal Mission and Missionary Margins." *Healthcare Forum Journal,* Jan/Feb. 1990, pp. 8–12.

Gray, B. H. *The Profit Motive and Patient Care.* Cambridge, Mass.: Harvard University Press, 1991.

Werhane, P. H. "The Ethics of Health Care as a Business." *Business and Professional Ethics Journal,* 1991, *9*(3,4), 7–20.

Policy Statements

Murphy, P. E. *Eighty Exemplary Ethics Statements.* Notre Dame, Ind.: University of Notre Dame Press, 1998.

Resource Allocation

ATS Bioethics Task Force. "Fair Allocation of Intensive Care Unit Resources." *American Journal of Respiratory and Critical Care Medicine,* 1997, *156,* 1282–1301.

Additional Resources

Catholic Health Association of the United States. *Organizational Integrity in Catholic Healthcare Ministry: The Role of the Leader.* St. Louis, Mo.: Catholic Health Association, 1998.

Index

Ethics term, perception of, 28
Ethnocentrism, *48*
Euthanasia issue, 309, 310–311
Evidence-based health care, shift
toward, 10, 331
Excellence, checklist for, *90*
Exclusion, 158, 159, 160
Executives, 149–160; code of ethics
for, 377–385; compensation for,
83, 122, 156; conflict of interest
involving, 149–160; discretion of,
260–265; education for, 69, 71,
72, 73; as models of behavior,
86–87; referring decisions to, 265,
269; research on decision making
of, 69, 71; role responsibilities of,
69, *70,* 253; support of, for ethics
mechanisms, 27–28. *See also*
Board of Directors
Expectations: of employees, 142–143;
unmet, disappointment over, 92–93
Expertise, overstepping bounds of,
12, 186–187, 188, 326–328
Explicity in resource allocation, 217
External financial relationships. *See*
Contractual relationships; Facility
ownership
External relationships: ethics statement addressing, 370; focus on,
35–36, 38; influence of, 261, 262;
obligation to promote good in, 52
External whistle-blowing, defined, 84

F

Facility ownership: and conflict of
interest, 101, 160, 163–164; standards addressing, 354, 355,
358–359
Fact-gathering process, 23, *24,* 60,
208–210; importance of, 29–30;
tools for, 30–38
"Facts" and judgment, 196
Fair-share contributions, 283–287
Faith-based organizations: advocacy
of, 288; sample ethics statements
of, 364, *365, 366,* 370–374

Families: and conflict of interest,
147, 151, *154, 155;* disclosing
clinical mistakes to, 312–313,
314; involvement of, in decisions,
209–210, 219, 237
Family employment, disclosing, *155*
Family matters: impact of, on job
performance, 171, 172; support
for, 173
Favors, accepting, *154*
Fear: of corporate integrity initiatives,
107, 108; of failure, 148, 235; and
fair-share language, 286; of litigation, 304; in removing life support, 237; of reporting, 73–74,
83, 84
Fear-based motivation, 80
Fear-driven recruitment, 121
Fee-for-service, 168
Financial incentives: for performance,
83, 110, 122–123; in recruitment,
161, 168, 337–338; of reimburse-
ment rates, 262, 263.
Financial interests, competing. *See*
Conflict of interest
Financial performance: meeting tar-
gets for, 255; monitoring, 254. *See
also* Profitability
Financial realities, 75, 79
Financial relationships. *See* Contrac-
tual relationships; Facility
ownership
Firing, 133–134, 138–139
Formal choices, 205
Formal structures, processes, and
relationships: focus on, 31–32,
33, 36, 38; influence of, 44, 46
Formulary committee, 215
For-profit motive, 325
For-profit regulation, 159
Fraud and abuse, 98–99, *100, 105;* in
billing, 98, 99, 104, 344; and hir-
ing decisions, 292–295
Free-market economy, result of,
161–162, 247, 249
Friedman, E., 84, 200